S0-AWR-401

Teacher's Resources

Nutrition, Food, and Fitness

Dorothy F. West, Ph.D.
*Food and Nutrition Author
and Educator*

Publisher
The Goodheart-Willcox Company, Inc.
Tinley Park, Illinois
www. g-w.com

2

Copyright © 2006

by

The Goodheart-Willcox Company, Inc.

Previous editions copyright 2004, 2000

All rights reserved. No part of this work may be reproduced,
stored, or transmitted for resale.

Manufactured in the United States of America.

Teacher's Resource Guide
ISBN-13: 978-1-59070-530-8
ISBN-10: 1-59070-530-0
Teacher's Resource Portfolio
ISBN-13: 978-1-59070-531-5
ISBN-10: 1-59070-531-9
Teacher's Resource CD
ISBN-13: 978-1-59070-532-2
ISBN-10: 1-59070-532-7

3 4 5 6 7 8 9 10 – 06 – 11 10 09 08 07 06

Contents

4

Part Three The Work of Noncaloric Nutrients

Part Four   Nutrition Management: A Lifelong Activity

Part Five   Other Aspects of Wellness

Part Six   Making Informed Choices

Introduction

Nutrition and wellness education can play a critical role in helping students improve their quality of life. Teaching students to make health-promoting choices can have short- and long-range benefits. As students adopt lifestyles focused on wellness, they can immediately begin to enjoy a sense of improved well-being. However, they will also be starting a positive ripple effect on the health of their future families and communities.

Your success in motivating students to develop healthful lifestyle habits may depend largely on your enthusiasm and your ability to reach students where they are. The following techniques may help you achieve your goals:

- Become aware of the underlying causes of students' nutritional problems, considering such factors as lifestyle and family environment. Support strengths of current eating habits and help students evaluate how choices can be improved.
- Help students clarify their values and beliefs about healthful lifestyles. Explore what food, nutrition, health, and fitness mean to students and their families.
- Help students develop wellness goals that are realistic, remembering that balance, variety, and moderation are the keys to a healthful lifestyle.
- Help students recognize the impact society's idealized body images have on self-acceptance. Focus on healthful eating and activity habits to achieve overall wellness.
- Offer students simple, clear, and powerful messages. Give examples of how positive choices can impact quality of life.
- Promote flexibility. In nutrition and wellness, there is very little that is rigid. Use the Dietary Guidelines for Americans and other nutrition and fitness recommendations as standards, not rules.
- Celebrate diversity. Acknowledge that choices among people can, and do, vary. There is no perfect diet or fitness program. All foods can fit into a healthful eating plan, and all physical activities can be part of an active lifestyle.
- Establish your credibility as a teacher of nutrition and wellness. You need to present yourself as more than someone who knows a lot of information. Students need to respect you as someone who understands the context in which youth and adults make health-related choices.

Along with your personal teaching style, quality resources can help you reach your goals in teaching nutrition and wellness. *Nutrition, Food, and Fitness* is a comprehensive text designed to help students make important decisions about nutrition and wellness with assurance and competence. Besides the student text, the *Nutrition, Food, and Fitness* learning package includes the *Teacher's Wraparound Edition, Student Activity Guide, Teacher's Resource Guide, Teacher's Resource Portfolio,* and *Teacher's Resource CD with* **Exam** *View® Test Generator Software.* Using these products can help you develop an effective nutrition and wellness program tailored to your students' unique needs.

Using the Text

The text, *Nutrition, Food, and Fitness,* is designed to help your students learn about nutrition and wellness. They will learn how to choose nutritious diets and incorporate physical activity into their daily lives. They will also study the significance of caring for their mental and social health as part of the total wellness picture.

The text is divided into 6 parts with a total of 25 chapters. The material is organized and presented in a logical sequence of topics for the study of nutrition and wellness. Although the text was written to be studied in its entirety, individual chapters and sections are complete enough to be studied independently.

The text is straightforward and easy to read. Hundreds of photographs and charts attract student interest and emphasize key concepts. References to the illustrations are included in the copy to help students associate the visual images with the written material. This helps reinforce learning.

The text includes an expanded table of contents to give students an overview of the wide variety of topics they will be studying. The glossary at the back of the book helps students learn terms related to nutrition and wellness. A complete index helps them find information they want quickly and easily.

Each chapter includes several features designed to help students study effectively and review what they have learned.

Learn the Language. A list of vocabulary terms appears at the beginning of each chapter. Terms are listed in the order in which they appear in the chapter.

These terms are in bold italic type throughout the text so students can recognize them while reading. Discussing these words with students will help them learn concepts to which they are being introduced. To help students become familiar with these terms, you may want to ask them to

- look up, define, and explain each term.
- relate each term to the topic being studied.
- match terms with their definitions.
- find examples of how the terms are used in current newspapers and magazines, reference books, and other related materials.

Objectives. A set of behavioral objectives are also found at the beginning of each chapter. These are performance goals students will be expected to achieve after studying the chapter. Review the objectives in each chapter with students to help make them aware of the skills they will be building as they read the chapter material.

Summary. A chapter summary is located at the end of each chapter. This section is a review of the major concepts covered in the entire chapter.

Check Your Knowledge. Review questions at the end of each chapter are included to cover the basic information presented. This section consists of a variety of true/false, completion, multiple choice, and short essay questions. It is designed to help students recall, organize, and use the information presented in the text. Answers to these questions appear in all the *Teacher's Resource* products.

Put Learning into Action. Suggested activities at the end of each chapter offer students opportunities to increase knowledge through firsthand experiences. These activities encourage students to apply many of the concepts learned in the chapter to real-life situations. Suggestions for both individual and group work are provided in varying degrees of difficulty. Therefore, you may choose and assign activities according to students' interests and abilities.

Explore Further. Suggestions for research projects are provided at the end of each chapter. These projects give students a chance to delve deeper into topics discussed in the text. These projects make excellent assignments for developing the analytical skills of gifted students. However, students at all levels can benefit from these investigative strategies.

Using the *Teacher's Wraparound Edition*

The *Teacher's Wraparound Edition* of *Nutrition, Food, and Fitness* is a special edition of the student text. It is designed with teaching strategies and classroom activities to make your students' study of the text more effective.

The introduction of the *Teacher's Wraparound Edition* begins with illustrated descriptions of the features in the various components of the *Nutrition, Food, and Fitness* teaching package. The introduction continues with several sections that provide useful background information for teaching food and nutrition classes, such as suggestions for teaching learners with special needs. A *Correlation of National Standards for Nutrition and Wellness with Nutrition, Food, and Fitness* is provided. This table shows how studying the text can prepare students to master competencies outlined in the National Standards for Family and Consumer Sciences Education. A *Scope and Sequence Chart* identifies major concepts presented in each chapter of the text. These materials are designed to assist you in developing lesson plans and evaluating student learning.

Teaching Elements

Teaching elements are located in the side margins throughout the *Teacher's Wraparound Edition.* Each type of element is labeled with a different colored bar. The following types of elements are provided in this edition:

Activity. These activities reteach or reinforce chapter concepts.

Discuss. These questions about text concepts reinforce learning as students focus on important points.

Enrich. These are more involved and challenging activities, including role playing, research assignments, and field trips.

Example. These examples illustrate important points in the chapter material.

Note. These are statistics, facts, historical notes, and notes to the teacher, which are provided to expand content or spark student interest.

Reflect. These questions are more personal than the discussion questions. They often ask students to apply content to their lives.

Resource. This related material comes from the *Student Activity Guide* or *Teacher's Resources.*

Vocabulary. These activities include defining, using words in sentences, using the glossary, and comparing terms to help reinforce students' use of chapter vocabulary.

Extension Activities

The *Teacher's Wraparound Edition* features an extension activity at the bottom of each page. These activities are designed to help students apply text information or extend learning beyond the scope of the text. Each page contains one of the following types of activities:

Across the Curriculum. These activities relate chapter content to other curriculum areas, such as math, language arts, and social studies.

Applied Science. These activities emphasize the important role scientific concepts play in chapter material.

Career Preparation. These activities help students relate what they are learning to the world of work.

Citizenship and Service. These activities encourage students' concern, appreciation, and involvement with the community at large to help them better understand their roles as citizens.

Family Enrichment. These activities promote stronger family relationships by encouraging students to apply what they have learned to their family lives.

FCCLA in Action. These individual and group projects coordinate with national programs and STAR Events offered by the Family, Career and Community Leaders of America organization.

Lesson Adaptation. These are suggestions for modifying teaching strategies to better meet the special needs of some students.

Problem Solving. These activities help students develop critical-thinking, decision-making, and problem-solving skills.

Technology in Use. These are suggestions for incorporating technology, particularly the Internet and computer software, into chapter lesson plans.

In addition, every chapter includes answers keys for the *Check Your Knowledge* review questions in the text.

Using the *Student Activity Guide*

The *Student Activity Guide* designed for use with *Nutrition, Food, and Fitness* helps students recall and review material presented in the text. It also helps them apply what they have learned as they make lifestyle choices that will affect their health.

The activities in the *Student Activity Guide* are divided into chapters that correspond to the chapters in the text. The pages of the guide are perforated so students can easily turn completed activities in to you for evaluation. The use of each activity in the *Student Activity Guide* is described in each of the *Teacher's Resource* products as a teaching strategy under the related instructional concept. Activities are identified by name and letter.

The *Student Activity Guide* includes different types of activities. Some have specific answers related to text material. You may want to use these exercises as introductory, review, or evaluation tools. Ask students to do the exercises without looking in the book. Then they can use the text to check their answers and answer questions they could not complete. Answers to these activities appear in all the *Teacher's Resource* products.

Other activities, such as case studies and surveys, ask for students' thoughts or opinions. Answers to these activities cannot be judged as right or wrong. These activities allow students to form ideas by considering alternatives and evaluating situations thoughtfully.

You can use these thought-provoking exercises as a basis for classroom discussion by asking students to justify their answers and conclusions.

Using the *Teacher's Resource Guide*

The *Teacher's Resource Guide* for *Nutrition, Food, and Fitness* suggests many methods of presenting the concepts in the text to students. It begins with a detailed introduction explaining how to use the various components in the teaching package. This section also contains several features designed to help you prepare meaningful lessons and increase the effectiveness of your classroom teaching. This information includes suggestions for teaching students of varying abilities, evaluating students, communicating with students, and promoting your program.

Correlation of National Standards for Nutrition and Wellness with *Nutrition, Food, and Fitness*

In 1998, the National Standards for Family and Consumer Sciences Education were finalized. This comprehensive guide provides family and consumer sciences educators with a structure for identifying what learners should be able to do. This structure is based on knowledge and skills needed for work life and family life, as well as family and consumer sciences careers. The National Standards Components include 16 areas of study, each with overall content of the area. Each comprehensive standard is then broken down into content standards that describe what is expected of the learner. Competencies further define the knowledge, skills, and practices of the content standards and provide the basis for measurement criteria.

By studying the text *Nutrition, Food, and Fitness*, students will be prepared to master the competencies for the area of study called *Nutrition and Wellness*. To help you see how this can be accomplished, a *Correlation of National Standards for Nutrition and Wellness with Nutrition, Food, and Fitness* has been included in each of the *Teacher's Resource products*. If you want to make sure you prepare students to meet the National Standards for Family and Consumer Sciences Education, this chart should be of interest to you.

Basic Skills Chart

Another feature of the *Teacher's Resource Guide* is a *Basic Skills Chart*. This chart has been included to identify those activities that encourage the development of the following basic skills: verbal, reading, writing, mathematical, scientific, and analytical. (Analytical skills involve the higher-order thinking skills of analysis, synthesis, and evaluation in problem-solving situations.) The chart includes activities from the "Put Learning into Action" section of the text, activities from the *Student Activity Guide,* and strategies from the *Teacher's Resources.* Incorporating a variety of these activities into your daily lesson plans will provide your students with vital practice in the development of basic skills. Also, if you find students in your classes are weak in a specific basic skill, you can select activities to strengthen that particular skill area.

Chapter-by-Chapter Resources

Like the *Student Activity Guide,* the *Teacher's Resource Guide* is divided into chapters that match the chapters in the text. Each chapter contains the following features:

Objectives. These are the objectives students will be able to accomplish after reading the chapter and completing the suggested activities.

Bulletin Boards. One or more bulletin board ideas are described for each chapter. Many of these ideas are illustrated for you. Putting up bulletin board displays can often be a stimulating student activity.

Teaching Materials. A list of materials available to supplement each chapter in the text is provided. The list includes the names of all the activities contained in the *Student Activity Guide* and all the masters contained in the *Teacher's Resources.*

Introducing the Chapter. These motivational exercises are designed to stimulate your students' interest in the chapter they will be studying. The activities help create a sense of curiosity that students will want to satisfy by reading the chapter.

Strategies to Reteach, Reinforce, Enrich, and Extend Text Concepts. A variety of student learning strategies is described for teaching each of the major concepts discussed in the text. Each major concept appears in the guide in bold type. The student learning experiences for each concept follow. Activities from the *Student Activity Guide* are identified for your convenience in planning daily lessons. They are identified with the letters *SAG* following the title and letter of the activity. (*Evaluating Health and Nutrition Information,* Activity D, SAG.)

The number of each learning strategy is followed by a code in bold type. These codes identify the teaching goals each strategy is designed to accomplish. The following codes have been used:

RT identifies activities designed to help you *reteach* concepts. These strategies present the chapter concepts in a different way to allow students additional learning opportunities.

RF identifies activities designed to *reinforce* concepts to students. These strategies present techniques and activities to help clarify facts, terms, principles, and concepts, making it easier for students to understand.

ER identifies activities designed to *enrich* learning. These strategies help students learn more about the concepts presented by involving them more fully in the material. Enrichment strategies include diverse experiences, such as demonstrations, field trips, guest speakers, panels, and surveys.

EX identifies activities designed to *extend* learning. These strategies promote thinking skills, such as critical thinking, creative thinking, problem solving, and decision making. Students must analyze, synthesize, and evaluate to complete these activities.

Chapter Review. These review activities are designed to help students summarize key information from the chapter. You can use these activities to help students check their learning and prepare for chapter tests.

Above and Beyond. This section gives suggestions for enrichment activities that require work beyond the average class assignments. Although these activities could enhance the learning of any student, they are recommended for gifted or above average students.

Answer Key. This section provides answers for review questions at the end of each chapter in the text, for activities in the *Student Activity Guide,* for the reproducible masters in the *Teacher's Resources,* and for the chapter tests.

Reproducible Masters. Several reproducible masters are included for each chapter. These masters are designed to enhance the presentation of concepts in the text. Some of the masters are designated as *transparency masters* for use with an overhead projector. These are often charts or graphs that can serve as a basis for class discussion of important concepts. You can also use them as student handouts. Some of the masters are designed as *reproducible masters.* You can give each student a copy of these activities, which encourage creative and critical thinking. They can also serve as a basis for class discussion. Some masters provide material not contained in the text that you may want students to know.

Chapter Test Masters. Individual tests with clear, specific questions that cover all the chapter topics are provided. Matching, true/false, and multiple choice questions measure student learning about facts and definitions. Essay questions are also provided in the chapter tests. Some of these require students to list information, while others encourage students to express their opinions and creativity. You may wish to modify the tests and tailor the questions to your classroom needs.

Using the *Teacher's Resource Portfolio*

The *Teacher's Resource Portfolio* for *Nutrition, Food, and Fitness* includes all the resources from the *Teacher's Resource Guide* plus a set of color transparencies. These materials come in a convenient three-ring binder with a handle for easy carrying and a hook and loop fastener to keep everything together. The binder format allows you to remove pages for easy copying. You can also insert additional resource materials of your own. Handy dividers organize materials into parts that correspond to the textbook so you can quickly find the items you need.

The color transparencies found in the *Teacher's Resource Portfolio* can help you add variety to your classroom lectures. You will find some transparencies useful in illustrating and reinforcing information presented in the text. Others will provide you with an opportunity to extend learning beyond the scope of the text. Attractive colors are visually appealing and hold students' attention. Suggestions for how you can use the transparencies in your classroom are included among the teaching strategies listed for each chapter.

Using the *Teacher's Resource CD with ExamView® Test Generator Software*

The *Teacher's Resource CD* includes all the contents of the *Teacher's Resource Portfolio* plus **Exam***View®* *Test Generator Software*. This format allows you to view and print pages exactly as they appear in the *Teacher's Resource Portfolio* from your computer. The color transparencies are included in PowerPoint format as well as PDF format. Lesson plans are also included.

To produce overhead transparencies, print transparency master pages onto acetate film designed for your printer. If you are printing a color transparency, you will need a color printer to produce a transparency that appears as it does on your screen. However, you can print color transparencies in gray scale using a black ink printer.

The **Exam***View®* *Test Generator Software* database includes all the test master questions from the *Teacher's Resources* plus an additional 25 percent new questions prepared just for this product. You can have the computer select questions randomly. You can also choose specific questions from the database and add your own questions to create customized tests. There is even an option to make different versions of the same test. Answer keys are generated automatically.

Using Other Resources

Learning in your class can be reinforced and expanded by exposing your students to a variety of viewpoints. Information may be obtained through various government offices and trade and professional organizations. Local sources of information might include cooperative extension offices and state departments of agriculture and health.

The Internet serves as an almost limitless source of information relating to topics students will study in your classroom. You will want to encourage students to utilize this technology. However, you need to caution them that not all the information they will find on the Internet is reliable. Coach students to verify information by checking multiple sources. Also, advise them to use the extensions at the ends of Web site addresses as keys to information sources. Government agency sites end in *.gov*, professional organization sites end in *.org*, and educational institution sites end in *.edu*. The extension *.com* identifies Web sites of commercial groups, which may exist mainly to promote business.

The following list includes additional sources of information and materials that may be of use to you and your students. Names, phone numbers, and Web site addresses are included. Please note that contact information may have changed since publication of this product.

Publications

Current magazines and journals are good sources of articles on various nutrition, food, and fitness topics. Having copies in the classroom will encourage students to use them for research and ideas throughout your course. The following publications may be helpful to you or your students:

American Health
ISSN 1523-3359
Choices Magazine
undp.org/dpa/choices
Consumer Reports
consumerreports.org
Developmental Psychology
(800) 374-2721
apa.org/journals/dev/currentTOC.html
Journal of Family and Consumer Sciences
(703) 706-4600
aafcs.org
Newsweek
newsweek.com
Time
time.com
What's New
(800) 555-5657
whats-new-mag.com

Trade and Professional Organizations*

American Association of Family and Consumer Sciences (AAFCS)
(703) 706-4600
aafcs.org

*Note: The phone numbers and Web site addresses listed may have changed since the publication of this product.

American Association for Vocational
   Instructional Materials
   (800) 228-4689
   aavim.com
American Council on Exercise (ACE)
   (800) 825-3636
   acefitness.org
American Diabetes Association
   (800) 342-2382
   diabetes.org
American Dietetic Association (ADA)
   (800) 877-1600
   eatright.org
American Heart Association
   (800) 242-8721
   amhrt.org
American Institute for Cancer Research
   (AICR)
   (800) 843-8114
   aicr.org
American Medical Association
   (312) 464-5000
   ama-assn.org
Association for Career and Technical
   Education (ACTE)
   (800) 826-9972
   acteonline.org
Bread for the World (BFW)
   (800) 822-7323
   bread.org
Center for Science in the Public Interest
   (CSPI)
   (202) 332-9110
   cspinet.org
Children's Defense Fund
   (202) 628-8787
   childrensdefense.org
Children's Nutrition Research Center
   (713) 798-4712
   bcm.tmc.edu/cnrc
Consumer Education for Teens
   wa.gov/ago/youth
Council of Better Business Bureaus, Inc.
   (703) 276-0100
   bbb.org
Dairy Council of Wisconsin
   (800) 325-9121
   dcwnet.org
Family, Career and Community Leaders of
   America (FCCLA)
   (703) 476-4900
   fcclainc.org
The Food Allergy Network
   foodallergy.org
Food and Agricultural Organization of the
   United Nations
   (800) 929-4040
   fao.org

Food for the Hungry
   (800) 248-6437
   fh.org/wcn/index.html
Food Marketing Institute
   (202) 452-8444
   fmi.org
Food Research and Action Center (FRAC)
   (202) 986-2200
   frac.org
Grocery Manufacturers of America
   (202) 337-9400
   gmabrands.com
Institute of Food Technologists
   (312) 782-8424
   ift.org
International Culinary and Nutrition Network
   icnn.com
International Food Information Council (IFIC)
   (202) 296-6540
   ific.org
JobWeb
   (800) 544-5272
   jobweb.org
Johns Hopkins Medicine Health Information
   (410) 955-8659
   hopkinsmedicine.org/healthinformation.html
Medline
   medline.cos.com
National Association of WIC Directors (NAWD)
   (202) 232-5492
   nwica.org
National Consumers League
   (202) 835-3323
   natlconsumersleague.org
National Fraud Information Center
   (800) 876-7060
   fraud.org
National Institute for Consumer Education
   (734) 487-2292
   nice.emich.edu
National Organization on Fetal Alcohol
   Syndrome
   (202) 785-4585
   nofas.org
The National Restaurant Association
   (202) 331-5900
   restaurant.org/index.html
Occupational Outlook Handbook
   bls.gov/oco/
Online Career Center
   (800) 666-7837
   occ.com/occ
Partnership for Food Safety Education
   (888) 723-3366
   fightbac.org
Public Voice for Food and Health Policy
   (202) 371-1840

Pure Food Campaign
(218) 226-4164
purefood.org

Safe Tables Our Priority (STOP)
(802) 863-0555
stop-usa.org

Shape Up America!
(240) 793-0908
shapeup.org

Students Against Destructive Decisions (SADD)
(877) 722-3462
saddonline.com

Tufts University Nutrition Navigator
navigator.tufts.edu

World Agricultural Outlook Board
(202) 720-5447
usda.gov/agency/oce/waob/waob.htm

World Health Organization
(202) 974-3000
who.int/home-page/

Government Agencies*

Sources of General Information

The Consumer Information Center (CIC) publishes the free *Consumer Information Catalog*, which lists hundreds of free and low-cost government booklets on many consumer topics. For copies of the catalog, contact the CIC online (www.pueblo.gsa.gov), call (719) 948-4000, or write to *Consumer Information Catalog*, Pueblo, CO 81009.

The Federal Information Center (FIC) can help you find information about U.S. Government agencies, services, and programs. The FIC can also tell you which office to contact for help with problems. You can contact the FIC during normal business hours by calling (800) 688-9889.

Consumer Product Safety Commission
(800) 638-2772
www.cpsc.gov

Department of Agriculture
(202) 720-2791
www.usda.gov

Agricultural Research Service
(301) 504-1638
ars.usda.gov

Center for Nutrition Policy and Promotion
(202) 418-2312
www.usda.govfcs/cnpp.htm

Food and Nutrition Services
(703) 305-2281
http://www.fns.usda.gov/fns/

Food and Nutrition Information Center of the National Agricultural Library
www.nal.usda.gov/fnic

Food Safety and Inspection Service
(800) 535-4555
www.fsis.usda.gov

Meat and Poultry Hotline
(800) 535-4555
www.fsis.usda.gov

School Meals Initiative for Healthy Children
(301) 435-0714
fns.usda.gov/tn/Initiative/index.htm

World Agricultural Outlook Board
(202) 720-5447
usda.gov/agency/oce/waob/waob.htm

Department of Education
(800) 872-5327
ed.gov

Safe and Drug-Free Schools Program
(202) 260-3954
www.ed.gov/offices/OESE/SFDS

Department of Health and Human Services
(877) 696-6775
www.dhhs.gov

Centers for Disease Control and Prevention (CDC)
(800) 311-3435
www.cdc.gov

Food and Drug Administration (FDA)
(888) 463-6332
www.fda.gov

Government Food Safety Information
foodsafety.gov

Government Healthfinder
healthfinder.gov

National Clearinghouse for Alcohol and Drug Information
(800) 729-6686
www.health.org

National Institute on Aging
(301) 496-1752
www.nia.nih.gov

National Institutes of Health
(301) 496-4000
www.nih.gov

National Institutes of Mental Health
(301) 443-4513

President's Council on Physical Fitness and Sports
(202) 690-9000
www.fitness.gov

Seafood Hot Line
(888) 723-3366

Weight-Control Information Network (WIN)
(301) 435-0714
niddk.nih.gov/health/nutrit/nutrit.htm

Department of Labor
(866) 4USA-DOL
www.dol.gov

Dictionary of Occupational Titles
www.wave.net/upg/immigration/dot_index.html

Occupational Information Network (O*NET)
online.onetcenter.org

Occupational Safety and Health
    Administration
    (202) 693-1999
    www.osha.gov
Federal Trade Commission (FTC)
    (877) 382-4357
    www.ftc.gov
Government Printing Office (GPO)
    (202) 512-1800
    www.gpo.gov
National Academy of Sciences
    (202) 334-2000
    www.nas.edu
Peace Corps
    (800) 424-8580
    peacecorps.gov

Educational Resources*

The following is a list of various companies that may serve as resources for additional teaching materials. Most provide videos and/or computer software. Many provide printed materials. Contact these organizations for their latest catalogs.

Cambridge Educational
    (800) 468-4227
    cambridgeeducational.com
The Health Connection
    (800) 548-8700
    healthconnection.org
Karol Media
    (800) 526-4773
    karolmedia.com
The Learning Seed
    (800) 634-4941
    learningseed.com
Meridian Education Corp.
    (800) 727-5507
    meridianeducation.com
Midwest Agribusiness Services, Inc.
    (800) 523-3475
Nasco
    (800) 558-9595
    enasco.com
RMI Media Productions
    (800) 821-5480
    rmimedia.com
Sax Family & Consumer Sciences
    (800) 558-6696
    www.artsupplies.com

Human Resources

A teacher of nutrition and wellness is often recognized as a team player in helping teens make nutrition and fitness decisions. A concerted effort to join forces with other interested groups and related professionals improves the chances of helping teens reduce at-risk health behaviors.

Involve families in the curriculum as much as possible. Invite family members to share health choices that have improved their quality of life. Family members and friends may be employed in health care services and may be available to offer information and resources for class use. Invite parents to listen to and offer feedback on student projects. Send newsletters and other materials developed by students home to keep parents informed about what your classes are studying.

Other people to involve in your program include community nutrition educators associated with health care facilities or the county extension services. Work with the foodservice staff in your school cafeteria to share resources. Ask these staff members if your students can display nutrition education materials in the cafeteria that might interest the whole student population.

Discuss curriculum building to present students with a nutrition and fitness message in an interdisciplinary environment. Consider sharing resources and developing projects with physical education teachers and sports team coaches. Invite teachers in the science department, including biology and chemistry teachers, to share their expertise. Working together may suggest the need for a curriculum advisory committee that focuses on nutrition and wellness across curriculum areas. Invite community nutrition advocates with responsibilities in a variety of agencies to be part of the committee. Together, you can present a strong message for promoting healthy lifestyle choices.

Teaching Techniques

You can make nutrition and wellness exciting and relevant by using a variety of teaching techniques. Below are some principles that will help you choose and use different teaching techniques in your classroom.

- Make learning stimulating. One way to do this is to involve students in lesson planning. When possible, allow them to select the modes of learning they enjoy most. For example, some students will do well with oral reports; others prefer written assignments. Some learn well through group projects; others do better working independently. You can also make courses more interesting by presenting a variety of learning activities and projects from which students may choose to fulfill their work requirement.
- Make learning realistic. You can do this by relating the subject matter to issues that concern young people. Students gain the most from learning when they can apply it to real-life situations. Case studies, role-playing, and drawing on personal experiences all make learning more realistic and relevant.
- Make learning varied. Try using several techniques to teach the same concept. Make use of outside resources and current events as they apply to material being presented in class. Students learn

through their senses of sight, hearing, touch, taste, and smell. The more senses they use, the easier it will be for them to retain information. Bulletin boards, videos, audio tapes, and transparencies all appeal to the senses.

- Make learning success-oriented. Experiencing success increases self-esteem and confidence. Guarantee success for your students by presenting a variety of learning activities. Key these activities to different ability levels so each student can enjoy both success and challenge. You will also want to allow for individual learning styles and talents. For instance, some students excel at organizing material, whereas others are artistic or analytical. Build in opportunities for individual students to work in ways and at projects that let them succeed and shine.

- Make learning personal. Young people become more personally involved in learning if you establish a comfortable rapport with them. Work toward a relaxed classroom atmosphere in which students can feel at ease when sharing their feelings and ideas in group discussions and activities.

Following are descriptions of various teaching techniques you may want to try. Keep in mind that not all methods work equally well in all classrooms. A technique that works beautifully with one group of students may not be successful with another. The techniques you choose will depend on the topic, your teaching goals, and the needs of your students.

One final consideration concerns student rights to privacy. Some activities, such as autobiographies, diaries, and opinion papers, may violate students' rights to privacy. You can maintain a level of confidentiality by letting students turn in unsigned papers in these situations. You may also encourage students to pursue some of these activities at home for personal enlightenment without fear of evaluation or judgment.

Helping Students Gain Basic Information

You can group teaching techniques according to different goals you may have for your students. One group of techniques is designed to convey information to students. Two of the most common techniques in this group are reading and lecture. Using a number of variations can make these techniques seem less common and more interesting. For instance, students may enjoy taking turns reading aloud as a change of pace from silent reading. You can energize lectures with the use of flip charts, overhead transparencies, and other visual materials. Classroom discussions of different aspects of the material being presented get students involved and help impart information.

Other ways to present basic information include the use of outside resources. Guest speakers, whether speaking individually or as part of a panel, can bring a new outlook to classroom material. You can videotape guest lectures to show again to other classes or to use for review. Along with videotapes, students enjoy films and filmstrips related to material being studied.

Helping Students Question and Evaluate

A second group of teaching techniques helps students develop analytic and judgment skills. These techniques help your students go beyond what they see on the surface. As you employ these techniques, encourage students to think about points raised by others. Ask students to evaluate how new ideas relate to their attitudes about various subjects.

Discussion is an excellent technique for helping students consider an issue from a new point of view. To be effective, discussion sessions require a great deal of planning and preparation. Consider the size of the discussion group and the physical arrangement. Since many students are reluctant to contribute in a large group, you may want to divide the class into smaller groups for discussion sessions. You will enhance participation if you arrange the room so students can see one another.

Discussion can take a number of forms. Generally it is a good idea to reserve group discussions involving the entire class for smaller classes. Buzz groups consisting of two to six students offer a way to get willing participation from students who are not naturally outgoing. They discuss an issue among themselves and then appoint a spokesperson to report back to the entire class.

Debate is an excellent way to explore opposite sides of an issue. You may want to divide the class into two groups, each taking an opposing side of the issue. You can also ask students to work in smaller groups and explore opposing sides of different issues. Each group can select students from the group to present the points for their side.

Helping Students Participate

Another group of teaching techniques is designed to promote student participation in classroom activities and discussion. There are many ways to involve students and encourage them to interact. Case studies, surveys, opinionnaires, stories, and pictures can all be used to boost classroom participation. These techniques allow students to react to or evaluate situations in which they are not directly involved. Open-ended sentences very often stimulate discussion. However, it is wise to steer away from overly personal or confidential matters when selecting sentences for completion. Students will be reluctant to deal with confidential issues in front of classmates.

The "fishbowl" can be a good way to stimulate class discussion. A larger observation group encircles an interactive group of five to eight students. The encircled students discuss a given topic while the others listen. Do not permit observers to talk or interrupt. Students can reverse positions at the end of a fishbowl session so some of the observers can become participants.

One of the most effective forms of small group discussion is the cooperative learning group. Match small groups of learners to complete a particular task or goal. Assign each person in the group a role. Measure the success of the group not only in terms of outcome, but in the successful performance of each member in his or her role.

In cooperative learning groups, students learn to work together toward a group goal. Each member is dependent upon others for the outcome. This interdependence is a basic component of any cooperative learning group. The value of each group member is affirmed as learners work toward their goal.

The success of the group depends on individual performance. Mix groups in terms of abilities and talents so there are opportunities for the students to learn from one another. Also, as groups work together over time, rotate roles so everyone has an opportunity to practice and develop different skills.

The interaction of students in a cooperative learning group creates a tutoring relationship. While cooperative learning groups may involve more than just group discussion, discussion is always part of the process by which cooperative learning groups function.

Helping Students Apply Learning

Some techniques are particularly good for helping students use what they have learned. Simulation games and role-playing allow students to practice solving problems and making decisions under nonthreatening circumstances. Role-playing allows students to examine others' feelings as well as their own. It can help them learn effective ways to react or cope when confronted with similar situations in real life.

Role-plays can be structured, with the actors following written scripts, or they may be improvised in response to a classroom discussion. Students may act out a role as they themselves see it being played, or they may act out the role as they presume a person in that position would behave. Students do not rehearse roles, and they compose lines on the spot. The follow-up discussion should focus on the participants' emotions and the manner in which the characters resolved the problem. Role-playing helps students consider how they would behave in similar situations.

Helping Students Develop Creativity

You can use some techniques to help students generate new ideas. For example, brainstorming encourages students to exchange and pool their ideas and to come up with new thoughts and solutions to problems. Do not allow evaluation or criticism of ideas.

The format of spontaneously expressing any opinions or reactions that come to mind lets students be creative without fear of judgment.

You can also promote creativity by letting students choose from a variety of assignments related to the same material. For example, suppose you wanted students to know what type of information to look for on product labels. You could ask them to contact a government agency to find out what the law requires on different labels. You might give them the choice of writing a case study involving the misreading of a label or a problem resulting from inadequate label information. Designing a product label or collecting a variety of labels and making a display would be options, too. Your students might even write a short story about a pantry full of cans without labels. Any teaching techniques you use to encourage students to develop their ideas will foster their creativity.

Helping Students Review Information

Certain techniques aid students in recalling and retaining knowledge. Games can be effective for drills on vocabulary and information. Crossword puzzles and mazes can make the review of vocabulary terms more interesting. Structured outlines of subject matter can also be effective review tools. Open-book quizzes, bulletin board displays, and problem-solving sessions all offer ways to review and apply material presented in the classroom.

Helping Students Value Diversity

Demographic data reminds teachers the makeup of the classroom is changing. With the changing mix of student ethnic and cultural backgrounds in the classroom comes a mix of differences in student expectations, lifestyles, needs, and values. The potential for misunderstanding can increase if approaches are not taken to build understanding and sensitivity to differences. Several of the following recommendations may be useful for enhancing the quality of the classroom environment to improve learning while living with diversity:

- Approach every student as a unique individual. Even though appearances, speech patterns, values, beliefs, and behaviors may be different, recognize many characteristics are shared by various cultural groups. Remember there are many individual differences even within groups.
- Understand a student's cultural behaviors, such as mannerisms and communication patterns, are not necessarily indicators of academic performance. Within each group there is a range of abilities, interests, and talents.
- Recognize your own discomfort when dealing with students who have diverse backgrounds. Be a role model of acceptance. Use inclusive language, structure teams for inclusion, coach students on

expected norms of behavior, stress a team atmosphere, and make it clear that everyone counts.

- Appreciate and utilize the different perspectives and lifestyle approaches to wellness. Go beyond tolerance to seeing diverse perspectives as assets.
- Use equal performance standards for all students. Help all students meet the standards.
- Provide feedback often and equally to all students. Give legitimate feedback regardless of race, sex, or other culturally related differences. Openly support the competencies and contributions of all students.
- Confront racist, sexist, or other stereotypical or discriminatory behavior exhibited by other students. Make your position clear by stating that neither you, nor the school, will tolerate discrimination.
- Be comfortable asking questions about preferred terminology or interaction. Since a teacher cannot be an expert in all groups, ask students to help you offer feedback without the use of inadvertent insensitive language that may have a negative impact on a student.

You, the teacher, ultimately hold the key for releasing the full potential of each student. Seek every opportunity to influence behaviors that promote students' abilities to learn from each other.

Helping Students Build Developmental Assets

Developmental assets refer to the "human capital" children and youth draw upon to grow up healthy, caring, and responsible. Nutrition education offers the opportunity to invest energies in helping students build upon these developmental assets. To support student growth, teachers are encouraged to set high performance levels for student learning and achievement. To expect less is to diminish the potential for growth.

Build upon the students' past experiences as you plan curriculum activities. Draw upon the students' friends and family members to respond to opinionnaires or questionnaires. Have students tell stories of their experiences. Students will begin to relate knowledge to their choices and sense positive use of time for creative and worthwhile projects. Provide a classroom environment that is supportive and welcoming. Make students feel valued in their contributions to classroom learning as they assist with the decision making and build commitment to group activities.

Some of the key assets valuable for youth development include the following:

- Social skills. Help students develop proactive communication, assertiveness skills, and responsiveness to others through pairing, small group discussion, and team projects.
- Positive sense of self-esteem. Success breeds success. Look for ways to build self-esteem by allowing students to experience small successes

in nutrition and fitness, one meal at a time or one day at a time.

- Problem-solving skills. Allow students to actively recognize their nutrition and fitness problems and give students opportunities to find solutions through problem-solving exercises. Actively involve students in decision making, rather than telling them what and how much to eat or what exercises to do.
- Positive values. Build upon caring, integrity, honesty, and justice values by creating learning experiences that involve contributions of service to the family, school, and/or community. Help students evaluate the needs of people locally and globally regarding the nutritional and health care issues of the world. Help students take action to help improve conditions for others.
- Positive sense of future. Promote expectations for long-term health by stressing the lifelong impact of present decisions.

Students will feel empowered when they realize they have the responsibility for making the choices that will directly affect their health.

Teaching Students of Varying Abilities

The students in your classroom represent a wide range of ability levels. Students with mental or learning disabilities who are mainstreamed require unique teaching strategies. You must not overlook gifted students, either. All the students in between will have individual needs to consider, too. Often you will be asked to meet the needs of all these students in the same classroom setting. Adapting daily lessons to meet the demands of all your students is a challenge.

To tailor your teaching to students with below-average learning abilities, consider the following strategies:

- Before assigning a chapter in the text, discuss and define the key words that appear at the beginning of each chapter. These terms are defined in the glossary at the back of the text. Ask students to write out the definitions and tell what they think the terms mean in their own words. You might want to invite students to guess what they think words mean before they look up the definitions. You can also ask them to use new words in sentences and to find the sentences in the text where the new terms are used.
- When introducing a new chapter, review previously learned information students need to know before they can understand the new material. Review previously learned vocabulary terms they will encounter again.
- Utilize the "Introducing the Chapter" section in the *Teacher's Resources* for each chapter. Students who have difficulty reading need a compelling

reason to read the material. These introductory activities can provide the necessary motivation. Students will want to read the text to satisfy their curiosity.

- Break the chapters into smaller parts, and assign only one section at a time. Define the terms, answer the *Check Your Knowledge* questions, and discuss the concepts presented in each section before proceeding to the next. It often helps to rephrase questions and problems in simple language and to repeat important concepts in different ways. Assign activities in the *Student Activity Guide* that relate to each section in the book. These reinforce the concepts presented. In addition, many of these activities are designed to improve reading comprehension.
- Ask students, individually or in pairs, to answer the *Check Your Knowledge* questions at the end of each chapter in the text. This will help students focus on the essential information contained in the chapter.
- Use the buddy system. Pair students who do not read well with those who do. Ask students who have mastered the material to work with those who need assistance. Also consider using parent volunteers to provide individual attention where needed.
- Select a variety of educational experiences to reinforce the learning of each concept. Look for activities that will help students relate information to real-life situations. Try to draw on the experiences of students at home, in school, and in the community.
- Give directions orally as well as in writing. You will need to explain assignments as thoroughly and simply as possible. Ask questions to be certain students understand what they are to do. Encourage them to ask for help if they need it. You will also want to follow up as assignments proceed to be sure no one is falling behind on required work.
- Use the overhead projector and the transparency masters included in the *Teacher's Resources.* A visual presentation of concepts will increase students' ability to comprehend the material. You may want to develop other transparencies to use in reviewing key points covered in each chapter.

If you have students with above-average learning abilities in your class, you will need to find ways to challenge them. These students require assignments that involve critical thinking and problem solving. They may enjoy helping you develop case studies and learning activities to use with the entire class. Because advanced students are more capable of independent work, they can use Internet and library resources to research topics in depth. Learning experiences listed in the *Basic Skills Chart* that involve analytical skills are appropriate for gifted students.

Evaluation Techniques

You can use a variety of evaluation tools to assess student achievement. Try using the reproducible forms, *Evaluation of Individual Participation, Evaluation of Individual Reports,* and *Evaluation of Group Participation,* included with the introductory material in the front of the *Teacher's Resources.* These rating scales allow you to observe a student's performance and rank it along a continuum. This lets students see what levels they have surpassed and what levels they can still strive to reach.

In some situations, it is worthwhile to allow students to evaluate their work. When evaluating an independent study project, for example, students may be the best judge of whether they met the objectives they set for themselves. Students can think about what they have learned and see how they have improved. They can analyze their strengths and weaknesses.

You may ask students to evaluate their peers from time to time. This gives the student performing the evaluation an opportunity to practice giving constructive criticism. It also gives the student being evaluated the opportunity to accept the criticism from his or her peers.

Tests and quizzes are also effective evaluation tools. You may give these in either written or oral form. In either case, however, you should use both objective and subjective questions to adequately assess student knowledge and understanding of class material.

Communicating with Students

Communicating with students involves not only sending clear messages, but also receiving and interpreting feedback. The following suggestions will encourage productive communication with your students:

- Recognize the importance of body language and nonverbal communication both in presenting material and interpreting student responses. Use eye contact, relaxed but attentive body position, natural gestures, and an alert facial expression as you present material. Look for the same body language from students as an indication of their attention. Voice is also an important nonverbal communicator. Cultivating a warm, lively, enthusiastic speaking voice will make classroom presentations more interesting. By your tone, you can convey a sense of acceptance and expectation to which your students will respond.
- Use humor whenever possible. Humor is not only good medicine, it opens doors and teaches lasting lessons. Laughter and amusement will reduce tension, make points in a nonthreatening and memorable way, increase the fun and pleasure in classroom learning, and break down stubborn

barriers. Relevant cartoons, quotations, jokes, and amusing stories all bring a light touch to the classroom.

- Ask questions that promote recall, discussion, and thought. Good questions are tools that open the door to communication. Open-ended inquiries that ask what, where, why, when, and how will stimulate thoughtful answers. You can draw out students by asking for their opinions and conclusions. Questions with yes or no answers tend to discourage rather than promote further communication. Avoid inquiries that are too personal or that might put students on the spot.

- Rephrase students' responses to be sure both you and other students understand what has been said. Paraphrasing information students give is a great way to clarify, refine, and reinforce material and ideas under discussion. For example, you might say, "This is what I hear you saying. . . Correct me if I'm wrong." Positive acknowledgment of students' contributions, insights, and successes encourages more active participation and open communication. Try comments like, "That's a very good point. I hadn't thought of it that way before." or, "What a great idea."

- Listen for what students say, what they mean, and what they do not say. Really listening may be the single most important step you can take to promote open communication. As students answer questions and express their ideas and concerns, try not only to hear what they say but to understand what they mean. What students leave unsaid can also be important. Make room for silence and time to think and reflect during discussion sessions.

- Share your feelings and experiences. The measure of what students communicate to you will depend in part on what you are willing to share with them. Express your personal experiences, ideas, and feelings when they are relevant. Do not forget to tell students about a few of your mistakes. Sharing will give students a sense of exchange and relationship.

- Lead discussion sessions to rational conclusions. Whether with an entire class or with individual students, it is important to identify and resolve conflicting thoughts. This will help students think clearly and logically. For example, in a discussion of the national hunger problem, students may think the government should provide more relief programs without passing costs on to taxpayers. Pointing out and discussing the inconsistencies in this position will lead to more logical approaches to both hunger relief and taxation.

- Create a nonjudgmental atmosphere. Students will only communicate freely and openly in a comfortable environment. You can make them comfortable by respecting their ideas, by accepting them for who they are, and by honoring their confidences. It is also important to avoid criticizing a student or discussing personal matters in front of others.

- Use written communication to advantage. The more ways you approach students, the more likely you are to reach them on different levels. Very often, the written word can be an excellent way to connect. Written messages can take different forms—a notice on the chalkboard, a note attached to homework, a memo to parents (with good news as well as bad), or a letter exchange involving class members.

- Be open and available for private discussion of personal or disciplinary problems. It is important to let students know they can come to you with personal concerns as well as questions regarding course material. You generally need to handle these discussions and disciplinary actions confidentially and in a private setting.

Promoting Your Program

You can make nutrition and wellness one of the most important course offerings in your school. You cover material every student and teacher can use. It pays to make the student body and faculty aware of your program. With good public relations you can increase your enrollment, gain support from administrators and other teachers, and achieve recognition in the community. The following suggestions can help you promote your program:

- Create visibility. It is important to let people know what is going on in nutrition and wellness classes. Ways to do this include announcements of projects and activities at faculty meetings and in school bulletins or newspapers, displays in school showcases or on bulletin boards, and articles and press releases in school and community newspapers. Talk up your program with administrators, other teachers, and students. Invite them to visit your classes.

- Interact within the school. Nutrition and wellness is related to many fields of learning. You can strengthen your program and contribute to other disciplines by cooperating with other teachers. For example, you can work with a health teacher to present information on digestive disorders, a physical education teacher to cover the benefits of exercise, or a chemistry teacher to discuss the molecular structure of carbohydrates. The more interaction you can generate, the more you promote the nutrition and wellness program.

- Contribute to the educational objectives of the school. If your school follows stated educational objectives and strives to strengthen specific skills, include these overall goals in your teaching. For example, if students need special help in developing verbal or writing skills, select projects and assignments that will help them in these areas. The *Basic Skills Chart* in the *Teacher's Resources* will give you ideas for activities that strengthen specific skills. Show administrators examples of work that indicate student improvement in needed skills.

- Serve as a resource center. Nutrition and wellness information is of practical use and interest to almost everyone. You can sell your program by making your department a resource center of nutrition and wellness materials related to weight management, menu planning, and food safety. Invite faculty members, students, and parents to tap into the wealth of nutrition and wellness information available in your classroom.

- Generate involvement and activity in the community. Real nutrition and wellness education takes place in the community. You are teaching concepts students can apply immediately where they live. You can involve students in community life and bring the community into your classroom through field trips, interviews with businesspeople and community leaders, surveys, and presentations from guest speakers. You may be able to set up cooperative projects between the school and community organizations around food safety, nutrition, social and mental health, and other topics.

- Connect with parents. If you can get them involved, parents may be your best allies in teaching and selling nutrition and wellness education. Let parents know when their children have done good work. Call on parents to share their experiences or to form a panel to discuss specific topics. Moms and dads have been through much of what you are preparing students to do. They have purchased and prepared foods, participated in exercise programs, and addressed weight management issues. Parents can be a rich source of real-life experience. Keep them informed on classroom activities and invite them to participate as they are able.

- Establish a student sales staff. Enthusiastic students will be your best salespeople. Encourage them to tell their parents and friends what they are learning in your classes. You might create bulletin boards or write letters to parents that focus on what students are learning in your classes. Ask students to put together a newsletter highlighting their experiences in nutrition and wellness education. Students could write a column from your department for the school paper.

We appreciate the contributions of the following Goodheart-Willcox authors to this introduction: "Teaching Techniques" from *Changes and Choices,* by Ruth E. Bragg; and "Evaluation Techniques" from *Contemporary Living,* by Verdene Ryder.

Evaluation of Individual Participation

Name_____   Date _____   Period _____

The rating scale below shows an evaluation of your class participation. It indicates what levels you have passed and what levels you can continue to try to reach.

1. Attentiveness

1	2	3	4	5
Completely inattentive.	Seldom attentive.	Somewhat attentive.	Usually attentive.	Extremely attentive.

2. Contribution to Discussion

1	2	3	4	5
Never contributes to class discussion.	Rarely contributes to class discussion.	Occasionally contributes to class discussion.	Regularly contributes to class discussion.	Frequently contributes to class discussion.

3. Interaction with Peers

1	2	3	4	5
Often distracts others.	Shows little interaction with others.	Follows leadership of other students.	Sometimes assumes leadership role.	Respected by peers for ability.

4. Response to Teacher

1	2	3	4	5
Unable to respond when called on.	Often unable to support or justify answers when called on.	Supports answers based on class information, but seldom offers new ideas.	Able to offer new ideas with prompting.	Often offers new ideas without prompting.

Total Points: _____ **out of 20**

Comments:

_____

_____

© Goodheart-Willcox

Evaluation of Individual Reports

Name_____   Date _____   Period _____

The rating scale below shows an evaluation of your oral or written report. It indicates what levels you have passed and what levels you can try to reach on future reports.

Report title_____Oral _____ Written _____

Criteria:

1. Choice of Topic

1	2	3	4	5
Slow to choose topic.	Chooses topic with indifference.	Chooses topic as assigned, seeks suggestions.	Chooses relevant topic without assistance.	Chooses creative topic.

2. Use of Resources

1	2	3	4	5
Unable to find resources.	Needs direction to find resources.	Uses fewer than assigned number of resources.	Uses assigned number of resources from typical sources.	Uses additional resources from a variety of sources.

3. Oral Presentation

1	2	3	4	5
No notes or read completely. Poor subject coverage.	Has few good notes. Limited subject coverage.	Uses notes somewhat effectively. Adequate subject coverage.	Uses notes effectively. Good subject coverage.	Uses notes very effectively. Complete coverage.

4. Written Presentation

1	2	3	4	5
Many grammar and spelling mistakes. No organization.	Several grammar and spelling mistakes. Poor organization.	Some grammar and spelling mistakes. Fair organization.	A few grammar and spelling mistakes. Good organization.	No grammar or spelling mistakes. Excellent organization.

Total Points: _____ out of _____

© Goodheart-Willcox

Evaluation of Group Participation

**Group
Members:**
_____   _____

_____   _____

_____   _____

_____   _____

The rating scale below shows an evaluation of the efforts of your group. It indicates what levels you have passed and what levels you can try to reach on future group projects.

1. Teamwork

1	2	3	4	5
Passive membership. Failed to identify what tasks needed to be completed.	Argumentative membership. Unable to designate who should complete each task.	Independent membership. All tasks completed individually.	Helpful membership. Completed individual tasks and then assisted others.	Cooperative membership. Worked together to complete all tasks.

2. Leadership

1	2	3	4	5
No attempt at leadership.	No effective leadership.	Sought leadership from outside group.	One member assumed primary leadership role for the group.	Leadership responsibilities shared by several group members.

3. Goal Achievement

1	2	3	4	5
Did not attempt to achieve goal.	Were unable to achieve goal.	Achieved goal with outside assistance.	Achieved assigned goal.	Achieved goal using added materials to enhance total effort.

Total Points: _____ out of 15

Members cited for excellent contributions to group's effort are:

_____   _____

_____   _____

Members cited for failing to contribute to group's effort are:

_____   _____

_____   _____

© Goodheart-Willcox

Correlation of National Standards

for

Nutrition and Wellness

with

Nutrition, Food, and Fitness

In planning your program, you may want to use the correlation chart below. This chart correlates the Family and Consumer Sciences Education National Standards with the content of **Nutrition, Food, and Fitness.** It lists the competencies for each of the content standards for Nutrition and Wellness. It also identifies the major text concepts that relate to each competency. Bold numbers indicate chapters in which concepts are found.

After studying the content of this text, students will be able to achieve the following comprehensive standard:

14.0 Demonstrate nutrition and wellness practices that enhance individual and family well-being.

Content Standard 14.1 Analyze factors that influence nutrition and wellness practices across the life span.	
Competencies	**Text Concepts**
14.1.1 Examine physical, emotional, social, psychological, and spiritual components of individual and family wellness.	**1:** What is wellness?; aspects of wellness; factors that affect wellness; nutrition and wellness **2:** Food is a reflection of culture; social influences on food choices; emotions affect food choices; the influences of agriculture, technology, economics, and politics **3:** Food, energy, and nutrients; the process of digestion; absorption of nutrients; metabolism; factors affecting digestion and absorption; digestive disorders **11:** Changing nutritional needs **12:** Energy input; energy output; energy imbalance; determining healthy weight **13:** Healthy people need a healthy weight; factors affecting your weight status; losing excess body fat; gaining weight **15:** Goals for physical activity; the benefits of physical activity; what is total fitness?; exercise and heart health; keys to a successful program; planning an exercise program **16:** The nutrient needs of an athlete; weight concerns of athletes; harmful performance aids **17:** Basic human needs; what is social health?; promoting positive social health; what is mental health?; promoting positive mental health; making positive life changes; seeking help for social and mental health problems **18:** Stress is a part of life; effects of stress on health; managing stress; preventing stress **19:** Drugs as medicine; drug misuse and abuse; stimulants; depressants; hallucinogens; drugs and athletes; getting help for a substance abuse problem **23:** Fitness trends

14.1.2 Compare the impact of psychological, cultural, and social influences on food choices and other nutrition practices.	1: Nutrition and wellness 2: Food is a reflection of culture; social influences on food choices; the influences of agriculture, technology, economics, and politics; nutrition knowledge affects food choices 13: Factors affecting your weight status 14: Probable causes of eating disorders 17: Basic human needs 21: Planning for nutrition 22: Factors that affect consumer food choices; being a consumer of fitness products and services; your consumer rights 23: Food preferences; fitness trends
14.1.3 Examine the governmental, economic, and technological influences on food choices and practices.	2: The influences of agriculture, technology, economics, and politics 20: People and public food safety 23: Are nonnutrient supplements safe?; bioengineering; functional foods; food safety advances 24: Economic reasons to care about world hunger; political reasons to care about world hunger; government policies; environmental factors
14.1.4 Investigate the impact of global and local events and conditions on food choices and practices.	2: The influences of agriculture, technology, economics, and politics 24: The hunger problem; why care about world hunger?; working toward national solutions; working toward global solutions; international organizations and programs
14.1.5 Examine legislation and regulations related to nutrition and wellness issues.	2: The politics of food 20: Government agencies 22: Using food labels; your consumer rights 24: National programs working toward hunger solutions

Content Standard 14.2 Evaluate the nutritional needs of individuals and families in relation to health and wellness across the life span.

Competencies	Text Concepts
14.2.1 Assess the effect of nutrients on health, appearance, and peak performance.	1: Nutrition and wellness 3: Food, nutrients, and energy; absorption of nutrients 5: Types of carbohydrates; the functions of carbohydrates; how your body uses carbohydrates; meeting your carbohydrate needs; health questions related to carbohydrates 6: What are lipids?; functions of lipids; lipids in the body; fats and heart health; fats and cancer; limiting fats and cholesterol in your diet 7: What is protein?; protein in the body; food sources of protein; how much protein do you need; the risks of too little or too much protein 8: What are vitamins?; the fat-soluble vitamins at work; the water-soluble vitamins at work; nonvitamins and other nonnutrients; are vitamin supplements needed?; preserving vitamins in foods 9: How minerals are classified; the macrominerals at work; the microminerals at work; minerals and healthful food choices 10: The vital functions of water; keeping fluids in balance 16: Nutrient needs of an athlete
14.2.2 Research the relationship of nutrition and wellness to individual family health throughout the life span.	11: Changing nutritional needs; pregnancy and lactation; infancy and toddlerhood; childhood; adolescence; adulthood
14.2.3 Assess the impact of food and diet fads, food addictions, and eating disorders on wellness.	12: Determining healthy weight 13: Healthy people need a healthy weight; factors affecting your weight status; losing excess body fat; gaining weight 14: Characteristics of eating disorders; probable causes of eating disorders; what help is available? 16: Weight concerns of athletes

14.2.4 Appraise sources of food and nutrition information, including food labels, related to health and wellness.	1: Evaluating research reports 4: Dietary Reference Intakes; Dietary Guidelines for Americans; the MyPyramid system; the Daily Values on food labels; using recommendations and guidelines 22: Using food labels

Content Standard 14.3 Demonstrate ability to acquire, handle, and use foods to meet nutrition and wellness needs of individuals and families across the life span.

Competencies	Text Concepts
14.3.1 Apply various dietary guidelines in planning to meet nutrition and wellness needs.	4: Dietary Reference Intakes; Dietary Guidelines for Americans; the MyPyramid system; the Daily Values on food labels; using recommendations and guidelines 6: Guidelines for food choices 10: Guidelines for fluid replacement 21: Planning for nutrition
14.3.2 Design strategies that meet the health and nutrition requirements of individuals and families with special needs.	5: Will too much sugar cause diabetes?; what is hypoglycemia?; what is lactose intolerance? 16: The nutrient needs of an athlete; weight concerns of athletes 21: Characteristics of family members
14.3.3 Demonstrate ability to select, store, prepare, and serve nutritious and aesthetically pleasing foods.	20: Shopping with safety in mind; storing foods safely; preparing foods safely 21: Planning for appeal; planning for nutrition; controlling food costs; saving time; meals away from home

Content Standard 14.4 Evaluate factors that affect food safety, from production through consumption.

Competencies	Text Concepts
14.4.1 Determine conditions and practices that promote safe food handling.	20: Common food contaminants; shopping with safety in mind; storing foods safely; keeping clean in the kitchen; preparing foods safely; packing food to go; when foodborne illness happens; people and public food safety
14.4.2 Appraise safety and sanitation practices throughout the food chain.	20: Common food contaminants; food producers; food processors and distributors; government agencies; food consumers
14.4.3 Determine how changes in national and international food production and distribution systems impact the food supply.	2: The economics of food; the politics of food 24: Government policies affecting world hunger; environmental factors affecting world hunger; recognize the hunger myths; focus on hunger solutions
14.4.4 Appraise federal, state, and local inspection and labeling systems that protect the health of individuals and the public.	20: U.S. Food and Drug Administration; U.S. Department of Agriculture and Food Safety and Inspection Service; National Marine Fisheries Service; U.S. Environmental Protection Agency; Federal Trade Commission; state and local agencies 22: Using food labels
14.4.5 Monitor foodborne illness as a health issue for individuals and families.	20: When foodborne illness happens; who is most at risk?; recognizing the symptoms; treating the symptoms; reporting foodborne illness
14.4.6 Review public dialogue about food safety and sanitation.	20: People and public food safety

Content Standard 14.5 Evaluate the impact of science and technology on food composition, safety, and other issues.	
Competencies	**Text Concepts**
14.5.1 Determine how scientific and technical advances impact the nutrient content, availability, and safety of foods.	**2:** Technology **20:** Storing foods safely; preparing foods safely **23:** Bioengineering; functional foods; competitive bacteria; DNA fingerprinting; active packaging; irradiation **24:** Research and technology advances as hunger solutions
14.5.2 Assess how the scientific and technical advances in food processing, storage, product development, and distribution impact nutrition and wellness.	**22:** Food processing; organic foods **23:** Bioengineering; functional foods; food safety advances **24:** Research and technology advances as hunger solutions
14.5.3 Determine the impact of technological advances on selection, preparation, and home storage of food.	**22:** Food processing **23:** Competitive bacteria; DNA fingerprinting; active packaging; irradiation
14.5.4 Assess the effects of food science and technology on meeting nutritional needs.	**22:** Food processing **23:** Bioengineering; functional foods; food safety advances **24:** Research and technology advances as hunger solutions

Basic Skills Chart

The chart below has been designed to identify those activities in *Nutrition, Food, and Fitness* text, *Student Activity Guide,* and *Teacher's Resources* that specifically encourage the development of basic skills. The following labels are used in the chart:

Text...*Put Learning into Action* activities at the end of each chapter in the text.

SAG...Activities in the *Student Activity Guide* (designated by letter).

TR...Strategies described in the *Teacher's Resources* (referred to by number).

Activities listed in the *Verbal* column include the following types: role playing, conducting interviews, oral reports, and debates.

Activities listed in the *Reading* column may involve reading in and out of the classroom. However, many of these activities are designed to improve reading comprehension of the concepts presented in each chapter. Some are designed to improve understanding of vocabulary terms.

Activities that involve written output are listed in the *Writing* column. The list includes activities that allow students to practice composition skills, such as letter writing, informative writing, and creative writing.

The *Math/Science* column includes activities that require students to use computation skills to solve typical problems they may come across in their everyday living. Activities that will enhance student understanding of scientific knowledge are also listed.

The final column, *Analytical,* lists those activities that involve the higher-order thinking skills of analysis, synthesis, and evaluation. Activities that involve decision making, problem solving, and critical thinking are included in this column.

	Verbal	Reading	Writing	Math/Science	Analytical
Chapter 1	Text: 1, 2, 4, 5 TR: 1, 3, 4, 6, 7, 8, 9, 10, 12, 14, 22, 23, 24, 25	Text: 5 SAG: B, D, E TR: 17, 18, 20, 21	Text: 2, 3, 5 TR: 25		Text: 4 SAG: A, C, E TR: 2, 5, 12, 15, 21, 23
Chapter 2	Text: 3 SAG: B, C TR: 1, 2, 3, 6, 7, 9, 10, 11, 15, 17, 18, 20, 21, 22, 24, 25, 26, 27, 28, 33, 37, 38	Text: 4 SAG: A, C, D, E TR: 15, 32, 34, 35, 36	Text: 1, 4, 5 SAG: D TR: 4, 16, 23		SAG: E TR: 5, 17, 29, 33, 36
Chapter 3	Text: 4 TR: 3, 6, 8, 14, 20, 23, 26, 28	SAG: A, B, D TR: 15, 22, 25, 29	Text: 3 TR: 27	Text: 1, 2 TR: 2, 4, 5, 9, 10, 12, 16, 17, 18, 19, 28	SAG: B, D TR: 22, 25, 27, 28
Chapter 4	Text: 1, 2 TR: 1, 2, 4, 6, 11, 12, 18, 20, 21, 22, 27, 28, 33, 34, 40	SAG: A, D TR: 3, 8, 9, 15, 17, 31, 32, 39	Text: 1, 3 TR: 12, 36, 37	Text: 3 SAG: B TR: 23, 25, 26	Text: 2 SAG: B, C, D TR: 14, 19, 25, 29, 30, 31, 35, 37, 39, 40

	Verbal	Reading	Writing	Math/Science	Analytical
Chapter 5	Text: 6 TR: 1, 3, 4, 5, 8, 14, 16, 18, 21, 22, 28, 29, 31, 35, 39, 42, 43	SAG: A, B, D, F TR: 7, 13, 31, 38, 40, 42	Text: 1, 5 SAG: E TR: 2, 18, 33, 37	Text: 4 SAG: C TR: 6, 12, 17, 23, 27, 34, 41	Text: 2, 3 SAG: A, F TR: 5, 7, 16, 18, 24, 25, 40, 43
Chapter 6	Text: 3, 5 TR: 1, 2, 4, 5, 6, 9, 12, 13, 16, 22, 25, 31, 32, 33, 34, 39	SAG: A, B, D, F TR: 8, 10, 18, 37, 38	Text: 1, 3, 4 SAG: E TR: 18, 36	Text: 2, 5 TR: 3, 7, 11, 15, 17, 20, 21, 24, 26, 34, 40, 41, 42	Text: 5 SAG: A, C, F TR: 8, 12, 19, 25, 29, 30, 38, 41, 42
Chapter 7	Text: 2, 4, 5 TR: 1, 2, 3, 4, 8, 12, 14, 16, 17, 21, 23, 28, 30, 32, 34	SAG: A, D, E, F, G TR: 15, 18, 19, 25, 26, 27, 29, 30, 33	Text: 1, 3 TR: 30, 31, 33, 35	TR: 4, 5, 6, 10, 20	Text: 2 SAG: B, C, G TR: 7, 8, 11, 14, 21, 29, 34
Chapter 8	TR: 1, 2, 3, 4, 6, 9, 10, 11, 12, 13, 16, 24, 26, 31, 34, 35, 37, 40	SAG: B, C, F TR: 13, 22, 23, 25, 27, 38, 39	Text: 1, 2, 3, 4, 5 SAG: D, E TR: 11, 15, 28, 29, 32, 35, 37, 39	TR: 6, 8, 10, 14, 15, 19, 20	Text: 3 SAG: A, F TR: 18, 21, 38
Chapter 9	Text: 1 TR: 1, 2, 3, 12, 14, 21, 27, 29, 34, 37, 38	SAG: A, B, C, D, E TR: 29, 30, 31, 33, 35, 36	Text: 1, 2, 3, 4 TR: 14, 28, 39	TR: 4, 5, 7, 8, 9, 13, 14, 15, 16, 17, 18, 24	Text: 2, 5 SAG: E TR: 19, 26, 36, 37, 38
Chapter 10	Text: 2 TR: 1, 2, 3, 7, 11, 13, 19, 20, 27	SAG: A, B, E TR: 14, 23, 24, 26	Text: 1 SAG: D TR: 5, 20, 25, 26	SAG: C TR: 5, 6, 9, 10, 12, 16, 18, 21	Text: 1 SAG: B, D, E TR: 14, 22, 24
Chapter 11	Text: 1, 6 TR: 1, 4, 5, 10, 12, 24, 26, 28, 29, 30, 31, 34, 37, 39, 40	Text: 2, 5 SAG: A, B, C, E, G TR: 3, 7, 9, 16, 17, 21, 32, 38	Text: 4, 5, 7 SAG: F TR: 35, 40	TR: 8, 20, 36	Text: 3 SAG: D, F, G TR: 11, 15, 18, 27, 30, 35, 38, 39
Chapter 12	TR: 1, 2, 3, 4, 7, 8, 9, 13, 15, 20	SAG: A, C, E TR: 14, 18, 21, 22	Text: 2, 3, 4 TR: 23, 24	Text: 1, 2, 4 SAG: B, D TR: 5, 6, 10, 11, 17	Text: 2 SAG: E TR: 21

	Verbal	Reading	Writing	Math/Science	Analytical
Chapter 13	Text: 1 TR: 1, 2, 4, 5, 6, 8, 12, 16, 18, 19, 23, 28, 29	SAG: B, F TR: 10, 26	Text: 1, 2, 3 SAG: A TR: 9, 24, 29	SAG: C TR: 13, 21	Text: 3 SAG: D, E, F TR: 8, 12, 15, 17, 20, 21, 25, 26
Chapter 14	Text: 2 SAG: C TR: 1, 2, 8, 10, 12, 19, 20, 23, 24	Text: 2, 27 SAG: A, C, D TR: 5, 7, 11, 15, 17, 22	Text: 1, 2 SAG: B TR: 15, 18, 23		SAG: C, D TR: 2, 9, 11, 19, 21, 22, 24
Chapter 15	Text: 1, 4 TR: 1, 2, 3, 4, 6, 7, 8, 9, 11, 13, 14, 15, 16, 19, 21, 23, 29, 32	SAG: B, D TR: 10, 23, 26, 27, 31, 32	Text: 2, 3, 6 SAG: A TR: 5, 10, 30	Text: 5 TR: 17	Text: 4, 6 SAG: D TR: 20, 22, 26
Chapter 16	Text: 1 SAG: C TR: 1, 2, 3, 4, 5, 8, 9, 11, 13, 17, 21, 23, 31, 32	SAG: A, B, D TR: 3, 7, 12, 14, 16, 18, 20, 21, 26, 29, 30, 31	Text: 1, 2 TR: 16, 22, 27, 28, 32, 33, 34	TR: 4, 11	Text: 1 SAG: B, D TR: 5, 22, 23, 26, 30
Chapter 17	Text: 2, 3 TR: 1, 2, 3, 9, 10, 12, 13, 17, 19, 20, 23, 25, 27, 29, 33	SAG: A, G TR: 7, 22, 34, 35, 38	Text: 1, 2, 3 SAG: B, C TR: 4, 11, 15, 18, 37		Text: 4 SAG: A, B, D, E, F, G TR: 5, 7, 8, 13, 14, 15, 21, 26, 28, 30, 31, 35, 37
Chapter 18	Text: 3 TR: 1, 2, 3, 4, 5, 6, 10, 11, 21, 24, 25	SAG: A, E, G TR: 8, 12, 17, 22, 23, 24, 25, 28	Text: 1, 2, 4 SAG: B, F TR: 12, 13, 18, 21		Text: 1, 2 SAG: C, D, F, G TR: 6, 7, 14, 15, 18, 20, 21, 23
Chapter 19	Text: 1, 2 TR: 1, 2, 3, 4, 5, 6, 8, 9, 10, 13, 15, 18, 22, 25, 26, 27, 28, 31, 32, 34, 37, 44, 45	Text: 3 SAG: B, C, F TR: 3, 7, 17, 19, 28, 41, 43, 44	Text: 4, 5 SAG: A TR: 12, 16, 19, 26, 38, 40, 46, 47	Text: 5 TR: 8, 22, 24	Text: 1 SAG: D, E, F TR: 2, 9, 16, 31, 39, 42, 43, 45

	Verbal	Reading	Writing	Math/Science	Analytical
Chapter 20	TR: 1, 2, 3, 9, 12, 16, 22, 25	Text: 1, 2 SAG: B, C, D TR: 6, 14, 21, 22, 23, 24	Text: 1 SAG: A TR: 5, 8, 11, 22, 24, 25	TR: 4	SAG: D TR: 9, 13, 21
Chapter 21	TR: 1, 2, 3, 4, 5, 10, 11, 12, 15, 16, 17, 20, 21, 22, 24, 25, 26, 27, 29, 33, 34, 35, 40, 41	Text: 3 SAG: F TR: 8, 28, 33, 37	Text: 1, 2 TR: 3, 42	SAG: D TR: 22, 23, 24	Text: 1 SAG: A, B, C, D, F TR: 3, 6, 8, 9, 13, 14, 16, 23, 24, 29, 31, 37, 38, 39, 41
Chapter 22	Text: 1, 2 TR: 1, 2, 3, 4, 5, 7, 8, 9, 10, 11, 12, 14, 15, 16, 17, 19, 20, 22, 25, 26, 27, 30, 32, 34, 35, 36, 41, 42	SAG: A, E TR: 6, 7, 11, 13, 18, 32, 38, 40	Text: 2, 4 SAG: C TR: 29, 42, 43	TR: 23, 24	Text: 3 SAG: B, D, E TR: 28, 30, 32, 33, 36, 39, 40
Chapter 23	Text: 1, 3 SAG: B TR: 1, 3, 5, 6, 8, 9, 10, 11, 13, 18, 19, 21, 22, 23, 24, 25, 26, 27, 28, 29, 34, 36	Text: 3 SAG: A, B, D TR: 2, 16, 17, 20, 27, 28, 32, 33, 35, 38	Text: 1 TR: 11, 16, 26, 38	Text: 2 TR: 24, 27	SAG: C, D TR: 4, 9, 15, 18, 19, 24, 31, 35
Chapter 24	Text: 2, 4 SAG: C TR: 1, 2, 3, 9, 10, 11, 14, 15, 16, 19, 22, 23, 25, 26, 28, 30, 32, 36, 38, 41	SAG: A, D, G TR: 4, 16, 18, 22, 28, 31, 35, 37, 38, 39	SAG: B, D TR: 13, 24, 29, 31, 34, 38, 40	Text: 1 TR: 8, 9, 21	Text: 4, 5 SAG: B, C, E, F, G TR: 1, 11, 12, 15, 20, 22, 24, 27, 30, 37, 39
Chapter 25	Text: 1, 4 TR: 1, 2, 3, 7, 8, 12, 14, 15, 20, 22, 23, 24, 25, 27, 28, 29, 32, 34, 36, 37, 38, 42, 44, 47	Text: 3 SAG: A, B, C, F TR: 4, 9, 10, 11, 28, 39, 40, 41	Text: 2, 5 TR: 11, 21, 30, 31, 35, 39, 43, 46		SAG: A, D, E, F TR: 9, 13, 16, 17, 25, 26, 27, 33, 34, 37, 41, 45

Making Wellness a Lifestyle

1

Objectives

After studying this chapter, students will be able to
- explain the physical, mental, and social aspects of wellness.
- list factors that contribute to disease.
- predict how lifestyle choices they make will affect their health.
- describe the relationship between nutrition and health.

Bulletin Boards

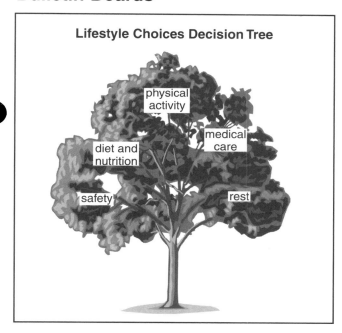

Lifestyle Choices Decision Tree

Title: *Lifestyle Choices Decision Tree*

Sketch a giant tree in the center of the bulletin board. Label branches of the tree with lifestyle choices that promote wellness, such as *diet and nutrition, medical care, safety, rest,* and *physical activity.* Have students work in pairs to cut out magazine pictures illustrating people engaged in healthy lifestyle activities. As students mount their pictures among the branches, they should be ready to explain why the pictures represent healthy behaviors.

Title: *Healthful Choices for Life's Long Haul*

Use black construction paper to form a highway going into the distance. Glue short pieces of white yarn to the construction paper to represent the centerline on the highway. Place signs along the highway labeled with age ranges from newborn to age 80 plus. Have students bring in family photos representing healthy people from each of these age ranges. Place the photos along the road to represent the complete life span. Ask students to add captions to each photo to describe the persons' healthy characteristics. If photos are not available, use magazine pictures instead.

Teaching Materials

Text, pages 10-25
  Learn the Language
  Check Your Knowledge
  Put Learning into Action
  Explore Further
Student Activity Guide, pages 7-12
  A. *Lifestyle Choices for Wellness*
  B. *Words in Wellness*
  C. *Behavior Change Contract*
  D. *Evaluating Health and Nutrition Information*
  E. *Backtrack Through Chapter 1*
Teacher's Resources
  Lifestyle Assessment, reproducible master 1-1
  The Wellness Continuum, color transparency CT-1
  Get in Gear with Wellness, transparency master 1-2
  Leading Causes of Death, transparency master 1-3
  Chapter 1 Test

Introducing the Chapter

1. Have students work in pairs to develop a list of factors that influence teens' health-related choices. Ask each pair to compile its list with another pair. After each group of four completes its expanded list, begin a large group discussion. Generate a comprehensive list of all the influences on adolescents' health-related choices. Then ask the class to suggest five specific ways teenagers can learn to increase individual responsibility for health-related choices.
2. *Lifestyle Assessment,* reproducible master 1-1. Have students take the assessment and score results. Discuss which of the risk factors students might reverse to improve health. You might also wish to give this questionnaire to students at the end of your course to help them evaluate lifestyle changes as a result of the course.

Strategies to Reteach, Reinforce, Enrich, and Extend Text Concepts

What Is Wellness?

3. **RF** Ask students to complete the following sentences: "When I am feeling at my very best I feel..." and "When I am feeling at my very worst I feel..." After students have completed their sentences, generate a laundry list of words to describe optimum health and health breakdown.

4. **RF** Have each student draw four horizontal lines across the width of a sheet of paper. Students should label the left end of each line *premature death* and the right end of each line *optimum health.* Have students mark the four lines to indicate where they think the following people fall along the wellness continuum: themselves, most teens, most adults, and most senior citizens. Have students compare their responses with classmates and discuss why there are variations.

5. **RF** *Lifestyle Choices for Wellness,* Activity A, SAG. Students are to identify lifestyle choices that contribute to premature death and lifestyle choices that contribute to optimum health. Then they are to answer follow-up questions.

Aspects of Wellness

6. **RT** *The Wellness Continuum,* color transparency CT-1. Use the transparency to illustrate that physical, mental, and social health are all components of wellness. Discuss how people can experience degrees of wellness for various factors related to each of these health areas. Ask students to give examples of other factors related to each health area.

7. **RT** *Get in Gear with Wellness,* transparency master 1-2. Use the transparency to explain to students how a balance among the three health areas can promote overall wellness. Ask students what lifestyle behaviors might contribute to health in each area. Write their responses in the appropriate gear on the transparency.

8. **RF** Have students list common stresses teens face daily. Discuss how these stresses affect teens' mental health and overall wellness.

9. **EX** Have students describe how being tired, skipping breakfast, and having a family argument about money can each affect physical, mental, and social health.

Factors That Affect Wellness

10. **ER** Have each student interview an adult who is over 60 years of age. Students should ask interviewees about their attitudes regarding health, health-promoting lifestyle habits, and family health histories. Ask students to share their findings in class as you discuss the impact of lifestyle choices on life expectancy.

11. **ER** Guest speaker. Invite a healthy person in his or her 80s to visit with the class. Encourage the person to describe factors that both helped and hindered his or her health throughout life.

12. **EX** Have students role-play a situation in which a teen offers a friend a cigarette. The friend should assertively refuse the cigarette. Following the role-play, discuss what the first teen might think of the friend for refusing the cigarette. Then discuss how people must assume personal responsibility for their health through their daily decisions. Also discuss how peer pressure may challenge a person's commitment to healthy lifestyle choices.

13. **ER** Field trip. Visit a work site wellness center. Ask a representative from the center to explain the purposes of the program to your students. The representative should also describe the characteristics of a healthy employee and what having healthy employees means to the organization.

14. **RT** *Leading Causes of Death,* transparency master 1-3. Discuss how lifestyle choices, environment, the health care system, and heredity could contribute to each of the causes of death listed on the transparency. Ask students why the leading causes of death might differ among various age groups.

15. **EX** *Behavior Change Contract,* Activity C, SAG. Students are to set goals for improving their health and then use the work sheet to keep track of their progress and evaluate the results of their efforts.

Nutrition and Wellness

16. **ER** Guest speaker. Invite a nutrition researcher to the class to discuss how new information is gained in the nutrition sciences. Relate the speaker's description of research methods to the scientific method described in the text.

17. **RT** Have students collect news articles that describe nutrition and health programs operating in the community. Make a display center of these articles.

18. **EX** *Evaluating Health and Nutrition Information,* Activity D, SAG. Students are to answer questions to help them analyze recent articles about health and/or nutrition research studies.

19. **ER** Guest speaker. Invite a representative from a local WIC program to speak to students about the nutritional needs of women with infants. Ask the speaker to describe how adolescents can become involved in their communities through a service learning project. Encourage students to volunteer.

Chapter Review

20. **RF** *Words in Wellness,* Activity B, SAG. Students are to use clues provided to complete a puzzle with key terms from the chapter.
21. **RF** *Backtrack Through Chapter 1,* Activity E, SAG. Students are to provide complete answers to questions and statements that will help them recall, interpret, apply, and practice chapter concepts.
22. **RF** Have each student write a question on one side of an index card about one of the concepts presented in the chapter. Students should write the answers to their questions on the backs of the cards. Divide the class into two teams. Select a moderator to read the questions and check for the correct answers. A question is directed to the first member of one team. If a correct answer is given, the next team member gets the next question. If an incorrect answer is given, the question is offered to the other team. One point is awarded for each correct answer. The team that correctly answers the most questions wins.

Above and Beyond

23. **ER** Have students prepare and present a program for teens on ways to deal with peer pressure and how to make health-promoting lifestyle choices. Students might develop skits, visual aids, or other strategies to show how health outcomes relate to daily individual choices.
24. **EX** Have students contact a social service agency to identify wellness needs of homeless people in the community. Have students work in groups to prepare proposals for service projects to address one of the health needs of the homeless. After receiving your approval for their proposals, students should carry out their service projects. When projects are completed, students should write reports or give oral presentations on the insights they have gained about the effects of homelessness on quality of life.
25. **ER** Have students compose songs, write poems, or create videotapes that incorporate the message of making lifestyle choices to promote health and maximize life expectancy. Arrange for students to present their creative works at a student, parent, or community gathering.

Answer Key
Text

Check Your Knowledge, page 24

1. Premature death lies at one end of the wellness continuum; optimum health lies at the other.
2. (List three:) medicine, physical therapy, diet, surgery, research
3. Irrational fears, stress, and depression may be signs of a mental health problem.
4. (List two:) learning how to use good communication to resolve interpersonal conflicts, seeking and lending support to others when needed, building a positive self-image
5. A teen's present actions and attitudes are shaping the person he or she will be in the future. It is hard to change a habit once it has been established.
6. (List three:) unhealthful lifestyle choices, poor environmental quality, inadequate health care, heredity
7. heart disease, cancer, stroke
8. (List five:) Eat three or more regularly spaced meals a day, including breakfast. Supply your body with needed nutrients. Sleep eight to nine hours each night. Maintain a healthy weight. Accumulate at least 60 minutes of moderate physical activity most days of the week. Do not smoke. Avoid drinking alcoholic beverages. Do not abuse drugs.
9. (Student response. See pages 19-20 in the text.)
10. over 45
11. (1) Make observations. (2) State a hypothesis. (3) Devise experiments to test the hypothesis to determine if it is true.
12. (List two:) Some people do not have enough money to acquire adequate nutrition. Others lack the information and skills needed to select a nutritious diet. Some may not know they need to make changes. Still others simply choose to ignore current nutrition recommendations.

Student Activity Guide

Words in Wellness, Activity B

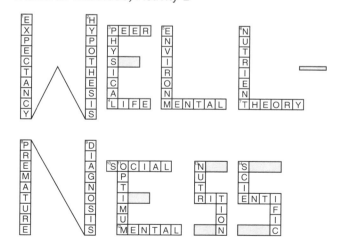

Backtrack Through Chapter 1, Activity E

1. (List four:) feel stronger; feel more alert; feel better about self; find it easier to cope with daily stresses; feel more satisfied with performance at home, school, work, play; begin to experience better relationships

2. physical health, mental health, social health
3. Holistic medicine is an approach to health care that focuses on all aspects of patient care—physical, mental, and social.
4. A risk factor is a characteristic or behavior that influences a person's chance of getting a disease.
5. decisions about smoking, decisions about nutrition, decisions about stress management, decisions about exercise
6. air pollutants, water pollutants, and food contaminants
7. (List one:) Patients fail to get regular checkups. Patients fail to seek medical care when symptoms appear. Patients fail to share information with physicians. Patients fail to follow physicians' advice.
8. (List two:) Some people take good health for granted. Some people do not notice the slow toll poor health habits take on their health. Some people fail to realize how addictive some poor health behaviors can be.
9. a branch of science that studies the incidence of disease in a population
10. (List three:) About one-third of the people in the United States eat an inadequate diet. One out of three adults is overweight. Popular lifestyles include less and less exercise. Important nutrients are missing from the diets of some groups of people. Fat, cholesterol, sodium, and sugar intake are higher than recommended.
11. (Student response. See pages 12-14 in the text.)
12. (Student response.)
13. (Student response.)
14. (Student response. See page 18 in the text.)
15. (Student response.)
16. Improved eating habits over the last 100 years has increased life expectancy in the United States.
17. (Student response.)
18. (Student response.)
19. (Student response.)
20. (Student response.)

Teacher's Resources

Chapter 1 Test

1.	I	19.	F
2.	F	20.	F
3.	J	21.	T
4.	C	22.	T
5.	A	23.	B
6.	B	24.	B
7.	H	25.	D
8.	G	26.	A
9.	K	27.	C
10.	E	28.	B
11.	T	29.	B
12.	F	30.	A
13.	F	31.	D
14.	T	32.	C
15.	T	33.	C
16.	T	34.	A
17.	T	35.	B
18.	F	36.	C

37. (List two:) physician makes incorrect diagnosis, physician makes diagnosis too late, health care facility lacks specialists, health care facility lacks needed equipment, health care facility is poorly managed, treatment is not given properly
38. (List three:) carpool or take public transportation, use nonpolluting cleaning products, handle food carefully to avoid contamination, contact local industries about their impact on the environment, write to government officials about environmental concerns, talk to employer about creating a safer work environment
39. (List three:) select a qualified physician, choose facilities that have a strong reputation, get regular checkups, see a doctor at the first sign of a problem, describe symptoms completely and accurately, ask physicians questions
40. (List two:) the audience to which the report is directed, who is relaying the information, the size of the study, the length of the study, the number of studies on this topic that have yielded similar results

Lifestyle Assessment

Name_____ Date _____ Period _____

This assessment will help you identify lifestyle choices that create health risks. The assessment has six sections: eating habits, physical activity and fitness, stress management, tobacco use, alcohol and other drug use, and safety. Complete one section at a time by circling the number corresponding to the answer that best describes your behavior. Then add the numbers you have circled to determine your total score for each section. The higher your score, the lower your health risk. Answer the questions honestly. Your answers will not be shared with anyone else.

	Almost Always	Some-times	Almost Never	Never
Eating Habits				
1. I eat a variety of foods each day, such as fruits, vegetables, whole grain breads and cereals, lean meats, dry beans or peanut butter, and dairy products.	3	2	1	0
2. I limit fatty foods.	3	2	1	0
3. I limit the amount of salt used in cooking and at the table.	3	2	1	0
4. I avoid eating too much sugar by limiting consumption of nondiet soft drinks, candy, and other sweets.	3	2	1	0
Your eating habits score				_____
Total points possible				12
Physical Activity and Fitness				
1. I maintain a healthy weight.	3	2	1	0
2. I accumulate an average of at least 60 minutes of moderate physical activity most days of the week.	3	2	1	0
3. I participate in individual, family, or team activities, such as swimming, tennis, and baseball, that increase my level of fitness.	3	2	1	0
Your exercise and fitness score				_____
Total points possible				9
Stress Management				
1. I am relaxed and cheerful.	3	2	1	0
2. I find it easy to relax and express my feelings freely.	3	2	1	0
3. I recognize and prepare for events or situations likely to be stressful for me.	3	2	1	0
4. I have close friends, relatives, or others whom I can talk to about personal matters and call on for help when needed.	3	2	1	0
5. I participate in group activities or hobbies I enjoy.	3	2	1	0
Your stress management score				_____
Total points possible				15

(Continued)

© Goodheart-Willcox

Name_____

	Almost Always	Some-times	Almost Never	Never
Tobacco Use				
1. I avoid smoking cigarettes.	3	2	1	0
2. I avoid use of smokeless tobacco products.	3	2	1	0

Your tobacco use score _____

Total points possible _____6_____

	Almost Always	Some-times	Almost Never	Never
Alcohol and Other Drug Use				
1. I avoid consumption of alcoholic beverages.	3	2	1	0
2. I avoid use of alcohol and other drugs as a way of handling problems in my life.	3	2	1	0

Your alcohol and
other drug use score _____

Total points possible _____6_____

	Almost Always	Some-times	Almost Never	Never
Safety				
1. I wear a seat belt when driving or riding in a vehicle.	3	2	1	0
2. I avoid riding in a vehicle with a driver who is under the influence of alcohol or other drugs.	3	2	1	0
3. I obey traffic rules and speed limits when driving.	3	2	1	0
4. I am careful when using appliances or power tools.	3	2	1	0
5. I wear appropriate protective equipment, such as a helmet and pads, when participating in sports activities.	3	2	1	0

Your safety score _____

Total points possible _____15_____

Your Total Health Assessment Score _____

Total Points Possible _____63_____

1. What do you think your total health assessment score says about you? _____

_____

_____

2. What are some lifestyle changes you might make to improve your score?_____

_____

_____

© Goodheart-Willcox

Get in Gear with Wellness

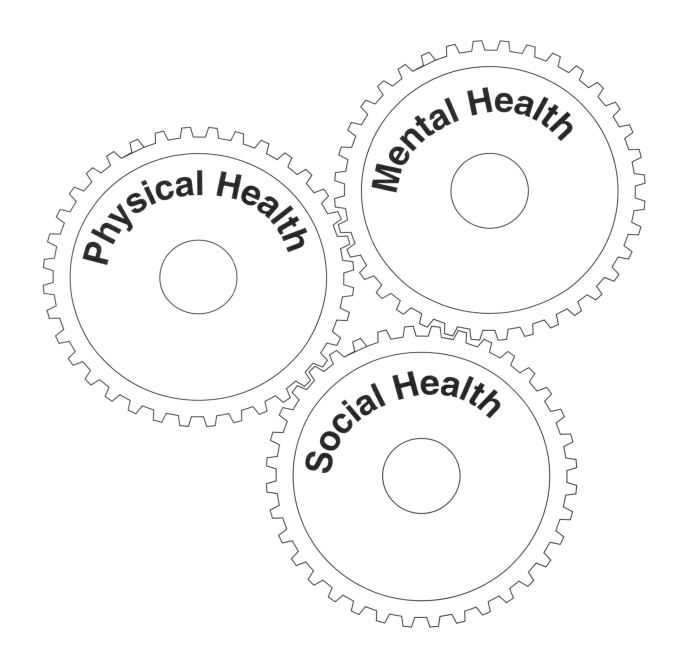

Transparency Master 1-3

Leading Causes of Death

Youth Ages 14-24

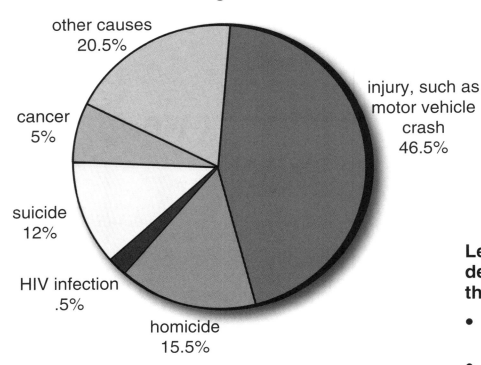

other causes
20.5%

cancer
5%

suicide
12%

HIV infection
.5%

homicide
15.5%

injury, such as
motor vehicle
crash
46.5%

**Leading causes of
death result from
these risk behaviors**

- Unintentional and
  intentional injuries
- Alcohol and other
  drug use
- Tobacco use
- Dietary behaviors
- Sexual behaviors
- Physical inactivity

Adults Ages 25 and Older

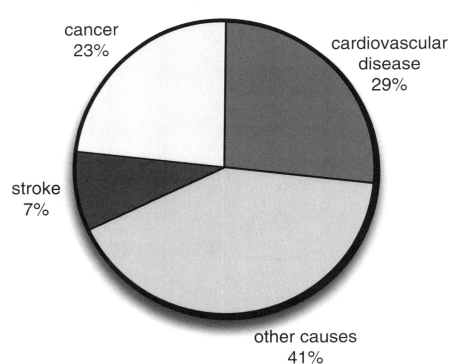

cancer
23%

stroke
7%

cardiovascular
disease
29%

other causes
41%

National Center for Health Statistics, 2002

© Goodheart-Willcox

Making Wellness a Lifestyle

Name_____

Date _____　　Period _____　　Score _____

Chapter 1 Test

Matching: Match the following terms and identifying phrases.

_____ 1. The fitness of the body.

_____ 2. The way a person feels about himself or herself, life, and the world.

_____ 3. A characteristic or behavior that influences a person's chance of being injured or getting a disease.

_____ 4. The state of the physical world, including the condition of water, air, and food.

_____ 5. The identification of a disease.

_____ 6. All the foods and beverages a person consumes.

_____ 7. The sum of the processes by which a person takes in and uses food substances.

_____ 8. A basic component of food that nourishes the body.

_____ 9. A principle that tries to explain something that happens in nature.

_____ 10. The average length of life of people living in the same environment.

A. diagnosis
B. diet
C. environmental quality
D. holistic medicine
E. life expectancy
F. mental health
G. nutrient
H. nutrition
I. physical health
J. risk factor
K. theory

True/False: Circle *T* if the statement is true or *F* if the statement is false.

T　F　11. A person's state of wellness is related to quality of life.

T　F　12. A person who is physically fit can be assumed to have achieved optimum health.

T　F　13. Learning how to use good communication to resolve conflicts with others is an example of a mental skill.

T　F　14. A construction worker faces greater environmental health risks than does a school teacher.

T　F　15. Physicians need information from patients to accurately diagnose medical problems.

T　F　16. Writing behavior change contracts can help people improve daily health patterns.

T　F　17. A hypothesis is a suggested answer to a scientific question.

T　F　18. The findings of a single scientific study can provide a sufficient basis for changing lifestyle behaviors.

T　F　19. Almost 50 percent of adults in the United States are more than 20 percent overweight.

T　F　20. Everyone in the United States has access to an adequate diet.

T　F　21. Education can help people understand and evaluate nutrition information reported in the media.

T　F　22. Nutritional choices influence the health of a nation's people.

© Goodheart-Willcox

(Continued)

Name_____

Multiple Choice: Choose the best response. Write the letter in the space provided.

_____23. Which of the following best describes the term *wellness?*
   A. A doctor's verification that a person is healthy.
   B. A person's high level of satisfaction with his or her appearance, lifestyle, and mental outlook.
   C. A physical state that comes from following a diet plan that includes only healthful foods.
   D. A state of health as described by friends.

_____24. Opposite premature death on the wellness continuum is _____.
   A. mental health
   B. optimum health
   C. physical health
   D. social health

_____25. The way a person relates to others refers to _____.
   A. environmental setting
   B. mental health
   C. physical health
   D. social health

_____26. A person who focuses on staying physically, mentally, and socially healthy practices an approach to wellness that can be described as _____.
   A. holistic
   B. inadequate
   C. simplistic
   D. unrealistic

_____27. Which factor is reported to have the greatest influence on people's state of health and wellness?
   A. Environmental quality.
   B. Heredity.
   C. Lifestyle choices.
   D. The health care system.

_____28. An example of a health-related factor over which a person has little control is his or her _____.
   A. environment
   B. heredity
   C. lifestyle behaviors
   D. All the above.

_____29. Which wellness factor is most associated with heredity?
   A. Having no physician living in the local vicinity.
   B. Having one parent diagnosed as a diabetic.
   C. Living near a hazardous waste dump.
   D. Living with a family member who smokes.

_____30. Who is primarily responsible for healthful lifestyle choices?
   A. An individual.
   B. A person's parents.
   C. Health care providers.
   D. Society.

_____31. Which of the following is *not* a practice recommended by health experts?
   A. Avoid drinking alcoholic beverages.
   B. Be physically active most days of the week.
   C. Maintain a healthy weight.
   D. Skip breakfast.

(Continued)

© Goodheart-Willcox

Name_____

_____32. Which of the following is *not* a common result of peer pressure among teens?
  A. Teens are encouraged to participate in health-promoting activities, such as sports.
  B. Teens are led to take part in activities that risk health, such as drinking alcohol.
  C. Teens ignore pressure from their friends.
  D. Teens who wish to make individual decisions face a challenge.

_____33. The primary purpose for setting new lifestyle goals and developing behavior change contracts is to _____.
  A. achieve and maintain a slim body
  B. avoid the need to take personal ownership for health choices
  C. make positive changes for improved health
  D. reduce the negative effects of risk-taking behaviors

_____34. Which of the following best represents an epidemiological research question?
  A. How does the rate of heart disease among people who consume high-fiber diets compare to the rate of heart disease among people who consume low-fiber diets?
  B. What is the average daily protein intake of Native Americans?
  C. Who tends to eat more fresh fruits and vegetables—teenage boys or teenage girls?
  D. All the above represent epidemiological research questions.

_____35. Why is the scientific method used?
  A. To determine the best way to live.
  B. To find answers to important questions.
  C. To influence people's behaviors.
  D. To save time in research.

_____36. Which of the following questions would researchers be most likely to consider when choosing what specific topic to study?
  A. Can this study definitively answer a question left unanswered by previous studies?
  B. Will the results of this study be applicable to all people in the United States?
  C. Will the desired number of participants be willing and able to complete the study?
  D. Researchers would consider all the above questions when choosing a research topic.

Essay Questions: Provide complete responses to the following questions or statements.

37. Describe two examples of how inadequate health care may contribute to a decreased state of wellness.

38. List three steps a person can take to help improve the quality of the physical environment.

39. Provide three guidelines a person can follow to help ensure he or she will receive quality health care.

40. What are two points to keep in mind when evaluating the reliability of a resource reporting nutrition information?

Factors Affecting Food Choices

Objectives

After studying this chapter, students will be able to
* explain how culture influences people's food choices.
* describe how family and friends influence food choices.
* analyze the effect of emotions on the way people eat.
* relate how agricultural resources, technology, economic factors, and politics affect the availability of food.

Bulletin Board

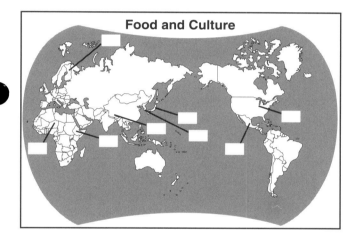

Food and Culture

Title: *Food and Culture*

Place a large world map in the center of the bulletin board. Have students identify their families' countries of origin. On index cards, write the names of students who have roots in a given country. Also write the names of a few dishes from that country. Then mount the index cards around the map. Use strings anchored with tacks to connect the cards to the appropriate countries.

Teaching Materials

Text, pages 26-42
  Learn the Language
  Check Your Knowledge
  Put Learning into Action
  Explore Further
Student Activity Guide, pages 13-18
  A. *Choices in Context*
  B. *How Do Friends Influence Food Choices?*
  C. *Food Choice Connection*
  D. *Food Supply*
  E. *Backtrack Through Chapter 2*
Teacher's Resources
  Origin of Common Foods, transparency master 2-1
  Food Helps Create Memories, reproducible master 2-2
  Factors That Influence Food Choices, color transparency CT-2
  Chapter 2 Test

Introducing the Chapter

1. Ask students to think about the best meal they have ever eaten. Ask them to describe the type of cuisine, who they ate with, and any other factors that made the meal enjoyable. Ask students whether they would be able to purchase the same meal in another country. Relate student responses to chapter concepts.
2. Ask students how they would feel about eating fried grasshoppers. Have students list factors that would influence their decisions about this food choice. Write responses on the chalkboard, underlining those that directly relate to information in the chapter.

Strategies to Reteach, Reinforce, Enrich, and Extend Text Concepts

Food Is a Reflection of Culture

3. **ER** Describe to students the analogy that each person is like a unique kind of bread. Each loaf has many common "ingredients" that are the same for all breads. However, each also has unique ingredients. Describe how these unique ingredients reflect the beliefs and social customs of a person's culture. Invite students to write "recipes" for their personal loaves, identifying the unique ingredients that make their "bread" slightly different from all others.
4. **ER** Have students develop brochures about their countries of origin to highlight unique aspects of their cultures, including cultural foods.
5. **RF** Use food features from magazines to create a display of pictures of international dishes. Ask students to analyze the pictures and write a two-

column list identifying ways foods of various cultures are alike and ways they are different. Discuss possible reasons why similarities and differences exist.

6. **RT** *Origin of Common Foods,* transparency master 2-1. On the world map used for the *Food and Culture* bulletin board, find the locations of foods listed on the transparency. Describe the characteristics of foods with which students are less familiar.

7. **ER** Field trip. Visit a grocery store with a large section of ethnic foods. Have each student copy the ingredient lists from three products he or she has never tried. Ask students to circle ingredients with which they are unfamiliar. Also arrange for the produce manager to explain the origins of the imported fruits and vegetables.

8. **ER** Guest speaker. Invite a historian to talk about food sources and patterns of eating in earlier civilizations.

9. **RF** Discuss diet patterns throughout history. Explain that people ate most foods raw before the development of various cooking methods. Then talk about how modern processing techniques have affected today's diet patterns. Ask students to predict eating trends for the next century.

10. **EX** Have students brainstorm a list of all the ethnic foods that come to mind. List student responses on the chalkboard.

11. **ER** Ask students to name their favorite ethnic cuisine. Tally responses on the chalkboard to determine which is the most popular ethnic cuisine. Discuss why people enjoy ethnic foods.

12. **ER** Guest speaker. Invite a chef from an ethnic restaurant to describe the characteristic preparation techniques, storage, shopping, and eating patterns of people from the culture expressed by the restaurant.

13. **EX** Guest speaker. Invite a parent or community member to demonstrate the making of a favorite ethnic food. Ask the person to tell where the ingredients can be purchased and how to serve and eat the food.

14. **EX** Panel discussion. Invite a panel of parents and/or teachers to discuss their experiences with foods while traveling internationally. Have panel members describe favorite foods and unusual foods. Also ask panel members how they coped with foods they did not recognize.

15. **ER** Have students use the Internet and/or library resources to explore food taboos of various cultures of the world. Students should investigate the origins of the taboos. Ask students to share their findings in class.

16. **EX** Ask students to write one-paragraph biographical descriptions of their families' food beliefs and habits. Tell students they must incorporate the following four terms into their paragraphs: *ethnic group, ethnic food, food norm,* and *food taboo.*

17. **ER** Plan a foods lab experience. Have each lab group prepare a recipe from a different region of the United States. Students may choose to search the Internet for recipes. Ask students to explain the characteristics of foods from their assigned region. Students should also evaluate the nutritional contributions of their food products as well as preparation time, cost per serving, and taste appeal.

18. **RT** Show students a food product labeled to indicate the product is kosher. Ask the class why this information is on the label and what it means.

19. **RF** Guest speaker. Invite a theologian to discuss the importance of food in the religions of the world. Ask the speaker to give examples of dietary laws that are followed by different religious groups.

Social Influences on Food Choices

20. **RT** Ask students what roles family members and friends play in shaping people's attitudes toward food. Use student responses to generate a list of all the social factors that influence a teen's food choices.

21. **RF** *How Do Friends Influence Food Choices?* Activity B, SAG. Students are to interview teens about the influence friends have on their food choices. Then students are to compile their findings and draw conclusions.

22. **ER** Have each student survey three teen friends about their favorite foods. Have all students compile their survey responses to identify the top 10 favorite foods among teens. Ask students why they think these particular foods are popular among teens.

23. **EX** *Food Helps Create Memories,* reproducible master 2-2. After reading the poem on the handout, students are to create their own poems or short stories about a role food has played in special times with family and friends. Compile student works in a class booklet or submit pieces to the school newspaper. You may wish to consider selling the booklet as a class fund-raiser.

24. **RF** Ask students what foods they would prepare or order to impress a boyfriend or girlfriend. Discuss their responses in relation to status foods.

25. **ER** Have each student watch television for a one-hour period. Students should note the day and time they watch. They should also keep a list of all the food commercials they see during their viewing periods. Students' lists should include the types of products, styles of commercials (humorous, informative, etc.), and length of commercials. Have students share their findings in class and discuss why certain foods are advertised more at some times than others.

Emotions Affect Food Choices

26. **RF** Have each student divide a sheet of paper into two columns. In the first column, have students list the words *sports event, date, celebration, illness, family gathering, excited, angry, bored, worried,* and *depressed.* In the second column, have students list a food that each item in the first column brings to mind. Have students compare their responses in small groups. As a class, discuss why certain foods often become associated with particular activities and feelings.

27. **RF** Ask students to give examples of situations in which food is used as a reward by individuals, parents, teachers, health professionals, and others. Discuss the possible consequences of using food in this way.

28. **ER** Ask for student volunteers to participate in a blind taste test comparing two similar food products. Food products might include generic and national brand canned peaches, homemade and purchased chocolate chip cookies, and low fat and regular hot dogs. Following the test, discuss the sources of people's individual food preferences.

29. **RF** *Choices in Context,* Activity A, SAG. Students are to read quotes about food choices and identify the factor influencing each choice.

The Influences of Agriculture, Technology, Economics, and Politics

30. **ER** Guest speaker. Invite a speaker from the county extension agency to discuss how soil quality, water supply, climate, education, and technology affect agricultural production.

31. **ER** Field trip. Arrange a field trip to a local supermarket. Ask the store manager to point out the latest food product developments, most popular imported food items, and newest packaging and marketing strategies. Also ask the manager to discuss factors that influence consumer product availability in the supermarket.

32. **EX** *Food Supply,* Activity D, SAG. Students are to choose a specific food item and use various resources to investigate how agriculture, technology, economics, and politics have influenced the availability of the food.

Nutrition Knowledge Affects Food Choices

33. **EX** Write food myths on index cards. Have a pair of students select a card and prepare a role-play situation. One student should express the myth and the other student should offer an appropriate response. Have other pairs of students repeat this exercise with the remaining cards. Following each role-play, discuss how the myth might have become popular and why accurate nutrition knowledge is important.

34. **ER** Have students prepare a display of resources and references that represent reliable sources of nutrition information.

Chapter Review

35. **RT** *Food Choice Connection,* Activity C, SAG. Students are to match terms with definitions from the chapter. Then they are to write mental connections called to mind by a list of foods.

36. **RF** *Backtrack Through Chapter 2,* Activity E, SAG. Students are to provide complete answers to questions and statements that will help them recall, interpret, apply, and practice chapter concepts.

37. **RF** *Factors That Influence Food Choices,* color transparency CT-2. Use the transparency to review how food choices can be affected by the cultural, social, and emotional factors shown in the inner ring. Emphasize how these factors affect people personally. Discuss the level of individual control people have over some of these factors. Then discuss the impact of agriculture, technology, economics, and politics on food choices. Focus on people's lack of direct control over these factors. Ask students to give examples of the various factors.

Above and Beyond

38. **EX** Divide students into lab groups and have each group plan and prepare a menu from a different culture. Each group should also prepare a presentation describing why its menu is representative of the chosen culture.

39. **EX** Have students prepare a display of foods from around the world. Each food product should be labeled with the name of the food, origin of the food, taste characteristics, and common uses in meal preparation.

Answer Key

Text

Check Your Knowledge, page 41

1. ingredients, seasonings, preparation methods
2. Each region reflects different ethnic heritages. Popular regional foods are often those that are associated with the ethnic heritage of the region.
3. an increasing number of working single parents, a rising family income for many dual-worker families, a smaller family size, increasing family mobility patterns
4. false

5. (List two:) People may choose to prepare foods in a way shown in a newspaper or magazine or on a television program. People may choose to buy foods reported to have certain health benefits. People are more likely to buy a product after hearing or seeing an ad for it over and over. Some people go on weight-loss diets to achieve the ideal of beauty portrayed by the media.
6. early in life
7. true
8. (List two:) emotions, genes, experiences with food
9. fertile soil, adequate water supply, favorable climate, technical knowledge, human energy
10. (List three:) modern farming machinery, faster food processing systems, rapid transportation, new foods, new packaging, new handling processes
11. Without adequate processing plants and storage facilities, up to 40 percent of crops may be lost to spoilage and contamination.
12. (List three:) Certain foods have magical powers. Taking vitamin and mineral supplements eliminates the need to eat nutritious foods. Naturally grown foods have greater nutritional value than other foods. Certain foods can cure diseases.

Student Activity Guide

Choices in Context, Activity A

1. cultural
2. media
3. social
4. historical
5. emotional
6. ethnic
7. regional
8. status
9. religious
10. individual preference

Food Choice Connection, Activity C

1. J
2. G
3. K
4. A
5. F
6. D
7. C
8. I
9. B
10. H

Backtrack Through Chapter 2, Activity E

1. (List three:) good taste of food, where they live, the people around them, available resources, experiences with food
2. (List four:) family members, friends, other people, schools, religious organizations, media
3. early settlers, Native Americans
4. a group of people who share common blood ties, land ties, or racial and religious similarities
5. Some members of religious groups view food customs as strict commandments. Others observe the customs to help keep traditions alive for future generations.
6. (List three:) beliefs about food, table manners, how to eat certain foods, food traditions, food likes and dislikes
7. feelings of good luck and happiness, feelings of frustration or disgust
8. weight management problems
9. agriculture, technology, economics, politics
10. The typical diet of a region usually is based on foods that grow well in that region.
11. (List four:) what land will be used for food production, what crops will be grown, how the economic resources of the country or region will be used, how food will be distributed, what standards must be met by imported foods, how food must be produced and processed
12. those that have been reviewed by registered dietitians
13. Becoming aware of how others affect the quality of your diet can help you improve your overall health.
14. to help put eating behaviors into a healthy perspective
15. (Student response.)
16. (Student response.)
17. (Student response.)
18. (Student response.)
19. (Student response.)
20. (Student response.)

Teacher's Resources

Chapter 2 Test

1. A	10. J	19. F	28. B
2. B	11. T	20. T	29. C
3. G	12. T	21. T	30. C
4. C	13. F	22. T	31. D
5. D	14. T	23. F	32. B
6. E	15. F	24. F	33. A
7. K	16. F	25. D	34. B
8. I	17. F	26. B	35. D
9. H	18. T	27. D	36. C

37. (List 10:) culture, historical influences, ethnic influences, food taboos, region, religion, family, friends, status of foods, media, emotions, individual preferences, agriculture, technology, economics, politics

38. (List two. Student response.)

39. People who develop negative feelings related to food are more likely to develop eating disorders or weight management problems.

40. (List three:) which land will be used for food production, what crops will be grown, how the country's economic resources will be used, how food will be distributed

Origin of Common Foods

Central America
Red peppers
Avocados
Squash
Pumpkin
Corn
Beans
Tomatoes
Turkeys
Pineapple

South America
Potatoes
Sweet potatoes
Peanuts
Cocoa

Africa
Watermelon
Okra

Europe
Cabbage
Apples
Pears
Lemons

Middle East
Sheep
Barley
Peas
Lentils
Wheat
Goats
Cattle
Grapes
Olives
Artichokes
Figs
Coffee

Asia
Cabbage
Turnips
Melons
Beets
Lettuce
Carrots
Oats
Almonds
Dates
Bananas
Tea
Onions
Cucumber
Eggplant
Peach
Rice
Soybeans
Pigs
Chickens
Oranges
Apricots

© Goodheart-Willcox

Reproducible Master 2-2

Food Helps Create Memories

Name_____   Date _____   Period _____

Read the following poem. Then write a poem or short story about the role food has played in special times with family and friends. Create a class booklet to share with others.

Tortillas

Watching
my best friend's
grandmother
shaping dough
cupping a soft mound
into a ball
clapping it flat
between
powdered palms
then smacking it
onto the counter,
flour
swirling around the kitchen
like snow.

She stacked them
on damp cheesecloth towels
steaming on the hot oven
gently
folding up the sides.
One towel-wrapped gift
for the families
of each of her children.
For days
we could picture her
leaning over the counter
and smell the warmth
of her baked creations.
"Mi hija."
She saw my heart
beneath my pale skin.

Amy Isom

_____

_____

_____

_____

_____

_____

_____

_____

_____

© Goodheart-Willcox

Factors Affecting Food Choices

Name_____

Date _____ Period _____ Score _____

Chapter 2 Test

Matching: Match the following terms and identifying phrases.

_____ 1. The beliefs and social customs of a group of people.

_____ 2. A food that is typical of a given racial, national, or religious culture.

_____ 3. Traditional food of the African American ethnic group.

_____ 4. Typical standard or pattern related to food and eating behaviors.

_____ 5. A social custom that prohibits the use of certain edible resources as food.

_____ 6. Food prepared according to Jewish dietary laws.

_____ 7. A belief or attitude that is important to someone.

_____ 8. A food that has a social impact on others.

_____ 9. A mainstay food in the diet.

_____ 10. The application of a certain body of knowledge.

A. culture
B. ethnic food
C. food norm
D. food taboo
E. kosher food
F. sacred food
G. soul food
H. staple food
I. status food
J. technology
K. value

True/False: Circle *T* if the statement is true or *F* if the statement is false.

T F   11. Food habits reflect people's values and beliefs.

T F   12. The cuisine of the United States is made up of both native foods and foods brought to America by early settlers.

T F   13. Consumer interest in ethnic foods is decreasing in the United States.

T F   14. Foods vary somewhat from one region of the United States to another because each region reflects different ethnic heritages.

T F   15. Family eating patterns seldom change over time.

T F   16. Eating three meals a day together continues to be a growing trend among families in the United States.

T F   17. Peers have little influence on their friends' eating behaviors.

T F   18. The purpose of food advertisements on television is to get people to buy food products.

T F   19. People develop most of their emotional responses to foods in adulthood.

T F   20. Genetic factors influence people's food preferences.

T F   21. The quality of soil in an area affects the types and amounts of food that can grow in the area.

T F   22. The nutritional status of people in a country depends on the country's economic ability to produce or buy food.

T F   23. Politics has little to do with food availability in the United States.

T F   24. Foods grown without chemical pesticides have greater nutritional value than other foods.

© Goodheart-Willcox

(Continued)

Name_____

Multiple Choice: Choose the best response. Write the letter in the space provided.

_____25. Culture is shaped and changed through _____.
A. contact with family members and friends
B. influence of the media
C. the introduction of new ideas
D. All the above.

_____26. What purposes do ethnic foods serve for a group of people?
A. Create a feeling of individuality for each member of the group.
B. Encourage ethnic pride.
C. Help people bond with members of other ethnic groups.
D. All the above.

_____27. In the United States, the practice of eating earthworms is an example of a food _____.
A. habit
B. norm
C. rule
D. taboo

_____28. Which statement below is the best example of how religion influences food choices?
A. Friends persuade a person to try a new food.
B. Hindu people do not eat beef.
C. Tacos and tortillas are popular in the Southwest.
D. The media promotes a new product.

_____29. Which of the following is *not* a trend affecting family eating patterns?
A. Family members are increasingly mobile.
B. More households are headed by working single parents.
C. Many dual-worker families have less income at their disposal.
D. The average family is smaller.

_____30. Offering friends a snack when they visit is an example of _____.
A. community expectations
B. family eating patterns
C. social influence on food choices
D. the status of food

_____31. Which of the following is the best example of a high-status food in the culture of the United States?
A. Hamburgers.
B. Noodle soup.
C. Pork and beans.
D. Steak.

_____32. More than half the food commercials children view on television are for _____.
A. dairy products
B. foods high in calories, sugar, fat, and salt
C. fresh fruits and vegetables
D. whole grain cereals

_____33. Which of the following is an example of using food to deal with emotions?
A. Eating when excited.
B. Eating when friends offer food.
C. Eating when hungry.
D. Eating when watching an advertisement for food.

(Continued)

© Goodheart-Willcox

Name_____

_____34. Refusing to give a child a snack because he or she would not share toys is an example of using food to _____.
  A. maintain the child's weight
  B. punish the child
  C. reward the child
  D. show love to the child

_____35. Using aseptic packaging to increase the shelf life of a perishable food is an example of applying _____.
  A. climate control
  B. nutrition knowledge
  C. political influence
  D. technological advances

_____36. The best source of reliable nutrition knowledge is _____.
  A. friends
  B. newspaper articles
  C. registered dietitians
  D. television

Essay Questions: Provide complete responses to the following questions or statements.

37. List 10 factors that influence people's food choices.

38. Give two examples of ways friends might influence food choices.

39. How can feelings related to food be harmful?

40. What are three decisions political leaders might make that can affect the nutritional status of a nation's people?

© Goodheart-Willcox

How Nutrients Become You

Objectives

After studying this chapter, students will be able to
- identify the six basic nutrient groups.
- distinguish the functions of the major parts of the digestive system.
- describe the processes of absorption and metabolism.
- explain factors affecting digestion and absorption.
- name common digestive disorders.

Bulletin Board

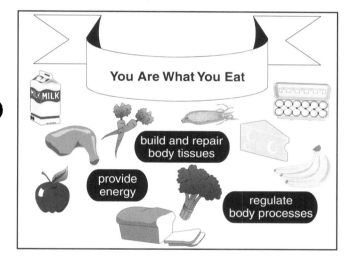

Title: *You Are What You Eat*

Place pictures of foods from each of the groups in the Food Guide Pyramid around the edge of the bulletin board. In the center of the pictures, place captions that describe the main functions of nutrients provided by healthful foods: *build and repair body tissues, regulate body processes,* and *provide energy.* Review with the students the importance of variety in the diet as one key component of a healthful lifestyle.

Teaching Materials

Text, pages 43–57
Learn the Language
Check Your Knowledge
Put Learning into Action
Explore Further

Student Activity Guide, pages 19–24
A. *Food Breakdown*
B. *What Could Be Wrong?*
C. *Digestive Disorders*
D. *Backtrack Through Chapter 3*

Teacher's Resources
The Body Shop, color transparency CT-3
Periodic Table of the Elements, reproducible master 3-1
When Needs Are Greatest, transparency master 3-2
Determining Energy Values, reproducible master 3-3
The Digestion Experiment, reproducible master 3-4
Nutrient Digestion in the Small Intestine, reproducible master 3-5
Chapter 3 Test

Introducing the Chapter

1. *The Body Shop,* color transparency CT-3. Use the transparency to compare and contrast a car's need for fuel with a body's need for healthful food.
2. Create a character by drawing a face on a piece of fresh produce, such as a potato. Use the character as you explain the body cannot use food directly to perform vital life functions. Instead, the body must break down food to obtain nutrients needed for growth, repair, maintenance, and energy.

Strategies to Reteach, Reinforce, Enrich, and Extend Text Concepts

Food, Nutrients, and Energy

3. **RF** Hold up a food item, such as an apple or a slice of bread, for students to see. Ask students to name the nutrients the food provides. List responses on the chalkboard under headings for the six major nutrient groups. Ask students why an unlimited supply of this food product would not sustain life.
4. **RT** Review the meanings of the terms *element, matter, atom, molecule,* and *compound.* Give examples of each. (You may wish to invite a chemistry teacher to serve as a guest speaker on these topics.)
5. **RF** *Periodic Table of the Elements,* reproducible master 3-1. Have students find and highlight on

the handout the elements essential to human health. (Remind students all elements essential to the diet may not yet be known.) The elements to identify include

- those found in vitamins, water, and energy-yielding nutrients: hydrogen (H), carbon (C), nitrogen (N), and oxygen (O)
- major minerals: sodium (Na), magnesium (Mg), phosphorus (P), sulfur (S), chlorine (Cl), potassium (K), and calcium (Ca)
- trace minerals: fluorine (F), chromium (Cr), manganese (Mn), iron (Fe), copper (Cu), zinc (Zn), selenium (Se), molybdenum (Mo), and iodine (I)

6. **RT** Have each student look up a favorite food in Appendix C or *Personal Best* software. Ask students to name nutrients for which values are listed in the appendix. List students' responses on the chalkboard. After all nutrients are listed, identify which nutrients are elements (minerals) and which are compounds (carbohydrates, fats, proteins, vitamins, and water).

7. **RT** *When Needs Are Greatest,* transparency master 3-2. Use the transparency to help illustrate the point that nutrient needs are greatest during periods of rapid growth. Discuss why eating a nutritious diet would be especially important during these periods.

8. **RF** Have each student interview a partner about how hunger affects his or her moods, attitudes, thinking, and physical performance. Each pair of students should identify at least four effects of hunger they have both experienced. In a class discussion, generate a comprehensive list of the effects of hunger and relate each effect to the importance of food as an energy source.

9. **RF** *Determining Energy Values,* reproducible master 3-3. Review with students the energy value per gram for fats, carbohydrates, and proteins. (You may also wish to review the energy value of alcohol.) Then have students use Appendix C or *Personal Best* software, to find the number of grams of carbohydrates, fats, and proteins in each of the food items listed on the worksheet. Have students calculate the number of calories provided by each of these nutrients and figure the total number of calories in each food.

The Process of Digestion

10. **RT** Cut four pieces of yarn, each in a different color to represent a different part of the digestive tract. Cut pieces as follows: mouth/esophagus—10 inches; stomach—8 inches; small intestine—20 feet; large intestine—3 feet, 6 inches. Tie pieces of yarn together, labeling each segment with the corresponding part of the digestive tract. Extend the yarn to its full length to help students visualize the average length of an adult digestive tract.

11. **RT** Ask students to refer to Diagram 3-7 on page 49 in the text as you review the functions of each organ in the digestive system.

12. **RF** Give each student two unsalted crackers. Have the students chew the crackers for two minutes without swallowing. Then ask students to compare how the crackers tasted at first with how they tasted after two minutes. Explain the change in taste from starchy to sweet was caused by the chemical action of the enzyme salivary amylase. This enzyme, which is found in the mouth, breaks down starch molecules in foods into simple sugar molecules.

13. **ER** Guest speaker. Explain to students when food accidentally enters the trachea instead of the esophagus, choking will occur. Invite the school nurse to demonstrate the abdominal thrust procedure for choking victims. Ask the nurse to demonstrate the procedure for infants as well as adults. Also ask the nurse to demonstrate how adults can self-administer the procedure when no one is available to provide assistance.

14. **ER** *Nutrient Digestion in the Small Intestine,* reproducible master 3-5. Have students work in groups of three to complete the chart and answer the questions about what happens to fats, proteins, and carbohydrates during digestion in the small intestine. Each student should be responsible for completing one column of the chart and sharing his or her responses with group members. Group members should work together to answer the questions so all students can develop an understanding of all chart content. When groups have completed their work, check for individual understanding by calling on students randomly to explain their answers.

15. **RF** *Food Breakdown,* Activity A, SAG. Students are to fill in the correct words describing the steps in the digestion process.

16. **ER** *The Digestion Experiment,* reproducible master 3-4. Discuss laboratory safety procedures. Then have lab groups complete the experiment as directed on the master. Students will be observing the effects of enzymes on a protein food. Following the experiment, discuss answers to the questions and review learning outcomes.

Absorption and Metabolism

17. **RT** Prepare the following materials for use in a demonstration that will illustrate the process of absorption. Spill coffee or juice on a smooth plastic cutting board and allow it to dry to form a visible stain. Label the cutting board *biological functions.* Label a dry paper towel *body* and a

glass of water *nutrients.* First, wipe the stain with the dry paper towel. Then sprinkle a few drops of water on the stain. Explain to students that, working alone, neither the "body" nor "nutrients" can perform the "biological function" of cleaning the stain. Lastly, dip the paper towel in the water and wipe the stained surface clean. Explain the body must absorb nutrients before it can use them to do its work. Ask students to give specific examples of work that nutrients help the body perform.

18. **ER**   Have groups of two to three students complete the following experiment to illustrate how villi promote absorption in the small intestine. Provide each group with two paper towels; two 8-inch square pans, each containing exactly 250 mL of water; and two graduated cylinders. Students should leave one towel unfolded. They should crease the second towel three times in an accordion-type fold. Students should dip the edge of the unfolded towel ½ inch into the water in one pan for 10 seconds. They should dip the folds of the second towel ½ inch into the water in the other pan for 10 seconds. After removing the towels from the water, students should use the graduated cylinders to measure the amount of water remaining in each pan. Explain that folding the towel allowed more surface area to come in contact with the water, thereby increasing the amount of water the towel was able to absorb. Similarly, the folds and villi lining the small intestine increase the surface area and speed the absorption of nutrients.

19. **ER**   For a demonstration that will illustrate the concept of metabolism, write the word *energy* on several small slips of paper. Place one slip inside each of three colors of plastic Easter eggs. Explain to students the three colors of eggs represent the three energy nutrients—carbohydrates, fats, and proteins. These nutrients have been absorbed through the digestive system and carried by the bloodstream to the cells. During metabolism, the cells break down the nutrients and release energy. As you describe this process, break the eggs apart and release the "energy" inside. Then reassemble the eggs in various two-tone combinations, explaining how the cells use components from nutrients to form other compounds needed by the body.

Factors Affecting Digestion and Absorption

20. **RF**   Invite students to share experiences of times when eating habits or emotions led to digestive difficulties. For each example, ask the class to suggest strategies that would help prevent or reduce the related difficulties.

21. **ER**   Guest speaker. Invite a registered dietitian to talk to the class about common food allergies and diet planning strategies used to address them.

22. **EX**   *What Could Be Wrong?* Activity B, SAG. Students are to answer questions about factors that could be affecting digestion and absorption in given cases.

Digestive Disorders

23. **RF**   Ask each student to visit a pharmacy and make a list of 10 OTC products sold to relieve digestive disorders. Have students note the brand name, cost, and related disorder for each product. As students share their findings in class, discuss the role a nutritious diet has in preventing digestive disorders.

24. **RF**   *Digestive Disorders,* Activity C, SAG. Students are to write descriptions of conditions, causes, and cures of listed digestive disorders.

Chapter Review

25. **RF**   *Backtrack Through Chapter 3,* Activity D, SAG. Students are to provide complete answers to questions and statements that will help them recall, interpret, apply, and practice chapter concepts.

26. **RF**   Have each student write questions on index cards about information from a different page of the chapter. Students should write answers on the backs of the cards. Draw a large tic-tac-toe grid on the board. Have two teams of students take turns answering the questions. When a team member answers correctly, he or she can mark an X or O on the grid. The first team to get three marks in a row wins.

Above and Beyond

27. **EX**   Have students write poems or short stories about the journey of a favorite food through the digestive tract. Ask students to describe what happens to the food as it passes through each part of the system. Instruct students to use illustrative words to describe sounds, colors, and textures as the food travels. Invite students to share their completed poems or stories with the class. Ask classmates to evaluate whether the description of the journey was accurate.

28. **EX**   Assign pairs of students an organ of the digestive tract. Have pairs conduct Internet research to learn more about the organs' locations, functions, and disorders. Have students use this information as one partner assumes the role of a journalist and the other partner assumes the role of the organ in a celebrity interview role-play.

29. **ER**   Have students collect information about conditions, causes, and cures of digestive disorders not discussed in the chapter. Such disorders might

include celiac disease, Crohn's disease, colitis, colon cancer, cholecystitis, hiatal hernia, irritable bowel syndrome, pancreatitis, and peritonitis. Sources of information might include physicians, journals, and the Internet. Have students compile their collected materials into a resource file. Then have the class create an advertisement for the school newspaper inviting interested persons to check the file if they are concerned about digestive distresses. You may also wish to make the file available to local care facilities, such as a senior citizens' center.

Answer Key

Text

Check Your Knowledge, page 56

1. The six nutrient groups are carbohydrates, fats, proteins, vitamins, minerals, and water. The three main functions of nutrients are to build and repair body tissues, regulate all body processes, and provide energy.
2. The energy value of food is measured in units called kilocalories.
3. Mechanical digestion happens as food is crushed and churned, such as through chewing. In chemical digestion, food is mixed with powerful enzymes and acids, which cause food to break apart and form simpler substances.
4. (List four:) breaks down starches; moistens mouth; brings out flavors of food; moistens, softens, and dissolves food; cleans teeth; neutralizes mouth acids
5. When you swallow food, the epiglottis closes, keeping food from entering the trachea. Breathing automatically stops when you swallow food to help prevent choking.
6. Mucus is a thick fluid that helps soften and lubricate food. It also helps protect the stomach from its strong acidic juices.
7. Proteases break down proteins into amino acids. Lipases break down fats into fatty acids, glycerol, and monoglycerides. Saccharidases break down carbohydrates into monosaccharides.
8. The main job of the large intestine is to reabsorb water.
9. The water-soluble nutrients include amino acids from proteins, glucose from carbohydrates, and water-soluble vitamins and minerals. The fat-soluble nutrients include fat-soluble vitamins as well as fatty acids and glycerol from fats. Capillaries in the villi lining the small intestine absorb water-soluble nutrients into the bloodstream and carry them to the liver through the portal vein. Lacteals in the villi absorb fat-soluble nutrients into the lymphatic system. These nutrients then make their way to the bloodstream.
10. Through metabolism, cells break down some nutrients to release energy, which is stored as ATP. When the body needs energy, chemical reactions break down ATP to release energy.
11. eating habits, emotions, food allergies, physical activity.
12. (List two. Student response. See pages 54-55 in the text.)

Student Activity Guide

Food Breakdown, Activity A

1. mastication
2. saliva
3. salivary amylase
4. mouth, stomach
5. epiglottis
6. peristalsis
7. gastric
8. chyme
9. pepsin
10. duodenum, jejunum, ileum
11. enzymes
12. bile
13. colon
14. elimination
15. feces

What Could Be Wrong? Activity B

1. food allergies
2. (Student response.)
3. (Student response.)
4. eating habits, emotions
5. (Student response.)
6. (Student response.)
7. physical activity
8. (Student response)
9. (Student response)
10. eating habits
11. (Student response.)
12. (Student response.)

Digestive Disorders, Activity C

(Student response. See pages 54-55 in the text.)

Backtrack Through Chapter 3, Activity D

1. elements—minerals; compounds—carbohydrates, fats, proteins, vitamins, and water
2. vitamins, minerals, and water
3. (Student response. See pages 44-45 in the text.)
4. A. four
   B. four
   C. nine
   D. seven
5. (Student response. See page 46 in the text.)
6. An enzyme is a type of protein produced by cells that causes specific chemical reactions.

7. The epiglottis prevents food from going down the windpipe.
8. Peristalsis is an involuntary series of squeezing actions by the muscles in the esophagus.
9. 2 to 3 hours
10. small intestine
11. 3 to 10 hours
12. Metabolism includes all the chemical changes that occur as cells produce energy and materials needed to sustain life.
13. ATP stands for adenosine triphosphate. It is the source of immediate energy found in muscle tissue.
14. (Student response. See page 52 in the text.)
15. A food allergy is a reaction of the immune system to some substance found in food. A food sensitivity is a reaction to food that does not involve the immune system.
16. (Student response. See page 53 in the text.)
17. (Student response. See page 54 in the text.)
18. Yes, because it might indicate a person has gastroesophageal reflux disease (GERD).
19. (Student response.)
20. (Student response. See page 52 in the text.)

Teacher's Resources

Determining Energy Values, reproducible master 3-3

1. A. 16 g × 4 cal/g = 64 cal
   B. 7 g × 9 cal/g = 63 cal
   C. 48 g × 4 cal/g = 192 cal
   D. 319 cal
2. A. 24 g × 4 cal/g = 96 cal
   B. 7 g × 9 cal/g = 63 cal
   C. 0 g × 4 cal/g = 0 cal
   D. 159 cal
3. A. 7 g × 4 cal/g = 28 cal
   B. 1 g × 9 cal/g = 9 cal
   C. 39 g × 4 cal/g = 156 cal
   D. 193 cal
4. A. 19 g × 4 cal/g = 76 cal
   B. 12 g × 9 cal/g = 108 cal
   C. 39 g × 4 cal/g = 156 cal
   D. 340 cal
5. A. 2.5 g × 4 cal/g = 10 cal
   B. .5 g × 9 cal/g = 4.5 cal
   C. 57.5 g × 4 cal/g = 230 cal
   D. 244.5 cal
6. raisins
7. spaghetti with meatballs
8. raisins
9. tuna
10. the energy value of food

The Digestion Experiment, reproducible master 3-4

1. beaker B
2. beaker A
3. The enzymes in the meat tenderizer broke down the protein in the egg white.
4. Enzymes cause chemical reactions that break food into smaller particles needed for use by the body.

Nutrient Digestion in the Small Intestine, reproducible master 3-5

1. A. amino acids
   B. monosaccharides
   C. fatty acids, glycerol, monoglycerides
2. A. proteases
   B. saccharidases
   C. lipases
3. 95 percent
4. salivary amylase; It helps chemically break down the starches in foods.
5. pepsin
6. duodenum, jejunum, ileum
7. The pancreas secretes bicarbonate, which neutralizes hydrochloric acid that has come into the small intestine from the stomach with partially digested food. The pancreas also produces digestive enzymes that aid in the chemical digestion that takes place in the small intestine.
8. The liver produces bile, which helps disperse fat in the water-based digestive fluids, giving enzymes in the fluids access to the fat for breakdown.
9. the large intestine
10. They are absorbed from the digestive tract into the circulatory or lymphatic system.

Chapter 3 Test

1.	L	20.	T
2.	F	21.	T
3.	M	22.	T
4.	O	23.	T
5.	C	24.	F
6.	B	25.	T
7.	G	26.	D
8.	A	27.	B
9.	N	28.	D
10.	H	29.	A
11.	D	30.	C
12.	K	31.	A
13.	J	32.	B
14.	I	33.	C
15.	E	34.	A
16.	F	35.	D
17.	T	36.	D
18.	T	37.	B
19.	F	38.	A

39. carbohydrates, fats, proteins, vitamins, minerals, water

40. Mechanical digestion happens as food is crushed and churned. This type of digestion involves chewing in the mouth and peristaltic action in the esophagus, stomach, and small intestine. Chemical digestion involves mixing food with acids and enzymes that help break down the food into simpler substances. This type of digestion begins with salivary amylase in the mouth and continues with gastric juices in the stomach and digestive enzymes in the small intestine.

41. Waste products of cell metabolism leave the body as urine through the kidneys, breath through the lungs, and perspiration through the skin.

42. (List three:) Choose a nutritious diet that includes a wide range of foods. Include good sources of fiber in the diet, such as fruits, vegetables, and whole grains. Avoid eating too quickly. Eat moderate amounts of food. Choose foods that are free from spoilage and contamination.

Periodic Table of the Elements

Name_____   Date _____   Period _____

Periodic Table of the Elements

In the periodic table the elements are arranged in order of increasing atomic number. Vertical columns headed by Roman numerals are called *Groups*. A horizontal sequence of elements is called a *Period*. The most active elements are at the top right and bottom left of the table. The staggered line (Groups IIIA-VIIA) roughly separates metallic from non-metallic elements.

Groups—Elements within a group have similar properties and contain the same number of electrons in their outside energy shell.
—The first group (IA) includes hydrogen and the alkali metals.
—The last (VIIA) contains the *inert gases*.
—Group VIIA includes the *halogens*.
—The elements intervening between groups IIA and IIIA are called *transition elements*.
—Short vertical columns without Roman numeral headings are called sub-groups.

Periods—in a given period the properties of the elements gradually pass from a strong metallic to a strong non-metallic nature, with the last number of a period being an inert gas.

LIGHT METALS

NON METALS

IA	IIA											IIIA	IVA	VA	VIA	VIIA	VIIIA
Hydrogen 1.0080 **H** 1																	Helium 4.003 **He** 2
Lithium 6.939 **Li** 3	Beryllium 9.012 **Be** 4											Boron 10.811 **B** 5	Carbon 12.01115 **C** 6	Nitrogen 14.007 **N** 7	Oxygen 15.999 **O** 8	Fluorine 18.998 **F** 9	Neon 20.183 **Ne** 10
Sodium 22.990 **Na** 11	Magnesium 24.312 **Mg** 12											Aluminum 26.981 **Al** 13	Silicon 28.086 **Si** 14	Phosphorus 30.974 **P** 15	Sulfur 32.064 **S** 16	Chlorine 35.453 **Cl** 17	Argon 39.948 **Ar** 18
Potassium 39.102 **K** 19	Calcium 40.08 **Ca** 20	Scandium 44.956 **Sc** 21	Titanium 47.90 **Ti** 22	Vanadium 50.942 **V** 23	Chromium 51.996 **Cr** 24	Manganese 54.938 **Mn** 25	Iron 55.847 **Fe** 26	Cobalt 58.933 **Co** 27	Nickel 58.71 **Ni** 28	Copper 63.54 **Cu** 29	Zinc 65.37 **Zn** 30	Gallium 69.72 **Ga** 31	Germanium 72.59 **Ge** 32	Arsenic 74.922 **As** 33	Selenium 78.96 **Se** 34	Bromine 79.909 **Br** 35	Krypton 83.80 **Kr** 36
Rubidium 85.47 **Rb** 37	Strontium 87.62 **Sr** 38	Yttrium 88.905 **Y** 39	Zirconium 91.22 **Zr** 40	Niobium 92.906 **Nb** 41	Molybdenum 95.94 **Mo** 42	Technetium (99) **Tc** 43	Ruthenium 101.07 **Ru** 44	Rhodium 102.91 **Rh** 45	Palladium 106.4 **Pd** 46	Silver 107.87 **Ag** 47	Cadmium 112.40 **Cd** 48	Indium 114.82 **In** 49	Tin 118.69 **Sn** 50	Antimony 121.75 **Sb** 51	Tellurium 127.60 **Te** 52	Iodine 126.90 **I** 53	Xenon 131.30 **Xe** 54
Cesium 132.90 **Cs** 55	Barium 137.34 **Ba** 56	57-71	Hafnium 178.49 **Hf** 72	Tantalum 180.95 **Ta** 73	Tungsten 183.85 **W** 74	Rhenium 186.21 **Re** 75	Osmium 190.2 **Os** 76	Iridium 192.2 **Ir** 77	Platinum 195.09 **Pt** 78	Gold 196.97 **Au** 79	Mercury 200.59 **Hg** 80	Thallium 204.37 **Tl** 81	Lead 207.19 **Pb** 82	Bismuth 208.98 **Bi** 83	Polonium (210) **Po** 84	Astatine (210) **At** 85	Radon (222) **Rn** 86
Francium 223 **Fr** 87	Radium (226) **Ra** 88	89-103	104	105	106	107	108	109	110	111	112	113	114	115	116	117	118

Lanthanum 138.91 **La** 57	Cerium 140.12 **Ce** 58	Praseodymium 140.91 **Pr** 59	Neodymium 144.24 **Nd** 60	Promethium (147) **Pm** 61	Samarium 150.35 **Sm** 62	Europium 151.96 **Eu** 63	Gadolinium 157.25 **Gd** 64	Terbium 158.92 **Tb** 65	Dysprosium 162.50 **Dy** 66	Holmium 164.93 **Ho** 67	Erbium 167.26 **Er** 68	Thulium 168.93 **Tm** 69	Ytterbium 173.04 **Yb** 70	Lutetium 174.97 **Lu** 71
Actinium 227 **Ac** 89	Thorium 232.04 **Th** 90	Protactinium (231) **Pa** 91	Uranium 238.03 **U** 92	Neptunium (237) **Np** 93	Plutonium (242) **Pu** 94	Americium (243) **Am** 95	Curium (247) **Cm** 96	Berkelium (249) **Bk** 97	Californium (251) **Cf** 98	Einsteinium (254) **Es** 99	Fermium (253) **Fm** 100	Mendelevium (256) **Md** 101	Nobelium (254) **No** 102	Lawrencium (257) **Lr** 103

KEY

Information	Color
Name of Element	Red
Atomic Weight	Blue
Atomic Symbol	Black
Atomic Number	Green

© Goodheart-Willcox

When Needs Are Greatest

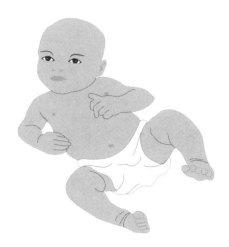

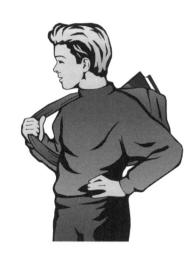

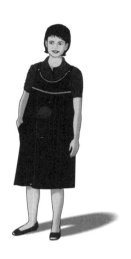

Infancy and
Early Childhood

Early Adolescence
(Ages 10-14)

Pregnancy

Why?

• Rapid growth requires nutrients to build tissues

• Higher rate of metabolism increases energy needs

© Goodheart-Willcox

Determining Energy Values

Name_____ **Date** _____ **Period** _____

Use Appendix C, *Nutritive Values of Foods,* to find the number of grams of carbohydrates, fats, and proteins in each of the food items listed. Calculate the number of calories provided by each of these nutrients and figure the total number of calories in each food. Then answer the questions that follow.

1. Canned white beans with pork and tomato sauce (1 cup)

   A. protein: _____ g × _____ cal/g = _____ cal

   B. fat: _____ g × _____ cal/g = _____ cal

   C. carbohydrate: _____ g × _____ cal/g = _____ cal

   D. total calories: _____

2. Tuna canned in oil (3 oz)

   A. protein: _____ g × _____ cal/g = _____ cal

   B. fat: _____ g × _____ cal/g = _____ cal

   C. carbohydrate: _____ g × _____ cal/g = _____ cal

   D. total calories: _____

3. Cooked macaroni (1 cup)

   A. protein: _____ g × _____ cal/g = _____ cal

   B. fat: _____ g × _____ cal/g = _____ cal

   C. carbohydrate: _____ g × _____ cal/g = _____ cal

   D. total calories: _____

4. Spaghetti with meatballs and tomato sauce, from home recipe (1 cup)

   A. protein: _____ g × _____ cal/g = _____ cal

   B. fat: _____ g × _____ cal/g = _____ cal

   C. carbohydrate: _____ g × _____ cal/g = _____ cal

   D. total calories: _____

5. Raisins (½ cup)

   A. protein: _____ g × _____ cal/g = _____ cal

   B. fat: _____ g × _____ cal/g = _____ cal

   C. carbohydrate: _____ g × _____ cal/g = _____ cal

   D. total calories: _____

6. Which food provides the fewest calories from protein? _____

7. Which food provides the most calories from fat? _____

8. Which food provides the most calories from carbohydrates? _____

9. Which food is lowest in total calories per serving? _____

10. What do calories measure? _____

© Goodheart-Willcox

The Digestion Experiment

Name_____ Date _____ Period _____

Objective: To show the functions of enzymes in the digestion process.

Supplies:

  2 150-mL beakers

  masking tape

  100 mL water

  2 mL meat tenderizer

  ½ hard-cooked egg, peeled

Procedure:

1. Label the beakers *A* and *B* with masking tape.
2. In beaker A, mix 50 mL of water with 2 mL of meat tenderizer. Stir until meat tenderizer is dissolved.
3. Pour the other 50 mL of water into beaker B.
4. Gently remove the yolk from the egg white half. Cut the egg white half in half lengthwise so there are two equal pieces. Place one piece in beaker A and the other in beaker B.
5. Place the beakers in a warm environment overnight.
6. Examine the beakers. Note any change in the egg in the chart below.

	Change Noted
Beaker A	
Beaker B	

Questions:

1. Which beaker showed the least degree of change? _____

2. Which beaker showed the greatest degree of change? _____

3. Why do you think these were your results? (Hint: the active ingredient in meat tenderizer is an enzyme.)

    _____

4. What conclusion about the function of enzymes in the digestion process can you draw from this experiment?

    _____

    _____

    _____

© Goodheart-Willcox

Nutrient Digestion in the Small Intestine

Name_____ **Date** _____ **Period** _____

Work in groups of three to complete the chart and answer the questions about what happens to fats, proteins, and carbohydrates during digestion in the small intestine. Each group member should be responsible for completing one column of the chart and sharing his or her responses with group members. Then work together to answer the questions.

	A. Proteins	B. Carbohydrates	C. Fats
1. End product(s) of digestion			
2. Enzymes involved			

3. What percentage of digestion occurs in the small intestine?_____

4. What enzyme is secreted in the mouth, and what role does it play in digestion?_____

_____

5. What enzyme begins to chemically break down protein in the stomach?_____

6. What are the three sections of the small intestine?_____

_____

7. What role does the pancreas play in digestion of foods in the small intestine? _____

_____

_____

_____

8. What role does the liver play in digestion of foods in the small intestine?_____

_____

_____

9. Where does chyme go when it leaves the small intestine? _____

10. What happens to nutrients after they have been digested in the small intestine?_____

_____

How Nutrients Become You

Name_____

Date _____   Period _____   Score _____

Chapter 3 Test

Matching: Match the following terms and identifying phrases.

_____ 1. The unit used to measure the energy value of food.

_____ 2. A complex protein produced by cells to speed a specific chemical reaction in the body.

_____ 3. Chewing.

_____ 4. A series of squeezing actions by the muscles in the gastrointestinal tract that helps move food through the tract.

_____ 5. A mixture of gastric juices and food formed in the stomach during digestion.

_____ 6. A digestive juice produced by the liver to aid fat digestion.

_____ 7. Solid wastes that result from digestion.

_____ 8. The passage of nutrients from the digestive tract into the circulatory system.

_____ 9. All the chemical changes that occur as cells produce energy and materials needed to sustain life.

_____ 10. A reaction of the immune system to certain proteins found in food.

_____ 11. Frequent expulsion of watery feces.

_____ 12. A difficulty in digesting food.

_____ 13. A burning pain in the middle of the chest caused by stomach acid flowing back into the esophagus.

_____ 14. Small crystals that form from bile in the gallbladder.

_____ 15. A disorder in which many abnormal pouches form in the intestinal wall.

A. absorption
B. bile
C. chyme
D. diarrhea
E. diverticulosis
F. enzyme
G. feces
H. food allergy
I. gallstones
J. heartburn
K. indigestion
L. kilocalorie
M. mastication
N. metabolism
O. peristalsis
P. ulcer

True or False: Circle *T* if the statement is true or *F* if the statement is false.

T   F   16. The simplest substances from which all matter is formed are called molecules.

T   F   17. Water is an example of a compound.

T   F   18. Lacking adequate nutrition during periods of growth may affect a person's learning abilities and behavior patterns.

T   F   19. The processes of digestion, absorption, and metabolism are not affected by the amounts of nutrients a person consumes.

T   F   20. The epiglottis keeps food from entering the trachea.

T   F   21. Liquids leave the stomach before solids.

T   F   22. ATP is the body's store of energy that is ready for immediate use.

(Continued)

© Goodheart-Willcox

Name_____

T F   23. Emotions, such as anger with a friend or tension over a test, can have a negative effect on digestion.

T F   24. The amount of physical activity a person gets has little effect on his or her digestion and metabolism.

T F   25. An ulcer can develop in the small intestine.

Multiple Choice: Choose the best response. Write the letter in the space provided.

_____26. Which of the following is one of the six nutrient groups?
  A. Chemicals.
  B. Compounds.
  C. Enzymes.
  D. Water.

_____27. Which function of nutrients is most related to a midmorning slump?
  A. Building new tissue.
  B. Providing energy.
  C. Regulating body processes.
  D. Repairing tissue.

_____28. Which of the following nutrients provides the greatest amount of energy?
  A. 250 mg of vitamin C.
  B. 22 g of carbohydrates.
  C. 20 g of protein.
  D. 13 g of fat.

_____29. Which statement best describes the process of digestion?
  A. Breakdown of food into simpler substances for the body to use.
  B. Collection of waste products that result from digestion.
  C. Passage of food from the digestive tract into the circulatory or lymphatic system.
  D. Transport of nutrients and oxygen to individual body cells.

_____30. About how long is the digestive tract, from beginning to end?
  A. 10 feet.
  B. 15 feet.
  C. 30 feet.
  D. 40 feet.

_____31. In which part of the digestive system does the least amount of digestion occur?
  A. Esophagus.
  B. Mouth.
  C. Small intestine.
  D. Stomach.

_____32. A thick fluid that helps soften and lubricate food in the stomach is called _____.
  A. bile
  B. mucus
  C. pancreatic juice
  D. pepsin

_____33. Which nutrients are acted upon by pepsin in the stomach?
  A. Carbohydrates only.
  B. Lipids only.
  C. Proteins only.
  D. Carbohydrates, lipids, and proteins.

(Continued)

© Goodheart-Willcox

Name_____

_____34. Which of the following best describes the pathway of food in the digestion process?
  A. Esophagus, stomach, small intestine.
  B. Large intestine, stomach, esophagus.
  C. Mouth, stomach, esophagus.
  D. Stomach, small intestine, esophagus.

_____35. What are the basic parts into which carbohydrates are broken down during digestion?
  A. Amino acids.
  B. Fatty acids.
  C. Glycerol.
  D. Monosaccharides.

_____36. Which part of the small intestine increases the surface area for absorption?
  A. Capillaries.
  B. Duodenum.
  C. Lacteals.
  D. Villi.

_____37. A person is likely to feel full longest after eating a meal high in _____.
  A. carbohydrates
  B. fats
  C. protein
  D. water

_____38. Which of the following is associated with the problem of constipation?
  A. Consuming a low-fiber diet.
  B. Drinking too much water.
  C. Following regular meal patterns.
  D. Getting too much exercise.

Essay Questions: Provide complete responses to the following questions.

39. Name the six basic types of nutrients you must obtain from the foods you eat.

40. What is the difference between mechanical digestion and chemical digestion? Where does each type of digestion take place?

41. How do the waste products of cell metabolism leave the body?

42. Identify three eating habits that would promote normal digestion and absorption.

© Goodheart-Willcox

Nutrition Guidelines

Objectives

After studying this chapter, students will be able to
- discuss how the Recommended Dietary Allowances (RDAs) and Dietary Reference Intakes (DRIs) are used.
- summarize the advice offered in the Dietary Guidelines for Americans, 2005.
- identify the recommended number of daily portions and portion sizes for each food group in MyPyramid.
- use percent Daily Values on food labels to evaluate a food's contributions to daily nutrient needs.
- describe how to evaluate a food's nutrient density.
- collect and analyze data about their current eating habits and use MyPyramid to plan nutritious menus.

Bulletin Board

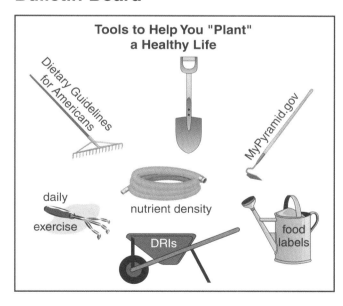

Tools to Help You "Plant" a Healthy Life

Dietary Guidelines for Americans

MyPyramid.gov

daily exercise

nutrient density

DRIs

food labels

Title: *Tools to Help You "Plant" a Better Diet*

Cover the bulletin board with light blue paper and a brown strip across the bottom to represent the sky and earth. Use brightly colored construction paper to make cutouts of common garden tools and place them on the board. Label the tools *DRIs, daily exercise, Dietary Guidelines for Americans, MyPyramid.gov, food labels,* and *nutrient density.*

Teaching Materials

Text, pages 58-72
Learn the Language
Check Your Knowledge
Put Learning into Action
Explore Further

Student Activity Guide, pages 25-30
A. *Tools for Healthful Eating*
B. *Snack Inspection*
C. *Personal Pyramid*
D. *Backtrack Through Chapter 4*

Teacher's Resources
Recommended Nutrient Intakes, color transparency CT-4
What Are Your Daily Needs? transparency master 4-1
Catch Nutrition Fever, reproducible master 4-2
Track Your Diet the Pyramid Way, reproducible master 4-3
Diet Analysis, reproducible master 4-4
Chapter 4 Test

Introducing the Chapter

1. Have a student define the word *tool*. Refer to the garden tools pictured on the *Tools to Help You "Plant" a Healthy Life* bulletin board. Ask students how garden tools may be similar to diet-planning tools.
2. Survey students to find out how many are familiar with or have used the following nutrition tools to help make eating decisions: DRIs, Dietary Guidelines for Americans, MyPyramid system, Daily Values on food labels, and nutrient density. Choose and plan class activities accordingly.
3. Have each student find a newspaper or magazine article related to nutrition. Ask students to identify the sources of any nutrition data cited in the articles. List these sources on the chalkboard. Star sources that can be considered tools for diet planning. Discuss the kinds of information that may be available from starred sources.
4. Ask students what value they think there may be in consuming a planned diet versus consuming an unplanned diet.

Strategies to Reteach, Reinforce, Enrich, and Extend Text Concepts

Dietary Reference Intakes

5. **RT** *Recommended Nutrient Intakes,* color transparency CT-4. Use the transparency to illustrate the four types of nutrient reference values that fall under the umbrella of DRIs (Dietary Reference Intakes). Distinguish the meaning and use of RDAs (Recommended Dietary Allowances), EARs (Estimated Average Requirements), AIs (Adequate Intakes), and ULs (Upper Tolerable Intake Levels). Discuss how using these reference values to plan and assess diets can help prevent chronic diseases as well as nutrient deficiency diseases.

6. **RT** Compare deficiency and toxicity as two extremes of health problems associated with vitamin consumption. Ask students to identify which DRIs relate most directly to each extreme.

7. **ER** Guest speaker. Invite a dietitian to discuss with the class how he or she uses the RDAs and the DRIs to assist clients in planning more healthful diets. Ask the speaker to discuss how the use of these diet-planning tools may change in the future as research reveals more about nutrient deficiency, disease prevention, and toxicity.

8. **RF** Have students practice finding and interpreting information in Appendix A, *Recommended Nutrient Intakes.* Ask them to find various pieces of information, such as the units used to measure vitamin A or the amount of iron needed by a 14- to 18-year-old female. Also ask them to suggest why recommendations for a given nutrient might differ between two age groups of people.

9. **ER** Have students find out how the DRIs are revised and who reviews them. Students may choose to consult with a registered dietitian, complete library research, or search the Internet for recent data from the Food and Nutrition Board of the Institute of Medicine, National Academy of Sciences.

Dietary Guidelines for Americans

10. **RT** Review the Dietary Guidelines for Americans with students. Explain how the guidelines interrelate, and discuss their total impact on healthful food choices and other wellness promoting lifestyle choices.

11. **RF** Ask students to give examples of their favorite snack foods that are high in fat, sugar, and/or salt. Write their responses on the chalkboard. Have students work in small groups to brainstorm lists of snack alternatives that are low in fat, sugar, and sodium. As a class, discuss the value of choosing foods that support the Dietary Guidelines.

12. **RF** Divide the class into small groups. Assign each group one of the following words: *variety, moderation, proportion.* Have each group write a set of sentences, each beginning with a different letter of the assigned word. Each sentence should offer a tip or describe a benefit associated with following the Dietary Guidelines.

13. **ER** Have each student create a poster that encourages teens to follow one or more of the Dietary Guidelines for Americans. Display posters in the classroom.

14. **RF** *Catch Nutrition Fever,* reproducible master 4-2. Have students respond to the yes-or-no questions and fill in the thermometer to assess how closely the students are following the Dietary Guidelines for Americans. Then have students answer the evaluation questions to explore ways to change health risks and promote wellness habits.

MyPyramid

15. **RT** Have students explore the MyPyramid food guidance system by logging on to MyPyramid.gov. They can generate their personal plan by clicking on the subject *MyPyramid Plan* and entering their age, gender, and physical activity. Have them print the PDF version of their results and use it along with the Web site to plan a one-week menu.

16. **RT** *What Are Your Daily Needs?* transparency master 4-1. Use the transparency to review the recommended daily amounts from each group in the MyPyramid system for various calorie levels. Relate body size, gender, age, and physical activity to calorie needs as you discuss who might fall under each calorie level. Point out to students that selections from the five major food groups must be low in fat to stay within specified calorie levels.

17. **RF** Have students collect a variety of pictures representing all of the food groups. Have them draw MyPyramid on their poster board. Students should select the approximate number and size of food portions from their pictures that would meet the daily needs for a 2,000-calorie plan. Food pictures should be placed in the appropriate food group band. Remind students to place high fat and/or high sugar foods near the top of their band and lowfat/low sugar foods near the bottom. Display the posters and have students evaluate them for variety, moderation, and proportion.

18. **RF** Survey students about how many portions they have each day from each group in MyPyramid. Discuss why some teens might be eating more or less than the recommended daily amounts.

19. **ER** *Personal Pyramid,* Activity C, SAG. Students are to label the groups of MyPyramid and give the recommended daily amounts for each group. Then they are to write the names of three of their favorite foods from each group in the appropriate spaces on the Pyramid.

20. **RF** Have students tally their food group eating patterns for one day. Ask students to record each time they consume a portion of a food from one of the food groups. Total the portion numbers for each food group. Have students identify where habit changes may be beneficial to health.

The Daily Values on Food Labels

21. **RF** Ask how many students read Nutrition Facts panels on food labels. Discuss what information on the panels interests students most.

22. **RF** Ask each student to bring a Nutrition Facts panel from a food product label to class. Have students work in pairs to list all the types of information presented on the panel.

23. **RF** Have students compare the reference values for a 2,000-calorie diet and a 2,500-calorie diet, as shown at the bottom of a Nutrition Facts panel. Ask students how the values for cholesterol and sodium differ from those of the other listed nutrients. Help students calculate the Daily Values for a 1,600-calorie and a 2,800-calorie diet.

24. **ER** Field trip. Visit a supermarket and have students use Nutrition Facts panels to hunt for food items with a little or a lot of a specific nutrient. Give each student a list of what to look for, such as a food that is very high in fiber or the cereal with the lowest amount of sodium.

25. **EX** *Snack Inspection,* Activity B, SAG. Students are to make predictions about the nutritional content of four snack foods. Then students are to compare the Nutrition Facts panels provided to evaluate the accuracy of their predictions and write conclusions.

26. **RF** Have each student plan a day's menus using only packaged foods that have Nutrition Facts panels. Tell students to estimate the number of servings of each food to be consumed. Then have students total all the percent Daily Values for listed nutrients to determine whether daily totals were greater or less than 100 percent for each of the nutrients. Ask students to suggest food substitutions that might improve the daily nutrient balance.

Nutrient Density

27. **RT** Explain the concept of nutrient density. Then show students two related food items, such as applesauce and an apple-filled snack pie. Ask the class which food they think is more nutrient dense

overall. Compare the Nutrition Facts panels of the two products to accurately compare the nutrient density.

28. **ER** Have teams of students use Appendix C or *Personal Best* software to prepare bar graphs illustrating the ratio of nutrients to energy supplied for each of two comparable foods. Possible food items include fruit juice and fruit drink or a cupcake and a granola bar. Teams should present their findings in class.

Using Food Recommendations and Guidelines

29. **RF** *Track Your Diet the Pyramid Way,* reproducible master 4-3. Students are to complete the chart to see how well their diets meet the recommendations of the MyPyramid system. Each day, students should list all the foods they eat for meals and snacks in the appropriate columns and rows. Then they should fill in a triangle at the top of the chart in the appropriate row to represent each portion they consume from one of the food groups. At the end of the week, blank triangles will indicate food groups in which students are falling short of the recommendations of MyPyramid.

30. **EX** *Diet Analysis,* reproducible master 4-4. Have students use Appendix C or *Personal Best* software to complete a diet analysis chart for the food diary on the handout. Then have students use Appendix B, *Recommended Nutrient Intakes,* to compare nutrient intakes with recommendations. Students should complete the activity by using Chapters 5 through 9 to identify food sources of nutrients that were lacking in the diet.

Chapter Review

31. **RF** *Backtrack Through Chapter 4,* Activity D, SAG. Students are to provide complete answers to questions and statements that will help them recall, interpret, apply, and practice chapter concepts.

32. **RF** *Tools for Healthful Eating,* Activity A, SAG. Students are to review chapter concepts by identifying true and false statements.

33. **EX** Divide students into groups according to which diet-planning tool they think works best for teens. Have each group prepare a presentation on the advantages and disadvantages of its diet-planning tool.

Above and Beyond

34. **ER** Refer to the *Using Other Resources* section in the front of this product for a list of Web sites. Have each student use addresses in the list to

search on the Internet for information about one of the diet-planning tools discussed in the chapter. Ask each student to share with the class one piece of information not found in the text.

35. **EX**   Have each student ask a friend or relative to keep a food diary for one to three days. Then students can use *Personal Best* software or a copy of the Diet Analysis Form from reproducible master 4-4 to analyze the day's nutrient contents. Remind students when presenting their analyses to emphasize that a one-day sample may not reflect a person's total eating pattern. When appropriate, students may wish to suggest food substitutes that would better meet nutrient needs.

36. **ER**   Have students write a nutrition column for each issue of the school newspaper. Each column could focus on how teens can use a different diet-planning tool to make more healthful food choices.

37. **EX**   Have students use the Dietary Guidelines for Americans to analyze the lunch menus from the school cafeteria. Have students compose a tactful letter to the cafeteria staff suggesting ways the nutritional value of the menus might be improved.

38. **EX**   Have students plan a Healthful Snacking Awareness Day at your school. Activities might include poster displays of healthful food choices, samples of healthful snacks, and demonstrations of ways to reduce fat, sugar, and salt in snack recipes.

39. **ER**   Have students use the Internet to review *Healthy People 2010,* which was developed by the U.S. Department of Health and Human Services. Have students use the objectives for Americans stated in this report to develop a bulletin board.

40. **ER**   Have students use the Internet to find food pyramids or similar eating plans for a variety of cultures. Discuss the similarities and differences among the various pyramids and eating plans.

Answer Keys

Text

Check Your Knowledge, page 71

1. false
2. The Dietary Guidelines for Americans were developed because the average American diet is too high in fats, cholesterol, and sugar. It is too low in the nutrients found in whole grains, vegetables, and fruits. Such dietary patterns are associated with heart disease, stroke, cancer, and liver disease, which are among the leading causes of death in the United States.
3. During your teen years, you should try to accumulate at least 60 minutes of moderate physical activity each day.
4. grains—6, vegetables—2.5, fruits—2, milk—3, meat—5.5
5. true
6. (Student response. See Chart 4-5 in the text.)
7. No more than 10 percent of total daily calories should come from saturated fat.
8. 2,000
9. A food that provides a greater percentage of nutrient needs than calorie needs has a high nutrient density.
10. (List two:) make sure the diary is complete, accurately estimate portion sizes, keep the diary for several days
11. Food composition tables are a reference guide listing the nutritive values of many foods in common servings, which can be used as a diet analysis tool.
12. (Student response. Give one tip for each food group. See Chart 4-10 in the text.)

Student Activity Guide

Tools for Healthful Eating, Activity A

1. T	11. F
2. F	12. T
3. F	13. T
4. T	14. T
5. F	15. T
6. F	16. T
7. T	17. T
8. F	18. T
9. T	19. T
10. T	20. F

Snack Inspection, Activity B

(Predictions and conclusions are student response.)
1. pretzels
2. snack mix
3. tortilla chips/snack mix
4. pretzels
5. potato chips/tortilla chips
6. snack mix
7. all zero
8. all zero
9. snack mix
10. snack mix
11. potato chips
12. tortilla chips
13. pretzels

Backtrack Through Chapter 4, Activity D

1. A. suggested levels of nutrient intake to meet the needs of most healthy people
   B. nutrient recommendation estimated to meet the need of half the healthy people in a group
   C. the recommended daily amount of a nutrient needed when no EAR can be established
   D. the maximum level at which a nutrient is unlikely to cause harm in most people
2. the Food and Nutrition Board
3. grains—6; vegetables—2.5; fruits—2; milk—3; meat and beans—5.5
4. the proportion of your diet that food group makes up
5. age, sex, body size, and activity level
6. the number of portions and the size of the portions
7. (See Figure 4-2 in the text.)
8. the percentages of a person's daily nutrient needs that one serving of the food provides
9. a comparison of the nutrients provided by a food with the calories provided by the same food
10. (Student response. See page 66.)
11. If you have a software program that includes a database of food composition tables, you can use it to analyze your diet. You enter information about your diet into the program, and the computer can create a detailed printout containing a nutrition analysis. Diet analysis can also be done on MyPyramid.gov.
12. You can use the MyPyramid system to create your personal food plan. Then you can plan meals and snacks for the entire day that include the recommended amounts from each group.
13. The DRIs contain numerical values regarding nutrient needs. You can use the DRIs to ensure you are consuming enough of various important nutrients.
14. By being aware of portion sizes, you can better ensure you are getting the right amount of needed nutrients.
15. (Student response. See page 62.)
16. (Student response.)
17. (Student response.)
18. (Student response.)
19. (Student response.)
20. (Student response.)

Teacher's Resources

Diet Analysis, reproducible master 4-4

Diet Analysis Form

Food Item	Food energy (cal.)	Protein (g)	Fat (g)	Saturated fat (g)	Cholesterol (mg)	Carbohydrate (g)	Dietary fiber (g)	Calcium (mg)	Iron (mg)	Potassium (mg)	Sodium (mg)	Vitamin A (µg)	Thiamin (mg)	Riboflavin (mg)	Niacin (mg)	Vitamin C (mg)
Milk	120	8	5	2.9	18	12	0	297	0.1	377	122	139	0.10	0.40	0.2	2
Eggs	160	12	12	3.2	548	2	0	56	2.0	130	138	156	0.08	0.28	Tr	0
Tuna	135	30	1	0.2	48	0	0	17	0.6	255	468	32	0.03	0.10	13.4	0
Bread	130	4	2	0.4	0	24	2	64	1.8	70	276	Tr	0.24	0.16	2.4	Tr
Cottage cheese	102.5	15.5	2	1.4	9.5	4	0	77.5	0.2	108.5	459	22.5	0.03	0.21	0.15	Tr
Banana	105	1	1	0.2	0	27	2	7	0.4	451	1	9	0.05	0.11	0.6	10
Diet cola	Tr	0	0	0	0	Tr	0	14	0.2	7	32	0	0	0	0	0
Beef	410	46	24	12.4	124	0	0	10	3.2	616	100	Tr	0.14	0.28	6.0	0
Applesauce	97.5	Tr	Tr	Tr	0	25.5	1.5	5	0.45	156	8	3	0.02	0.04	0.25	2
Potatoes	225	4	9	2.2	4	35	4	55	0.5	607	620	42	0.18	0.08	2.3	13
Fruit punch	170	Tr	0	0	0	44	0	30	0.8	96	30	4	0.06	0.08	Tr	122
Ice cream	185	5	6	3.5	18	29	Tr	176	0.2	265	105	52	0.08	0.35	0.1	1
Totals	1840	125.5	62	26.4	769.5	202.5	9.5	808.5	10.45	3138.5	2359	459.5	1.01	2.09	25.4	150
RDA or AI	2368	46	92[1]	26[2]	less than 300	130	36	1300	15	2000	less than 2400	700	1	1	14	65
Greater than (>) or less than (<) the recommended level	<	>	<	<	<	>	<	<	<	>	<	<	>	>	>	>

[1]Recommended calorie intake × 35 percent ÷ 9 calories per gram
[2]Recommended calorie intake × 10 percent ÷ 9 calories per gram

Chapter 4 Test

1. D	18. T
2. I	19. T
3. A	20. T
4. K	21. F
5. G	22. F
6. J	23. D
7. C	24. A
8. B	25. D
9. H	26. A
10. F	27. B
11. F	28. D
12. T	29. C
13. T	30. C
14. T	31. D
15. T	32. A
16. F	33. C
17. F	34. A

35. to prevent diseases caused by a lack of nutrients and chronic diseases linked to nutrition
36. (Student response. See pages 68-69 in the text.)
37. (Student response should include 10 portions from the grains group; 3.5 portions from the vegetable group; 2.5 portions from the fruit group; 3 portions from the milk group; and 7 portions from the meat and beans group.)

What Are Your Daily Needs?

How many portions do you need each day?

Calorie level	about 1,600	about 2,000	about 2,400
Grains group	5	6	8
Vegetable group	2	2½	3½
Fruit group	1½	2	2
Milk group	3	3	3
Meat and beans group	5	5½	6½

There are 12 levels based on age, gender, and activity level. Go to <u>MyPyramid.gov</u> to find the food plan that is based on your needs.

© Goodheart-Willcox

Catch Nutrition Fever

Name_____ Date _____ Period _____

Check the *Yes* or *No* column to indicate whether each statement describes you. Starting at the bottom of the thermometer, fill in one square for each yes response. Then answer the questions at the bottom of the page.

	Yes	No	
	____	____	1. My diet includes grain foods, vegetables, fruits, milk and milk products, and meat and meat alternatives every day.
	____	____	2. My body weight is in an appropriate proportion to my height and physical build.
Nutrition Fever	____	____	3. My weekly schedule includes at least 60 minutes of moderate physical activity each day.
	____	____	4. My diet includes at least six daily portions of grain foods, such as breads, cereals, rice, and pasta.
Heating Up	____	____	5. My diet includes at least two and a half daily portions of vegetables.
	____	____	6. My diet includes at least two daily portions of fruits.
	____	____	7. I take steps when selecting, preparing, and storing food to keep it safe to eat.
Cool as a Cucumber	____	____	8. I regularly trim the fat from meats and remove the skin from poultry.
	____	____	9. I choose nonmeat protein sources, such as dry beans and peas, often.
	____	____	10. I regularly select lowfat and fat free dairy products.
	____	____	11. I limit my intake of high-fat snacks and desserts, dressings, spreads, and cooking oils.
	____	____	12. I limit my intake of soft drinks, jams, jellies, candies, and desserts.
	____	____	13. I read labels to examine the sodium content of foods.
	____	____	14. I limit the amount of salt I add to foods during preparation and at the table.
	____	____	15. I completely avoid consuming alcohol.

16. Which no responses are easy to change? Explain your response. _____
_____

17. Which no responses are hard to change? Explain your response. _____
_____

18. What can you do today to improve your food and activity choices and follow the Dietary Guidelines for Americans more closely? _____

© Goodheart-Willcox

Track Your Diet the Pyramid Way

Name _____　Date _____　Period _____

Complete this chart to help you see how well your diet meets the recommendations of MyPyramid for a 2,000-calorie plan. Each day, write all the foods and amounts you eat for meals and snacks in the appropriate columns and rows. At the top of the chart, fill in a triangle in the appropriate row to represent each portion you consumed from one of the food groups. For instance, if you eat an apple, fill in a triangle in the fruit row for that day. At the end of the week, if you have only a few blank triangles, you are doing a good job of following MyPyramid. If you have several blank triangles, however, look for ways to add foods from the missing groups to your diet. Remember, your diet pattern based on your gender, age, and activity level may require more or less portions than this plan.

Group/portions	Sunday	Monday	Tuesday	Wednesday	Thursday	Friday	Saturday
Milk 3 cups	△△△	△△△	△△△	△△△	△△△	△△△	△△△
Meat 5.5 ounces	△△△△△△	△△△△△△	△△△△△△	△△△△△△	△△△△△△	△△△△△△	△△△△△△
Vegetable 2.5 cups	△△△	△△△	△△△	△△△	△△△	△△△	△△△
Fruit 2 cups	△△	△△	△△	△△	△△	△△	△△
Grain 6 ounces	△△△△△△	△△△△△△	△△△△△△	△△△△△△	△△△△△△	△△△△△△	△△△△△△
Breakfast							
Snack							
Lunch							
Snack							
Dinner							
Snack							

© Goodheart-Willcox

Diet Analysis

Name_____   Date _____   Period _____

LaRonda is a 16-year-old female. Complete the accompanying chart to help you analyze her diet for one day. Fill in the first column with the food items from the food diary below. Then use Appendix C, *Nutritive Values of Foods,* to fill in the columns identifying the nutrient composition of each item. Be sure to adjust nutrient amounts appropriately for LaRonda's portion sizes. Figure the total amount of each nutrient LaRonda consumed. Use Appendix B, *Recommended Nutrient Intakes,* to fill in the AI or RDA for each nutrient recommended for LaRonda's age and gender group. Finally, fill in the last line to indicate whether LaRonda's intake of each nutrient was greater than (>) or less than (<) the recommended amount. After completing the chart, answer the questions at the bottom of the page. (You may wish to use diet analysis software instead of the accompanying chart to help you analyze LaRonda's diet.)

Food Diary

Breakfast
Milk, lowfat (2%)—1 cup
Eggs, hard-cooked—2

Lunch
Tuna, canned, water pack—3 ounces
Bread, wheat—2 slices
Cottage cheese, lowfat (2%)—½ cup
Banana—1
Diet cola—12 ounces

Dinner
Beef roast, relatively lean—6 ounces
Applesauce, sweetened—½ cup
Potatoes, mashed—1 cup
Fruit punch—12 ounces
Ice cream, vanilla, hardened—1 cup

In the space below, list the nutrients for which LaRonda's diet provided less than the recommended amount. Then refer to Chapters 5 through 9 in the text to help you list a good food source for each of these nutrients.

_____

_____

_____

_____

_____

(Continued)

© Goodheart-Willcox

Diet Analysis Form

Food Item	Food energy (cal.)	Protein (g)	Fat (g)	Saturated fat (g)	Cholesterol (mg)	Carbohydrate (g)	Dietary fiber (g)	Calcium (mg)	Iron (mg)	Potassium (mg)	Sodium (mg)	Vitamin A (µg)	Thiamin (mg)	Riboflavin (mg)	Niacin (mg)	Vitamin C (mg)
Totals																
RDA or AI			[1]	[2]	less than 300					2000	less than 2400					
Greater than (>) or less than (<) the recommended level																

[1]Recommended calorie intake × 35 percent ÷ 9 calories per gram
[2]Recommended calorie intake × 10 percent ÷ 9 calories per gram

© Goodheart-Willcox

Nutrition Guidelines

Name_____

Date _____   Period _____   Score _____

Chapter 4 Test

Matching: Match the following terms and identifying phrases.

_____ 1. A set of nutrient reference values that can be used to plan and assess diets for healthy people.

_____ 2. Suggested levels of nutrient intake to meet the needs of most healthy people.

_____ 3. A value set for nutrients for which research is too inconclusive to determine an RDA.

_____ 4. The maximum level at which a nutrient is unlikely to cause harm to most people.

_____ 5. A food guidance system used to help people plan healthy diets and physically active lifestyles according to the Dietary Guidelines for Americans.

_____ 6. A unit of measured food, such as cups or ounces.

_____ 7. A set of recommendations focusing on nutritious diet, healthy weight, adequate exercise, and food safety.

_____ 8. Recommended nutrient intakes, which are based on daily calorie needs, used as references on food labels.

_____ 9. A comparison of the nutrients provided by a food with the calories provided by the food.

_____ 10. A record of the kinds and amounts of all foods and beverages consumed for a given time.

A. Adequate Intake (AI)

B. Daily Values

C. Dietary Guidelines for Americans

D. Dietary Reference Intake (DRI)

E. Estimated Average Requirement (EAR)

F. food diary

G. MyPyramid system

H. nutrient density

I. Recommended Dietary Allowance (RDA)

J. portion size

K. Upper Tolerable Intake Level (UL)

True/False: Circle *T* if the statement is true and *F* if the statement is false.

T F 11. According to MyPyramid, the food groups should represent equal proportions of your diet.

T F 12. Active people usually require more food group portions per day than inactive people.

T F 13. One portion of milk is equal to one cup of milk.

T F 14. Serving size must be indicated on a food label.

T F 15. Physical activity is an essential part of a weight management plan.

T F 16. Researchers have identified an existing food that contains all the nutrients in the amounts most people need.

T F 17. Safe foods are those that are grown without the use of chemical pesticides.

T F 18. A person following the Dietary Guidelines for Americans is likely to choose fat free milk over whole milk on a regular basis.

T F 19. *Low nutrient density* is a useful term for describing the quality of a food.

T F 20. A three-day food diary reflects eating patterns more accurately than a one-day food diary.

T F 21. A diet analysis is designed to tell a person if he or she needs to lose weight.

T F 22. Poultry pieces with skin on are lower in fat than skinless meat pieces.

(Continued)

© Goodheart-Willcox

Name_____

Multiple Choice: Choose the best response. Write the letter in the space provided.

_____23. How many daily portions from the milk group do most teens need?
  A. None.
  B. One.
  C. Two.
  D. Three.

_____24. Which food item can be placed in the vegetables section of MyPyramid?
  A. Peas.
  B. Grapes.
  C. Meat.
  D. Yogurt.

_____25. Mark ate 2 cups of spaghetti for dinner. How many portions from the grains group did he consume?
  A. One.
  B. Two.
  C. Three.
  D. Four.

_____26. Which characteristic best describes the average American diet?
  A. Too high in fats, cholesterol, and sugar.
  B. Too high in nutrients found in vegetables.
  C. Too high in vitamins, minerals, and fiber.
  D. Too low in sodium.

_____27. According to the Dietary Guidelines for Americans, choosing and preparing foods with less salt may help reduce the risk of _____.
  A. cancer
  B. high blood pressure
  C. overweight
  D. tooth decay

_____28. A person who chooses a diet of many different foods within each food group is practicing the principle of _____.
  A. balance
  B. excess
  C. moderation
  D. variety

_____29. Percent Daily Values on a Nutrition Facts panel are based on a typical diet of how many calories?
  A. 1,600.
  B. 1,800.
  C. 2,000.
  D. 2,500.

_____30. A Nutrition Facts panel indicates one serving of a food product supplies 2 grams of dietary fiber, which is 8 percent of the Daily Value. How many servings of that product would a person need to eat to consume 100 percent of the Daily Value for fiber?
  A. 4 to 5 servings.
  B. 8 to 9 servings.
  C. 12 to 13 servings.
  D. 16 to 17 servings.

(Continued)

© Goodheart-Willcox

Name_____

_____31. Two ounces of potato chips supply 302 calories (15% of daily needs) and 2 grams of protein (4% of daily needs). What can you conclude about nutrient density?
   A. Potato chips are a health food.
   B. Potato chips are a junk food.
   C. Potato chips have high nutrient density for protein.
   D. Potato chips have low nutrient density for protein.

_____32. A 3-ounce serving of meat is about the size of a _____.
   A. deck of playing cards
   B. golf ball
   C. paperback book
   D. soda cracker

_____33. What information will a food composition table provide?
   A. Food groups and number of servings in each.
   B. Foods that make the most nutritious choices.
   C. Nutritive values of foods in common serving sizes.
   D. Percentage of calories each food provides for a day.

_____34. Which of the following is the most healthful choice when selecting and preparing foods from the grains group?
   A. Add only half the recommended amount of butter or margarine when preparing pasta and rice mixes.
   B. Add salt to cooking water when preparing pasta.
   C. Choose bread, rice, and pasta less often than cakes and doughnuts.
   D. Choose instant hot cereals instead of regular and quick-cooking products.

Essay Questions: Provide complete responses to the following questions or statements.

35. What is the purpose of the Dietary Reference Intakes?

36. Explain how to analyze a diet without the use of a computer.

37. Plan a day's menus that include the appropriate number of portions from MyPyramid for a teenage male (2,800 calories).

© Goodheart-Willcox

Carbohydrates: The Preferred Body Fuel

5

Objectives

After studying this chapter, students will be able to
- describe the three types of carbohydrates.
- list the functions of carbohydrates.
- explain how the body uses carbohydrates.
- use food labels to meet their carbohydrate needs.
- evaluate the role of carbohydrates in a variety of health issues.

Bulletin Boards

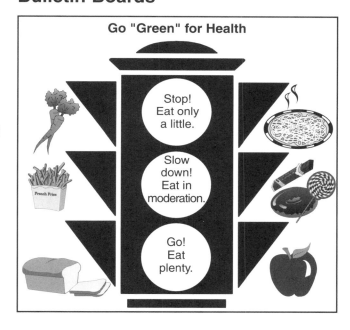

Go "Green" for Health

Stop! Eat only a little.

Slow down! Eat in moderation.

Go! Eat plenty.

French Fries

Title: *Go "Green" for Health*

Place a large cutout of a traffic light on the bulletin board. Label the red light *Stop! Eat only a little.* Label the yellow light *Slow down! Eat in moderation.* Label the green light *Go! Eat plenty.* Place pictures of carbohydrate-rich foods around the traffic light. Place a red, yellow, or green circle beside each picture to indicate the nutrient density of the food. For instance, you might put a red circle beside a candy bar, a yellow circle beside white rice, and a green circle beside raw carrots.

Title: *Each Day the Carbohydrate Way*

Under the title, write the name of the current month. Then write the names of the days of the week across the board. Make a cutout of an apple for each day of the month and arrange the cutouts under the days of the week to accurately represent this month's calendar. Write the appropriate date on each apple. Each day, place a small picture or write the name of a different carbohydrate-rich food on the apple for that day. To increase student awareness of the variety of carbohydrate sources available, be sure to choose some less-familiar foods and examples that represent a variety of cultures.

Teaching Materials

Text, pages 74-90
- *Learn the Language*
- *Check Your Knowledge*
- *Put Learning into Action*
- *Explore Further*

Student Activity Guide, pages 31-38
- A. *Carbohydrates in Action*
- B. *Using Carbohydrates*
- C. *Meeting Carbohydrate Needs*
- D. *Fuel for the Body*
- E. *Carbohydrate Headlines*
- F. *Backtrack Through Chapter 5*

Teacher's Resources
- *Testing for Sugar and Starch*, reproducible master 5-1
- *Starch and Fiber Survey,* reproducible master 5-2
- *Recommended Calorie Distribution,* transparency master 5-3
- *Planning High-Fiber Menus,* reproducible master 5-4
- *From Healthy Teeth to a Happy Smile,* color transparency CT-5
- Chapter 5 Test

Introducing the Chapter

1. Tell students that fruits and vegetables are a good source of carbohydrates. Then go around the room asking each student to name a fruit or vegetable beginning with a different letter of the alphabet.
2. Have each student write on an index card one myth they have heard about carbohydrate foods, such as starches make you fat or sugar causes diabetes. Collect the cards and save them for use in checking knowledge and understanding at the end of the unit.

Strategies to Reteach, Reinforce, Enrich, and Extend Text Concepts

Types of Carbohydrates

3. **RF** Make a three-column chart on the chalkboard. Head the columns *Monosaccharides, Disaccharides,* and *Polysaccharides.* Ask students to name food sources of each. Write correct responses in the appropriate columns.

4. **RF** Display one tablespoon of sugar and one tablespoon of flour on separate plates. Ask students what the two ingredients have in common and what makes each unique. (Both ingredients are refined carbohydrates. Sugar is a simple carbohydrate that contains almost no nutrients. Flour is a complex carbohydrate that contains protein, B vitamins, and iron.)

5. **ER** Divide the class into small groups. Give each group a tray of randomly arranged carbohydrate-rich foods, such as an apple, honey, sugar, white bread, milk, whole wheat bread, sugared cereal, bran cereal, nuts, and dry beans. Ask students to group the foods that provide primarily simple carbohydrates on the left side of the tray. Have students group the foods that provide primarily complex carbohydrates on the right side of the tray. Have students further separate the simple carbohydrates into sources of monosaccharides and disaccharides. Have students use Appendix C or *Personal Best* software to determine the dietary fiber content of one serving of each food. Ask students to also note any other nutrients these carbohydrate foods provide in significant amounts.

6. **ER** *Testing for Sugar and Starch,* reproducible master 5-1. Have lab groups complete the experiments as directed on the master. Students will be identifying food items that contain sugar and starch. Following the experiment, discuss results and answers to the questions.

7. **RF** *Carbohydrates in Action,* Activity A, SAG. Students are to complete a chart identifying types of carbohydrates and where they are found. Then students are to answer questions to help them plan an advertisement for a food product that is a good source of complex carbohydrates.

The Functions of Carbohydrates

8. **RF** Ask students to divide a sheet of paper into 4 sections. In each section, ask students to creatively illustrate each of the following functions of carbohydrates: produce energy, spare proteins, break down fats, provide bulk in the diet. Have partners exchange papers and interpret each others drawings.

9. **RT** Have each student make a list of all the activities he or she does in a day. After students have completed their lists, explain that each activity requires energy, and carbohydrates are the best source of that energy.

10. **RT** Use an analogy to illustrate the protein-sparing function of carbohydrates. Tell students to imagine you have a hand-powered generator hooked up to a lightbulb. Sitting beside this equipment is a pile of children's building blocks. Explain that your hands represent protein. They can be used to turn the crank on the generator and provide energy for the lightbulb. They can also be used to build a wall with the blocks. Explain that a battery represents carbohydrates. The battery can be hooked up to the lightbulb to provide energy more efficiently than the generator. However, it cannot be used to build the wall. Once the battery (carbohydrates) is being used to provide energy, your hands (protein) are free to do the work of building that only they can do.

11. **ER** Guest speaker. Invite a physician, county extension nutritionist, or registered dietitian to speak to the class about cancer prevention and dietary patterns. Ask the speaker to focus on recent research findings on the role of fiber in disease prevention.

12. **RF** Fill two beakers with water. Place 1 teaspoon of oat bran in one beaker and 1 teaspoon of wheat bran in the other. Stir both mixtures for one minute. Discuss why the oat bran dissolves and the wheat bran does not. Review the health benefits of both soluble and insoluble fiber.

How Your Body Uses Carbohydrates

13. **RF** *Using Carbohydrates,* Activity B, SAG. Students are to choose the answer that best completes each statement about carbohydrate use in the body.

14. **EX** Ask students to describe how their bodies feel after doing something, such as exercising, that requires a lot of physical energy. Then have the class brainstorm a list of tips for using carbohydrates to refuel the body. Tips should focus on what foods to eat and when to eat them.

Meeting Your Carbohydrate Needs

15. **RF** Discuss why sugar is popular and plentiful in most people's diets.

16. **ER** Have each student make a list of the food choices available in a vending machine in your community. Ask students to share their findings in class, noting where the machines are located and who is most likely to use them. Have students determine what percentage of the foods in

vending machines are high in sugar and low in complex carbohydrates. Discuss why vending machine choices might be limited mostly to foods high in simple carbohydrates. Debate whose responsibility it is to determine what is placed in vending machines. Should it be up to food manufacturers, vending machine companies, businesses where machines are placed, government, or consumers?

17. **ER**   Guest speaker. Invite a registered dietitian to speak to the class about the advantages of a diet with adequate amounts of starch and fiber. Have the dietitian discuss how to calculate recommended carbohydrate intake based on daily calorie needs.

18. **EX**   *Starch and Fiber Survey,* reproducible master 5-2. Have each student use the handout to survey three teens about their intakes of starch and fiber. Have the class compile and analyze their findings. Students should determine which gender does a better job of meeting starch and fiber needs. Students should also evaluate how familiar teens are with serving sizes and sources of fiber. Have the class summarize their findings in an article for your school newspaper.

19. **RF**   Have students make a list of ways teens can increase the fiber in their diets.

20. **RF**   Have students use Appendix C or *Personal Best* software to generate a list of foods from each food group that are high in fiber. Have students place a star beside food items that provide 3 or more grams of fiber per serving. Post the list on the board for student reference.

21. **RT**   *Recommended Calorie Distribution,* transparency master 5-3. Use the transparency to illustrate the recommended distribution of daily calories according to many health and nutrition experts. Compare this distribution with a typical diet in the United States and a very high carbohydrate diet, which might be typical of a developing country. Ask students how they think the typical U.S. diet measures up to current health recommendations. Also ask students why they think distributions vary from culture to culture.

22. **RF**   Ask students to identify which groups in MyPyramid include sources of carbohydrates. Review the recommended number of servings from each group. Emphasize that as calorie needs increase, serving recommendations increase for the carbohydrate-rich bread, cereal, rice and pasta; vegetable; and fruit groups.

23. **RF**   *Meeting Carbohydrate Needs,* Activity C, SAG. Students are to complete a chart identifying their food group sources of carbohydrates for one day. Then they are to complete calculations to figure the total number of grams of carbohydrate they consumed and answer evaluation questions.

24. **EX**   *Planning High-Fiber Menus,* reproducible master 5-4. Have students plan menus for one day that are rich in carbohydrates and high in fiber. Students should identify the serving size of each food item listed in their menus. Have students refer to Appendix C or *Personal Best* software to determine the grams of fiber provided by each food item. Then ask students to evaluate the fiber content of their menus by answering the questions at the bottom of the page.

25. **RF**   Have students compare two bread labels to determine which type of bread is highest in fiber content. Have students read ingredient lists to establish a relationship between fiber content and predominant ingredients. Note that labels can be misleading. A loaf of bread labeled *wheat bread* is not necessarily high in whole grains.

26. **RF**   Have students use Nutrition Facts panels to compare the number of grams of sugars in various beverages, such as 100 percent fruit juice, fruit juice drink or cocktail, and fruit-flavored soda. Have students review the ingredient lists on these products as you discuss the difference between naturally occurring sugars and added refined sugars.

27. **ER**   Have students use Nutrition Facts panels to find the grams of sugars per serving for pairs of food items from each group in MyPyramid, such as presweetened and unsweetened breakfast cereals, glazed and unglazed carrots, syrup-packed and juice-packed pineapple, plain and fruit-flavored yogurt, pinto beans and baked beans. Also have students find the grams of sugars for several popular foods from the fats, oils, and sweets section of the Pyramid, such as soft drinks and candy bars. For each item, have students convert grams of sugar into teaspoons of sugar (4 grams of sugar equal one teaspoon). Then have students create posters illustrating the number of teaspoons of sugar in servings of these food items.

28. **RF**   Ask each student to bring in a food label. Have students form groups based on how their labels fit into MyPyramid. Have group members identify the types of added carbohydrates that appear on the ingredient lists of the food labels. As a class, discuss which food group seems to include the most added carbohydrates overall. Identify the types of products within each group that were high in added carbohydrates. Discuss what functions the added carbohydrates serve in each food.

Health Questions Related to Carbohydrates

29. **RF**   Ask students how they would respond if they heard an adult say "The reason I am overweight today is because my mother made such great

spaghetti and macaroni when I was a kid." Have students identify the reasons starches are not necessarily the source of excess calories.

30. **RT** *From Healthy Teeth to a Happy Smile,* color transparency CT-5. Use the transparency to review tips for good dental hygiene.

31. **ER** Ask students to contact their dentists or use the Internet to find more information about oral hygiene. Have students share their findings in class.

32. **ER** Guest speaker. Invite a dentist or dental hygienist to speak to the class about factors that contribute to the development of healthy teeth and how teeth can be maintained over a lifetime.

33. **ER** Have students prepare a factual pamphlet for parents about sugar and hyperactivity. The pamphlet should include tips on planning snacks and meals that are high in nutrients and add variety to a child's diet. Have a registered dietitian review the pamphlet so students can make any necessary corrections before copying the pamphlet and distributing it to parents in your community.

34. **ER** Guest speaker. Invite a diabetic educator to explain the food exchange system used by people with diabetes mellitus to control blood glucose levels throughout the day. Ask the speaker to address the symptoms, causes, and treatment for hypoglycemia.

35. **ER** Have students contact the United Dairy Industry of America to learn about the recommendations offered to people who are lactose intolerant.

36. **ER** Have students prepare a display of products for people with lactose intolerance. The display should also include some suggestions for meeting calcium needs without the use of milk.

37. **ER** *Carbohydrate Headlines,* Activity E, SAG. Students are to write brief rebuttals debunking myths about carbohydrates.

Chapter Review

38. **RT** *Fuel for the Body,* Activity D, SAG. Students are to complete the crossword puzzle using terms from the chapter.

39. **RF** Distribute the myth cards students prepared in strategy 2. Have students work with partners to write why the myths are false based on information in the text and other resources. Ask partners to share their responses with the class.

40. **RF** *Backtrack Through Chapter 5,* Activity F, SAG. Students are to provide complete answers to questions and statements that will help them recall, interpret, apply, and practice chapter concepts.

41. **EX** Have students develop a carbohydrate trivia game that could be played to review chapter information. Question categories may include functions, use by the body, meeting needs, related health concerns, and dietary recommendations.

Above and Beyond

42. **ER** Have students investigate the differences between soluble and insoluble fiber. Ask students to prepare posters or oral reports identifying food sources and health benefits of each.

43. **EX** Have each student suggest a way to increase the fiber content of a recipe of his or her choice. Divide students into lab groups and have each group choose to prepare one of the high-fiber recipes. Have the class taste and evaluate all the food products.

Answer Key

Text

Check Your Knowledge, page 89

1. (List two each:) monosaccharides—glucose, fructose, galactose; disaccharides—sucrose, lactose, maltose
2. Simple carbohydrates are monosaccharides, which are made up of single sugar molecules, and disaccharides, which are made up of two sugar molecules. Complex carbohydrates are polysaccharides, which have a larger, more intricate structure made up of many sugar molecules.
3. If the diet does not provide enough carbohydrates, the body will draw mainly upon proteins for fuel needs.
4. (List two:) Fiber helps you feel full. Fiber slows the rate at which the stomach empties. Fibrous food sources are usually lower in calories than foods high in fat.
5. true
6. Two-thirds of the body's glycogen is stored in the muscles for use as an energy source during muscular activity. The liver stores the other one-third of the glycogen for use by the rest of the body.
7. Naturally occurring sugars are generally accompanied by other nutrients in foods. Refined sugars contribute no nutrients other than simple carbohydrates, thereby reducing the nutrient density of foods to which they are added.
8. a minimum of 600 calories
9. (List three:) whole grain breads and cereals, vegetables, fruits, dry beans
10. the type of food, when you eat it

11. In Type I, or insulin-dependent diabetes, the pancreas is not able to make insulin. This type of diabetes occurs most often in children and young adults. People with Type I diabetes must take daily injections of insulin to maintain normal blood glucose levels. In Type II, or noninsulin-dependent diabetes, body cells do not respond well to the insulin the pancreas makes. This type of diabetes is much more common, and it usually occurs in adults over age 40. Type II diabetes can often be controlled with diet and exercise.

12. Lactose intolerance is caused by a lack of the digestive enzyme lactase, which is needed to break down lactose, the main carbohydrate in milk.

Student Activity Guide

Carbohydrates in Action, Activity A

1. polysaccharide; plant foods
2. monosaccharide; fruits, honey
3. monosaccharide; bonded to glucose in milk sugar (lactose)
4. monosaccharide; blood
5. disaccharide; milk
6. disaccharide; grains
7. polysaccharide; grain products, starchy vegetables
8. disaccharide; table sugar, beet sugar, cane sugar, molasses, maple syrup

(Students may justify other sources for many of the carbohydrates.)

Using Carbohydrates, Activity B

1. B
2. B
3. A
4. B
5. A
6. B
7. B
8. A
9. A
10. A
11. A
12. B
13. A
14. B

Fuel for the Body, Activity D

Crossword answers:
- 1. DIABETES MELLITUS
- 1 Down. DISACCHARIDE
- 2. INSOLUBLE
- 3. S (CARIES)
- 4. P
- 5. CARIES
- 6. M
- 7. HYPOGLYCEMIA
- 8. STARCH
- 9. SUGARS
- 10. STARCH
- 11. G
- 12. HORMONE
- 13. SIMPLE
- 14. FIBER
- 15. INSULIN
- 17. COMPLEX
- 18. REFINED
- 19. GLUCOSE
- 20. CARBOHYDRATES

Backtrack Through Chapter 5, Activity F

1. sugars, starches, and fiber
2. carbon, hydrogen, and oxygen
3. The body splits disaccharides into monosaccharides during digestion.
4. (List four each:) simple—table sugar, candy, syrups, soft drinks
   complex—breads, cereals, rice, pasta, vegetables
5. provide energy, spare proteins, assist in the breakdown of fats, provide bulk in the diet
6. (List three:) appendicitis, heart and artery disease, colon cancer, diabetes mellitus
7. naturally occurring sugars and refined sugars
8. no more than 25 percent; a minimum of 20 percent
9. 4
10. (List six:) excessive hunger; excessive thirst; weakness; irritability; nausea; changes in eyesight; slow healing of cuts; drowsiness; numbness in legs, feet, or fingers

11. because the body can use carbohydrates so efficiently as a fuel supply
12. If the diet does not provide enough carbohydrates, the body will draw upon proteins for fuel needs. This will keep the body from using proteins for their more vital functions of building and maintaining cell structures.
13. Fiber absorbs water, which softens stools, and helps prevent constipation. Softer stools are easier to pass, reducing the likelihood of hemorrhoids. Some fibers form gels that add bulk to stools, which helps relieve diarrhea.
14. Simple sugars are often found in foods that provide few nutrients. Complex carbohydrates are generally found in foods that also supply vitamins, minerals, and fiber. Complex carbohydrates also have greater satiety value.
15. by reading food labels to see if added sugars appear near the beginning of the ingredient list
16. Particles from sugars and starches eaten between meals tend to remain in the mouth for longer periods. Bacteria feed on these food particles and produce acid that eats away tooth enamel, which can lead to dental caries.
17. choosing nondairy sources of calcium, consuming small amounts of milk with meals, consuming milk alternates like yogurt and cheese
18. males—38 grams; females—36 grams
19. (Student response.)
20. (Student response.)

Teacher's Resources

Testing for Sugar and Starch, reproducible master 5-1

Results of sugar test
    apple—color change
    banana—color change
    cream cheese—no color change
    milk—color change
Results of starch test
    apple—no color change
    canned corn—color change
    cream cheese—no color change
    rice—color change

Chapter 5 Test

1. B	10. E	19. T	27. B
2. A	11. F	20. F	28. A
3. B	12. D	21. F	29. D
4. B	13. T	22. F	30. B
5. A	14. T	23. T	31. A
6. A	15. F	24. F	32. A
7. B	16. T	25. B	33. C
8. A	17. T	26. C	34. A
9. B	18. F		

35. Supplements do not offer the range of nutritional benefits provided by food sources of fiber. For instance, whole grain breads and cereals, vegetables, and fruits offer a variety of vitamins and minerals as well as fiber.
36. (Student response. See page 84 in the text.)
37. (Student response. See page 84 in the text.)

Testing for Sugar and Starch

Name_____ Date _____ Period _____

Part I: Test foods for sugar

Objective: To identify food sources of simple carbohydrates.

Supplies:

3　g apple, crushed
3　g banana
3　g cream cheese
5　mL milk
4　test tubes
20　mL water
　　Benedict's solution
　　eyedropper
　　Bunsen burner

Procedure:

1. Place the apple, banana, cream cheese, and milk in separate test tubes.
2. Mix 5 mL of water with the food in each test tube.
3. Add 10 drops of Benedict's solution to each test tube.
4. Heat the tubes gently over the flame of a Bunsen burner. Do not let the mixtures boil. (CAUTION: Keep test tubes slanted while heating to avoid spattering of the hot liquid.)
5. The Benedict's solution provides an accurate test for the presence of sugars. If sugar is present in a solution, the Benedict's solution will change color to yellow and then orange. Record your results in the chart below.

Food Item	Change Noted
Apple	
Banana	
Cream cheese	
Milk	

Which of the above results did you find most surprising? Explain your answer._____

_____

_____

(Continued)

© Goodheart-Willcox

Name_____

Part II: Test foods for starch

Objective: To identify food sources of complex carbohydrates.

Supplies:

3   g apple, crushed
3   g canned corn, crushed
3   g cream cheese
3   g white rice
4   test tubes
     water
     Bunsen burner
     tincture of iodine
     eyedropper

Procedure:

1. Place the apple, corn, cream cheese, and rice in separate test tubes. Fill the tubes half-full with water and mix.
2. Heat the test tubes over the flame of a Bunsen burner until the mixtures are boiling. Let them boil for 3 minutes, then cool.
3. Add 2 drops of iodine to each test tube. A blue or purple color shows the presence of starch. Record your results.

Food Item	Change Noted
Apple	
Corn	
Cream cheese	
Rice	

Which of the above results did you find most surprising? Explain your answer._____

_____

_____

_____

_____

© Goodheart-Willcox

Starch and Fiber Survey

Name_____ Date _____ Period _____

Use the following questions to survey three teens about their intakes of starch and fiber. Record the letters that correspond to the teens' responses in the chart below. Compile your results with those of your classmates and analyze your findings. Summarize your findings in an article for your school newspaper.

1. What is your gender?   A. male   B. female

2. What do you consider to be a serving of cooked cereal, rice, or pasta?   A. ½ cup   B. ¾ cup   C. 1 cup   D. 2 cups   E. other

3. What do you consider to be a serving of bread?   A. 1 slice   B. 2 slices   C. other

4. What do you consider to be a serving of vegetables?   A. ½ cup   B. ¾ cup   C. 1 cup   D. 2 cups   E. other

5. How many servings of breads, cereals, rice, and pasta do you eat each day?   A. 1 to 2   B. 3 to 5   C. 6 to 9   D. 10 to 11   E. 12 or more

6. How many servings of starchy vegetables, such as potatoes, corn, dried beans, or peas, do you eat each day?   A. less than 1   B. 1   C. more than 1

7. How many servings of other vegetables do you eat each day?   A. 1 to 2   B. 3 to 4   C. 5 or more

8. How many servings of whole fruits do you eat each day?   A. 1 to 2   B. 3 to 4   C. 5 or more

9. Which of the following do you think is the best source of fiber?   A. meat   B. baked beans   C. orange juice   D. broccoli   E. whole wheat bread

10. How likely are you to choose whole grain breads or cereals instead of refined breads or cereals?   A. very likely   B. somewhat likely   C. not likely

Survey Responses

Questions	Person 1	Person 2	Person 3
1.			
2.			
3.			
4.			
5.			
6.			
7.			
8.			
9.			
10.			

© Goodheart-Willcox

Recommended Calorie Distribution

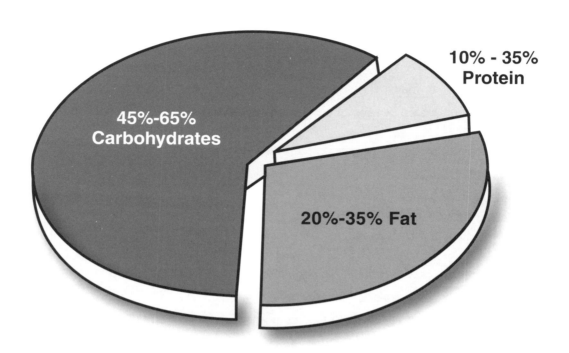

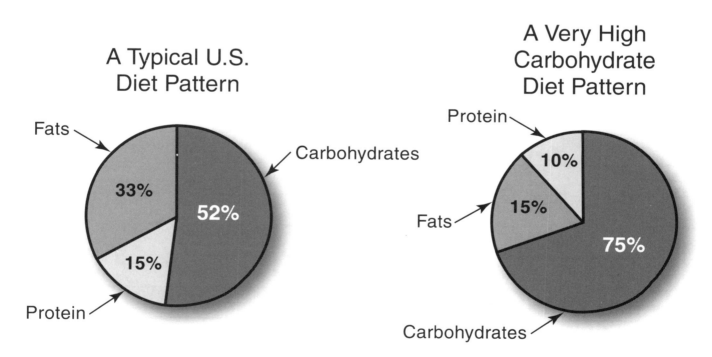

© Goodheart-Willcox

Planning High-Fiber Menus

Name_____   Date _____   Period _____

Plan menus for one day that are rich in carbohydrates and high in fiber. Identify the portion size of each food item listed in your menus. Refer to Appendix C, *Nutritive Values of Foods,* to determine the grams of fiber provided by each food item. Then answer the questions at the bottom of the page.

Meal	Food Items	Portion Sizes	Fiber per Serving (g)
Breakfast			
Snack			
Lunch			
Snack			
Dinner			
Snack			

1. What is your age? _____

2. According to the formula given in the text, how many grams of fiber should you include in your diet each day? _____

3. How did the amount of fiber provided by your menus compare with your daily fiber needs? _____
_____

4. Which three foods in your menus provided the most fiber?_____
_____

5. From which groups in the MyPyramid system did your richest fiber sources come? _____
_____

6. What adjustments might you make to your menus to make them meet your fiber needs better?_____
_____
_____

© Goodheart-Willcox

Carbohydrates: The Preferred Body Fuel

Name_____

Date _____ Period _____ Score _____

Chapter 5 Test

Matching: Match the types of carbohydrates on the left with the classifications on the right.

_____ 1. disaccharide

_____ 2. fiber

_____ 3. glucose

_____ 4. monosaccharide

_____ 5. polysaccharide

_____ 6. starch

_____ 7. sugars

A. complex carbohydrate

B. simple carbohydrate

Matching: Match the following health conditions with their definitions.

_____ 8. Tooth decay.

_____ 9. A lack of or an inability to use the hormone insulin, which results in a buildup of glucose in the bloodstream.

_____ 10. A low blood glucose level.

_____ 11. An inability to digest lactose, the main carbohydrate in milk, due to a lack of the digestive enzyme lactase.

_____ 12. A condition in which a person seems to be in constant motion and is easily distracted.

A. dental caries

B. diabetes mellitus

C. hemorrhoids

D. hyperactivity

E. hypoglycemia

F. lactose intolerance

True/False: Circle *T* if the statement is true or *F* if the statement is false.

T F   13. Nearly all carbohydrates come from plant sources.

T F   14. A diet that includes too little carbohydrate prevents the body from using proteins to build and maintain cell structures.

T F   15. People who are trying to lose weight should avoid the bulk of a diet rich in fiber.

T F   16. One source of soluble fiber is oat bran.

T F   17. Hormones are chemicals produced in the body and released into the bloodstream to regulate specific body processes.

T F   18. The liver can store unlimited amounts of glycogen.

T F   19. Complex carbohydrates have greater satiety value than simple carbohydrates.

T F   20. Candy bars are the main source of sugar in teen diets.

T F   21. Reduced fat and fat free products are generally low in added sugar.

T F   22. Refined sugars have more calories per gram than starchy foods.

T F   23. A baby's teeth can be harmed by allowing the child to sleep with a bottle of milk.

T F   24. Children can become addicted to the taste of sugar.

(Continued)

© Goodheart-Willcox

Name_____

Multiple Choice: Choose the best response. Write the letter in the space provided.

_____25. Which of the following foods is *not* a good source of dietary fiber?
A. Apple.
B. Chicken.
C. Lentils.
D. Popcorn.

_____26. Why are carbohydrates the body's preferred source of energy?
A. They are inexpensive to buy.
B. They are plentiful in the diet.
C. They can be used efficiently as fuel.
D. They spare fats.

_____27. Meg decided to follow a very high protein diet to lose weight. She was avoiding nearly all carbohydrate foods. What health condition is she most at risk of developing?
A. Diabetes mellitus.
B. Ketosis.
C. Lactose intolerance.
D. Starvation.

_____28. Which carbohydrate provides the most bulk to the diet?
A. Fiber.
B. Fructose.
C. Lactose.
D. Sucrose.

_____29. Research has indicated that diets high in fiber may reduce the risk of _____.
A. colon cancer
B. heart and artery disease
C. hemorrhoids
D. All the above.

_____30. What form must all carbohydrates be in for cells to use them as an energy source?
A. Fructose.
B. Glucose.
C. Glycogen.
D. Insulin.

_____31. What happens to a person's blood glucose level after eating?
A. It rises.
B. It falls.
C. It is not affected.
D. It rises or falls depending on gender.

_____32. Which group in MyPyramid is the best source of foods high in starch?
A. The grains group.
B. The fruit group.
C. The meat and beans group.
D. The milk group.

© Goodheart-Willcox

Name_____

_____33. The ingredient list on a package of vanilla pudding reads as follows: sugar, wheat flour, starches, added flavorings. Which ingredient is present in the largest amount?
   A. Flavorings.
   B. Starches.
   C. Sugar.
   D. Wheat flour.

_____34. Due to lactose intolerance, Lupe does not drink milk. Which nutrient is most likely to be deficient in her diet because of this eating pattern?
   A. Calcium.
   B. Carbohydrates.
   C. Vitamin C.
   D. Water.

Essay Questions: Provide complete responses to the following questions or statements.

35. Explain why it is better to get fiber through food sources than from a supplement.

36. How can you use a food label to help you meet your carbohydrate needs?

37. How would you respond if someone asked you, "Should I cut starchy foods out of my diet because they are fattening?"

© Goodheart-Willcox

Fats: A Concentrated Energy Source

6

Objectives

After studying this chapter, students will be able to
- describe the characteristic differences between saturated and unsaturated fatty acids.
- list five functions of lipids in the body.
- summarize how the body digests, absorbs, and transports lipids.
- explain the role fats play in heart health.
- identify 10 heart-health risk factors.
- make food choices that follow recommended limits for dietary fats and cholesterol.

Bulletin Board

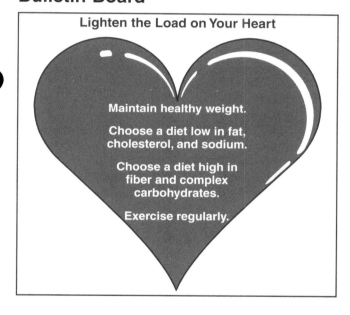

Lighten the Load on Your Heart

Maintain healthy weight.

Choose a diet low in fat, cholesterol, and sodium.

Choose a diet high in fiber and complex carbohydrates.

Exercise regularly.

Title: *Lighten the Load on Your Heart*

Use red construction paper to make a cutout of a large heart and place it in the center of the bulletin board. Within the cutout, place tips for improving heart health, such as *Maintain healthy weight. Choose a diet low in fat, cholesterol, and sodium. Choose a diet high in fiber and complex carbohydrates. Exercise regularly.*

Teaching Materials

Text, pages 91-109
Learn the Language
Check Your Knowledge
Put Learning into Action
Explore Further

Student Activity Guide, pages 39-48
  A. *Facing Fats*
  B. *What's My Job?*
  C. *Recognize the Risks*
  D. *Heart of the Matter*
  E. *Letters from Lowfat Lane*
  F. *Backtrack Through Chapter 6*
Teacher's Resources
  Comparison of Dietary Fats and Oils, color transparency CT-6
  An Emulsion Experiment, reproducible master 6-1
  How Lipids Are Carried in Your Body, transparency master 6-2
  Smart Heart Ways to Beat Heart Disease, transparency master 6-3
  How Do You Score on Fat? reproducible master 6-4
  Options for Lowering Fat Intake, reproducible master 6-5
  Chapter 6 Test

Introducing the Chapter

1. Have students sample two versions of a food item such as yogurt. One sample should be fat free and the other should be traditional. Have students choose which of the comparable products they think tastes best. Discuss why consumers are interested in fat free food products. Also discuss how the availability of more lowfat and fat free foods is affecting today's consumer.
2. Ask students to identify the groups of MyPyramid in which fats are most and least concentrated. Identify common high-fat and lowfat foods in each food group.
3. Remind students that 4 grams of fat equal one teaspoon. Have each student use Appendix C or *Personal Best* software to find the number of grams of fat in a favorite food. Then give each student an empty baby food jar. Have students label their jars with the names of their food items and the number of grams of fat. Have students put the appropriate number of teaspoons of shortening in the jars to represent the amount of fat in the food items. Display the labeled jars for all students to see.
4. To explore the concepts of choices and tradeoffs, have students brainstorm lower-fat alternatives for any high-fat foods identified in strategy 3.

Strategies to Reteach, Reinforce, Enrich, and Extend Text Concepts

What Are Lipids?

5. **RF** *Comparison of Dietary Fats and Oils,* color transparency CT-6. Use the transparency to illustrate the proportions of saturated, monounsaturated, and polyunsaturated fats in different fats and oils. Review how the differences relate to the physical properties of the lipids. Ask students to notice which products contain cholesterol or trans-fatty acids. Review the concept of rancidity as you discuss why oils are often hydrogenated. Ask students how each product might be used in food preparation.

6. **RF** Show students a solid stick of butter and a jar containing liquid corn oil. Ask students to identify the similarities and differences between the two products.

7. **ER** *An Emulsion Experiment,* reproducible master 6-1. Have lab groups complete the experiment as directed on the master. Students will be observing the emulsifying effects of phospholipids. Following the experiment, discuss answers to the questions and review learning outcomes. Relate the results of this experiment to the emulsifying role of bile during the digestion of fats.

8. **RF** *Facing Fats,* Activity A, SAG. Students are to complete a chart identifying the prevalent type of fatty acid and state at room temperature for various types of fats. Then students are to answer questions about triglycerides and other lipids.

Functions of Lipids

9. **RF** Ask students to respond to the statement "Because fats are so high in calories, I would be better off to avoid them completely."

10. **RF** *What's My Job?* Activity B, SAG. Students are to complete a chart by listing functions lipids perform in the body and examples of each function. Then students are to match descriptions of processes involving lipids with appropriate terms.

Lipids in the Body

11. **RT** *How Lipids Are Carried in Your Body,* transparency master 6-2. Use the transparency to illustrate for students the pathway of lipids to and from the liver.

12. **RF** Have students compare the body's ability to store carbohydrates as glycogen with the body's ability to store fats in adipose tissue. Ask students how the functions of these two energy sources differ.

Fats and Heart Health

13. **RF** Review the meaning of the term *risk factor.* List risk factors for coronary heart disease on the chalkboard. Identify which factors are controllable and which are not. Also identify the factors that pose the greatest risks. Encourage students to find out how people are changing their behaviors to control risk factors.

14. **RT** Discuss the difference between dietary cholesterol and blood cholesterol. Also connect LDL with artery clogging tendencies and HDL with artery clearing processes.

15. **ER** Guest speaker. Invite a cardiologist to explain the meaning of the various components of a blood lipid profile. Also ask the speaker to address basic diagnosis and treatment options as related to heart disease.

16. **RF** Put slips of paper labeled *good news* and *bad news* in a container. Have each student draw a slip of paper and give a positive or negative effect of cholesterol, accordingly.

17. **RT** Obtain a model of five pounds of body fat. Discuss where most excess body fat is stored. Review with the class how to calculate a dietary calorie adjustment for weight loss.

18. **ER** Have students conduct Internet research before writing reports on the effects of stress and other personality factors on heart health.

19. **ER** *Recognize the Risks,* Activity C, SAG. Students are to identify factors that increase the risk for coronary heart disease and then answer questions about the controllability of the factors.

20. **RT** Review with students how to calculate recommended limits for grams of fat and saturated fat based on daily calorie needs (calories $\times$ .35 = total fat calories per day $\div$ 9 calories per gram = daily limit for total grams of fat; calories $\times$ .1 = saturated fat calories per day $\div$ 9 calories per gram = daily limit for grams of saturated fat.)

21. **ER** Guest speaker. Invite a registered dietitian to speak to the class about the effects of diet on heart health.

22. **RF** *Smart Heart Ways to Beat Heart Disease,* transparency master 6-3. Use the transparency to review practices that help prevent heart disease. Ask students to identify behavior guidelines for following each practice.

Fats and Cancer

23. **ER** Guest speaker. Invite a representative from the American Cancer Society to speak about the latest research on diet and cancer prevention. You might also want to ask the speaker to address smoking and other lifestyle factors that are linked to cancer. Ask the representative to bring brochures, posters, and videos you can use as resources.

24. **ER** Field trip. Visit a local hospital to show students the equipment used to conduct cancer screenings, such as mammograms. Discuss the importance of self-testing.

25. **ER** Have students debate the pros and cons of fats in the diet. Members of each debate team should be prepared to support their points with information from the text or other resources.

Limiting Fats and Cholesterol in Your Diet

26. **RF** Have students look again at the jars prepared in strategy 3. Have students calculate the number of calories that come from fat in each food. Have students use Appendix C or *Personal Best* software to identify the amount of saturated fat and cholesterol in each food. Students should also calculate the percentage of calories in each food that come from fat by dividing calories from fat by total calories per serving.

27. **RF** Display a variety of food products, some with visible fat and some with invisible fat. Have students read product labels to identify the source and amount of fat in each product.

28. **RF** Demonstrate how invisible fat can become visible by placing a cupcake on a paper towel for 15 minutes. Hold up the paper towel for students to see the fat that has transferred from the food to the towel.

29. **RF** *How Do You Score on Fat?* reproducible master 6-4. Have students answer the questions to evaluate their fat intake. Discuss alternatives to high-fat foods in the diet.

30. **RF** Write the names of a variety of food items from each of the food groups on index cards. Have each student draw a card. Students should use Appendix C or *Personal Best* software to look up the number of fat grams per serving in the food items and write the numbers on the cards. Have students line up according to the fat content of their food items, from lowest to highest. Ask students to evaluate the taste, cost per serving, and ease of preparation of the foods at each end of the line.

31. **RF** Discuss how making gradual changes in eating habits can improve a person's success in adopting a lower-fat diet. Ask students to give examples of gradual changes people might make.

32. **RF** Use Chart 22-11 on page 384 of the text to review nutrient content claims related to fats. Have students compare Nutrition Facts panels from traditional and reduced-fat versions of products such as canned soup, mayonnaise, potato chips, and ice cream. Be sure students compare total calories per serving as well as fat grams. Summarize by asking students why paying attention to serving size remains important when eating reduced-fat foods.

33. **ER** Create a display of foods that contain fat replacers. Divide the class into small groups. Have groups review the ingredient lists to identify the fat replacers. Then have groups list consumer guidelines for using fat replacers in the diet.

34. **ER** *Options for Lowering Fat Intake,* reproducible master 6-5. Divide the class into small groups. Assign each group a recipe that includes several of the original ingredients listed on the handout. Have groups use substitutions suggested on the handout to reduce the fat content in their assigned recipes. Have students calculate the fat gram savings in the modified recipes. You may wish to have groups prepare original and modified recipes to compare taste, texture, and appearance.

35. **ER** Have students prepare a display of tasty, lowfat, nutrient-dense foods from each food group that teens and adults can grab on the run. If possible, arrange the display in conjunction with a parent meeting to help give parents ideas of healthful snacks they can keep on hand for their teens.

36. **EX** *Letters from Lowfat Lane,* Activity E, SAG. Students are to respond to letters asking health-related questions about fats.

Chapter Review

37. **RF** *Heart of the Matter,* Activity D, SAG. Students are to complete a word puzzle using terms from the chapter.

38. **RF** *Backtrack Through Chapter 6,* Activity F, SAG. Students are to provide complete answers to questions and statements that will help them recall, interpret, apply, and practice chapter concepts.

Above and Beyond

39. **ER** Have groups of students prepare one-page fact sheets titled "Buying and Preparing Heart-Healthy Foods" for distribution to parents. Have students use computer graphics to illustrate key points. Evaluate creativity as well as accuracy of content in the fact sheets.

40. **EX** Have students create a class Web site on the Internet that informs people about diet and other lifestyle behaviors related to the prevention of heart disease and cancer. The Web site should also include links to other reliable Web sites that will provide more information on this topic.

41. **ER** Have students plan plant-based menus for one day. Have them conduct research to identify the cancer-protective nutrients and phytochemicals their menus provide. Conduct a food lab to prepare the foods and evaluate the appeal of a plant-based diet.

42. **EX** Have each student obtain a copy of a menu from a local restaurant. Have students use Appendix B or *Personal Best* software to identify food items on the menus that contain less than 3 grams of fat per serving. Students should choose a complete lowfat meal from their menus.

Answer Key

Text

Check Your Knowledge, pages 108-109

1. triglycerides, phospholipids, sterols
2. (List two for each:) saturated fatty acids—beef fat, lard, butterfat, coconut oil, palm oil; monounsaturated fatty acids—olive oil, peanut oil; polyunsaturated fatty acids—corn oil, safflower oil, soybean oil
3. hydrogenation
4. When oils are hydrogenated, some of the unsaturated fatty acids in the oils change their molecular shapes, forming trans-fatty acids.
5. (List three:) egg yolks, organ meats, crab, lobster
6. (List five:) provide essential fatty acids; provide a concentrated source of energy; carry fat-soluble vitamins; form cell membranes; help make hormones, vitamins, and other secretions; hold in body heat; protect vital organs from shock
7. Lipoproteins carry large fat particles in the bloodstream. The water-soluble proteins in lipoproteins allow fats to remain dispersed in the water-based blood. This helps the fats move efficiently through the blood vessels to the tissues where they are needed.
8. A heart attack occurs when there is a buildup of plaque in the arteries feeding the heart muscle. A stroke occurs when there is a buildup of plaque in the arteries leading to the brain.
9. People over age 65 are at increased risk for CHD. Males have a greater risk for CHD than females until age 50.
10. true
11. amounts of cholesterol, HDL, LDL, and triglycerides in the blood
12. 300 mg of cholesterol per day
13. fish oils
14. Eating a high-fat diet may promote the development of colon, prostate, breast, and other types of cancers. Choosing a diet that includes a variety of fruits, vegetables, and grains and maintaining a healthy weight are cancer-protective lifestyle choices.
15. when they are over the age of two
16. (List five. Student response. See page 107 in the text.)

Student Activity Guide

Facing Fats, Activity A

1. saturated, solid
2. polyunsaturated, liquid
3. monounsaturated, liquid
4. polyunsaturated, liquid
5. saturated, solid
6. saturated, liquid
7. monounsaturated, liquid
8. saturated, solid
9. polyunsaturated, liquid
10. to improve a food's keeping quality
11. No, each involves about the same health risks related to heart disease.
12. A phospholipid is a lipid that has a phosphorous-containing compound in its chemical structure.
13. egg yolks, chocolate, and commercially baked products
14. Emulsifiers are used to keep a fat suspended within a watery substance.
15. In the body, cholesterol can make sex hormones and bile acids.
16. animal fat, because cholesterol is found only in animal foods—it is not found in plant foods, such as vegetable oil

What's My Job? Activity B

(Examples are student response.)
    provide essential fatty acids
    gives concentrated energy
    serves as an internal blanket (insulates the body)
    cushions vital organs
    dissolves and carries vitamins A, D, E, and K
    are an essential part of cell structure

Matching
1. C
2. A
3. E
4. B
5. D
6. M
7. G
8. N
9. F
10. L
11. K
12. I
13. J

Recognize the Risks, Activity C

1. sixty years old
2. male
3. African American

4. father has high blood pressure
5. overweight
6. chain smoker
7. high-fat diet
8. sedentary lifestyle
9. irritable, impatient personality
10. normal-stress work
11. high blood pressure
12. diabetic
13. high serum cholesterol
14. age, race, sex, and family history
15. smoking, inactivity, stress and personality type, overweight, diabetes, high blood pressure, high serum cholesterol
16. (Student response.)

Heart of the Matter, Activity D

1. EMULSIFIER
2. HEART ATTACK
3. TRANS-FATTY ACID
4. MONOUNSATURATED
5. ADIPOSE
6. RANCID
7. PHOSPHOLIPIDS
8. CORONARY HEART
9. LECITHIN
10. OMEGA
11. ESSENTIAL
12. UNSATURATED
13. LIPOPROTEIN
14. SATURATED
15. FATTY ACID
16. CHOLESTEROL
17. LIPID
18. HIGH-DENSITY
19. POLYUNSATURATED
20. HYDROGENATION
21. VERY LOW
22. TRIGLYCERIDES
23. HYPERTENSION
24. ATHEROSCLEROSIS
25. BLOOD LIPID
26. PLAQUE
27. STROKE
28. CHYLOMICRON
29. FAT REPLACER

Backtrack Through Chapter 6, Activity F

1. three fatty acids attached to glycerol
2. those from animals
3. to convert liquid oils into solid fats, improve keeping quality
4. It allows the oil in the mayonnaise to stay suspended in the vinegar, creating the texture of mayonnaise.
5. because the body already produces these nutrients

6. Sterols include some hormones, vitamin D, and cholesterol.
7. through the bloodstream
8. coronary heart disease (CHD)
9. Female hormones provide some protection against heart disease for young women.
10. smoking, inactivity, stress and personality type, overweight, diabetes, high blood pressure, high serum cholesterol
11. Exercise helps people manage weight, reduces stress, control cholesterol, and strengthen the heart muscle.
12. Excess fat in the diet has been linked to the development of certain kinds of cancer.
13. The word lipid encompasses all fats, oils, phospholipids, and cholesterol.
14. HDL picks up cholesterol in the body and transports it back to the liver as a waste product. LDL carries cholesterol through the bloodstream to the body cells.
15. (Student response. See page 96 in the text.)
16. Cholesterol is termed either "good" or "bad" based upon its effect on the body. HDL rids the body of cholesterol, so it is called "good." LDL distributes cholesterol in the body, so too much of it is considered "bad."
17. No (Explanation is student response. See page 102 in the text.)
18. (Student response.)
19. (Student response.)
20. (Student response.)

Teacher's Resources

An Emulsion Experiment, reproducible master 6-1

1. The oil and vinegar will remain separate layers. The mixture including the egg yolk should be blended.
2. The egg yolk acted as an emulsifier, keeping the oil particles suspended in the vinegar.
3. lecithin
4. In the body, bile acts as an emulsifier. Bile breaks fats into tiny droplets and keeps them suspended in the digestive fluid, which improves the absorption of the fat.

Chapter 6 Test

1. H	11. B	21. F	31. C
2. Q	12. E	22. F	32. D
3. N	13. A	23. T	33. C
4. J	14. C	24. F	34. B
5. F	15. I	25. T	35. A
6. P	16. T	26. F	36. C
7. L	17. T	27. T	37. B
8. G	18. T	28. D	
9. D	19. F	29. B	
10. O	20. T	30. B	

38. uncontrollable (list three:) age, gender, race, family history

controllable (list six:) smoking, high blood pressure, high blood cholesterol, diabetes mellitus, overweight, inactivity, stress, and personality

39. Choosing a diet that includes a variety of fruits, vegetables, and grains is a cancer-protective lifestyle choice. These foods contain fiber and certain chemicals that have anticancer effects. Maintaining a healthy weight is a cancer-protective factor, too. This is because having a high percentage of body fat increases the risks of some types of cancer.

40. (List three:) Eat more fruits, vegetables, whole grains, and fat free dairy products. Eat no more than 6 ounces of cooked fish, skinless poultry, or lean meat a day. Go easy on fried foods. Limit visible fats. Choose lean cuts of meat, trim all visible fat before cooking, and use lowfat cooking methods.

An Emulsion Experiment

Name_____ Date _____ Period _____

Objective: To observe the action of emulsifying agents on fats.

Supplies:

60	mL vinegar
2	medium clear mixing bowls
500	mL salad oil
	electric mixer
1	egg yolk

Procedure:

1. Pour 30 mL of vinegar in one mixing bowl. Add 250 mL of salad oil a few drops at a time, beating constantly with an electric mixer at medium speed. Observe what happens as you are mixing and write your observations in the table below.
2. Let the mixture stand for 5 minutes. Record your observations after 1 minute and at the end of 5 minutes in the table below.
3. Place the egg yolk and 30 mL of vinegar in the other bowl. Beat at medium speed until well blended.
4. Add 250 mL of oil carefully, a few drops at a time, while beating constantly. Make sure the droplets of oil spread evenly through the egg yolk. In the table below, record your observations during the beating process.
5. Let the mixture stand for 5 minutes. Record your observations after 1 minute and at the end of 5 minutes in the table below.

Observations			
	During mixing	**1 minute after mixing**	**5 minutes after mixing**
Oil and vinegar			
Oil, vinegar, and egg yolk			

Questions:

1. What differences did you observe between the mixture with egg yolk and the mixture without yolk? _____

   _____

2. Why do you think this happened? _____

   _____

3. What substance found in egg yolk acts as an emulsifier? _____

4. How do your observations relate to the function of bile in the body? _____

   _____

   _____

© Goodheart-Willcox

How Lipids Are Carried in Your Body

Small Intestine
triglycerides are broken down
lipids are absorbed
some are packaged as chylomicrons

Liver
cholesterol and triglycerides
are packaged into VLDL

HDL carry cholesterol and
other lipids from body cells
back to liver to be
processed as waste

VLDL lose triglycerides
and become LDL, which
carry cholesterol and
other lipids to body cells

Body Cells
break down fatty acids for
energy or rebuild them into
triglycerides for storage

© Goodheart-Willcox

Smart Heart Ways to Beat Heart Disease

Maintain healthy weight

Choose a diet low in saturated fats and cholesterol and moderate in total fats

Be physically active

Lower total cholesterol
Reduce LDL—clogs arteries
Increase HDL— removes cholesterol

Lower triglyceride levels

Maintain normal blood pressure (120/80)

Do not smoke

© Goodheart-Willcox

How Do You Score on Fat?

Name_____ **Date** _____ **Period** _____

Check the boxes that reflect your eating behaviors. Then see how your diet rates.

How often do you eat…

	Seldom or never	1–2 times a week	3–5 times a week	Once a day	More than once a day
1. fried foods such as French fries, fried chicken, or fried fish	☐	☐	☐	☐	☐
2. fatty meats such as bacon, sausage, hot dogs, luncheon meats, steaks, and heavily marbled roasts	☐	☐	☐	☐	☐
3. whole milk, ice cream, or high-fat cheese such as Cheddar, Swiss, American, and Colby	☐	☐	☐	☐	☐
4. high fat desserts or snacks such as pies, cakes, cookies, and candy bars	☐	☐	☐	☐	☐
5. salad dressings (regular, not low fat) or mayonnaise	☐	☐	☐	☐	☐
6. whipped cream, sour cream, or cream cheese	☐	☐	☐	☐	☐
7. butter or margarine	☐	☐	☐	☐	☐

Several checks in the last two columns indicate that you may have a high fat intake. What steps can you take to cut back on fat intake?

_____

_____

_____

_____

_____

© Goodheart-Willcox

Options for Lowering Fat Intake

Original Ingredient	Fat Grams	Substitution Options	Fat Grams in Substitute
1 oz. hard cheese	9	1 oz. reduced-fat cheese 1 oz. fat free cheese 1 oz. fat free processed cheese	5 0 0
1 oz. cream cheese	10	1 oz. lowfat cream cheese (Neufchâtel) 1 oz. fat free cream cheese 1 oz. lowfat cottage cheese (1%)	5 0 0
1 whole egg	5	¼ cup egg substitute 2 egg whites	0 0
1 cup whole milk	8	1 cup 1% milk ⅓ cup powdered fat free milk + ⅔ cup water 1 cup fat free milk	3 0 0
1 cup sour cream	40	1 cup lowfat (1%) cottage cheese (puréed) 1 cup fat free sour cream 1 cup nonfat plain yogurt	2 0 0
1 cup mayonnaise	176	1 cup lowfat mayonnaise ½ cup nonfat plain yogurt + ½ cup nonfat cottage cheese (puréed) 1 cup fat free mayonnaise	16 0 0
1 cup whole-milk ricotta	32	1 cup part skim ricotta 1 cup regular cottage cheese 1 cup lowfat (1%) cottage cheese 1 cup fat free ricotta 1 cup fat free cottage cheese	24 10 2 0 0
1 cup heavy cream	90	1 cup evaporated whole milk 1 cup evaporated fat free milk	19 0
1 stick butter or margarine	98	½ cup applesauce + 3 T. canola oil	42
¼ cup oil (for baking)	56	2 T. applesauce or banana, prune, or pumpkin purée + 2 T. canola oil	28
1 cup cream soup	27	½ cup defatted broth + ½ cup evaporated fat free milk thickened with ½ T. cornstarch	0
1 cup regular ice cream	14	1 cup lowfat ice cream 1 cup sherbet 1 cup fat free frozen yogurt 1 cup fat free ice cream	6 4 0 0

1 oz. chocolate	15	4 t. cocoa powder + 2 t. brown sugar
		  + 2 T. evaporated fat free milk, heated
		  to boiling; stir to dissolve cocoa
			0

1 cup nuts	70	½ cup nuts, lightly dry roasted to bring out their flavor	35

© Goodheart-Willcox

Fats: A Concentrated Energy Source

Name_____

Date _____   Period _____   Score _____

Chapter 6 Test

Matching: Match the following terms and identifying phrases.

_____ 1. A group of compounds that includes triglycerides, phospholipids, and sterols.

_____ 2. The major type of fat found in foods and in the body.

_____ 3. A fatty acid that has no double bonds in its chemical structure.

_____ 4. A fatty acid that has only one double bond between carbon atoms in a carbon atom chain.

_____ 5. The process of breaking the double carbon bonds in unsaturated fatty acids and adding hydrogen.

_____ 6. A fatty acid with an odd molecular shape that forms when oils are hydrogenated.

_____ 7. A class of lipids that have a phosphorus-containing compound in their chemical structures, which allows them to combine with both fat and water.

_____ 8. A phospholipid made by the liver and found in many foods.

_____ 9. A substance, such as a phospholipid, that can mix with water and fat.

_____ 10. A class of lipids that have complex molecules made of rings of carbon atoms with attached chains of carbon, hydrogen, and oxygen.

_____ 11. A white, waxy lipid made by the body that is part of every cell.

_____ 12. A fatty acid needed by the body for normal growth and development that cannot be made by the body.

_____ 13. Tissue in which the body stores lipids.

_____ 14. A ball of triglycerides thinly coated with cholesterol, phospholipids, and proteins formed to carry absorbed dietary fat to body cells.

_____ 15. Fat droplets coated by proteins so they can be transported in the bloodstream.

A. adipose tissue
B. cholesterol
C. chylomicron
D. emulsifier
E. essential fatty acid
F. hydrogenation
G. lecithin
H. lipid
I. lipoprotein
J. monounsaturated fatty acid
L. phospholipids
M. polyunsaturated fatty acid
N. saturated fatty acid
O. sterols
P. trans-fatty acid
Q. triglycerides

True/False: Circle *T* if the statement is true or *F* if the statement is false.

T   F   16. Most foods contain a mixture of saturated, monounsaturated, and polyunsaturated fatty acids.

T   F   17. Peanuts are a good source of monounsaturated fatty acids.

T   F   18. Lipids that are high in unsaturated fatty acids tend to be liquid at room temperature.

T   F   19. Cholesterol can be found in some fruits and vegetables.

T   F   20. Lipids help carry dissolved vitamins A, D, E, and K in the body.

(Continued)

© Goodheart-Willcox

Name_____

T F   21. Lecithin helps break fats into tiny droplets and keep them suspended in watery digestive fluid.

T F   22. Plaque buildup in blood vessels generally begins at about age 40 among people who consume high-fat diets.

T F   23. Cigarette smokers have a much higher risk of dying from a heart attack than nonsmokers.

T F   24. Low density lipoproteins (LDL) are considered the "good cholesterol."

T F   25. Overweight people often have a combination of heart-health risk factors.

T F   26. The American Heart Association recommends taking fish oil pills daily to get enough omega-3 fatty acids.

T F   27. Changing eating habits to reduce fat and cholesterol is often easier for teens than it is for adults.

Multiple Choice: Choose the best response. Write the letter in the space provided.

_____28. If Sue's daily diet provided 67 grams of fat, how many calories from fat did she consume?
    A. 67 calories.
    B. 268 calories.
    C. 469 calories.
    D. 603 calories.

_____29. A buildup of plaque in arteries leading to the brain may result in _____.
    A. a heart attack
    B. a stroke
    C. atherosclerosis
    D. high blood pressure

_____30. Which of the following is an uncontrollable heart-health risk factor?
    A. diabetes mellitus
    B. family history
    C. high blood cholesterol
    D. high blood pressure

_____31. The second number in a blood pressure reading measures diastolic pressure, which is the _____.
    A. amount of blood the heart pumps in one beat
    B. number of heart beats per minute
    C. pressure on the arteries when the heart is between beats
    D. pressure on the arteries when the heart muscle contracts

_____32. Which of the following is a benefit of exercise that has a positive impact on heart health?
    A. Exercise helps people control cholesterol.
    B. Exercise helps people manage weight.
    C. Exercise helps people reduce stress.
    D. All the above.

_____33. Carin has a recommended daily intake of 2,300 calories. What is Carin's recommended daily calorie limit from total fats?
    A. 280.
    B. 560.
    C. 805.
    D. Carin can stay healthy with no fats in her diet.

(Continued)

© Goodheart-Willcox

Name_____

_____34. Jamie requires about 2,000 calories per day to maintain her energy balance. What is Jamie's recommended daily limit for grams of saturated fat?
   A. 9 grams.
   B. 22 grams.
   C. 53 grams.
   D. 162 grams.

_____35. Which food is a source of invisible fats and oils?
   A. Cookies.
   B. Fat free vegetable dip.
   C. Mayonnaise on a sandwich.
   D. Sugar.

_____36. Fat replacers are best used in the diet to _____.
   A. cut down on food costs
   B. lose weight
   C. reduce fat in the diet
   D. replace a regular diet

_____37. Which food is a better choice for a person on a low-cholesterol, lowfat diet?
   A. Au gratin potatoes.
   B. Baked potato with skin.
   C. French fries.
   D. Fried hash browns.

Essay questions: Provide complete responses to the following questions or statements.

38. Name three uncontrollable and six controllable heart-health risk factors.

39. Describe two lifestyle choices and explain how they can help protect against cancer.

40. Describe three guidelines for making food choices that will help a person limit his or her dietary fat and cholesterol.

© Goodheart-Willcox

Proteins: The Body's Building Blocks

Objectives

After studying this chapter, students will be able to
* explain the difference between essential and nonessential amino acids.
* discuss the functions of protein.
* identify animal and plant food sources of protein.
* calculate their daily protein needs.
* describe problems associated with protein deficiencies and excesses.

Bulletin Board

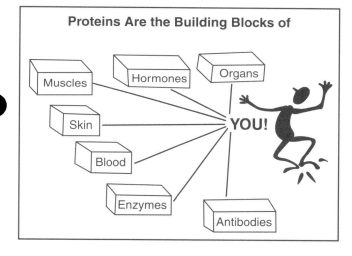

Proteins Are the Building Blocks of

Muscles   Hormones   Organs

Skin   YOU!

Blood

Enzymes   Antibodies

Title: *Proteins Are the Building Blocks of YOU!*

Place a large cutout of a person on the bulletin board. Beside the person, place large cutouts of blocks. Label the blocks with various body tissues and compounds made from proteins, such as muscles, organs, skin, blood, enzymes, hormones, and antibodies. Use lines to connect blocks with the person.

Teaching Materials

Text, pages 110–124
> *Learn the Language*
> *Check Your Knowledge*
> *Put Learning into Action*
> *Explore Further*

Student Activity Guide, pages 49–56
> A. *Building Blocks of Proteins*
> B. *A Billboard for Proteins*
> C. *Animal vs. Plant Proteins*

D. *Complementary Proteins—A "Good Match"*
E. *Protein Balance*
F. *Not Too Little—Not Too Much*
G. *Backtrack Through Chapter 7*

Teacher's Resources
> *Testing Foods for Protein,* reproducible master 7-1
> *Health Benefits of a Vegetarian Diet,* color transparency CT-7
> *Estimating Your Protein Intake,* reproducible master 7-2
> *A Look at Protein Supplements,* transparency master 7-3
> Chapter 7 Test

Introducing the Chapter

1. Show students pictures of a variety of protein foods, such as pinto beans, lentils, tofu, cheese, milk, eggs, nuts, meat, poultry, and fish. Explain that all these foods are good sources of protein. Ask students to identify the group from MyPyramid in which each food belongs.

2. Give each student a label with a Nutrition Facts panel from a different food item. Use food items from each of the food groups. Include some foods with no protein content. Instruct students not to share information about the protein content of their food items. Ask students to line up from high protein food sources to low protein food sources. Students must guess their positions in line by guessing the protein content of the foods on both sides of them. Then ask students to share label information and re-form their line to accurately reflect protein content. Discuss what factors students considered when guessing the protein content of foods.

3. Have students write down 10 words that come to mind when they hear the word *protein.* List responses on the chalkboard. Relate responses to chapter concepts.

Strategies to Reteach, Reinforce, Enrich, and Extend Text Concepts

What Is Protein?

4. **RT** Have students review the amino acid diagram on page 111 of the text. List the chemical components of protein on the board. Ask students

how the chemical composition of proteins compares to the compositions of carbohydrates and fats.

5. **RT** Discuss the difference between essential and nonessential amino acids.

6. **ER** *Testing Foods for Protein,* reproducible master 7-1. Have lab groups complete the experiment as directed on the master. Students will be observing a chemical reaction indicating the presence of protein in foods. Following the experiment, discuss answers to the questions and review learning outcomes. (You should be able to obtain Biuret solution from the chemistry lab.)

Protein in the Body

7. **RF** *A Billboard for Proteins,* Activity B, SAG. Students are to list the six basic functions of protein in the body. Then they are to design a billboard to advertise one of the functions.

8. **EX** Have two teams of students debate the statement "Proteins are more important than carbohydrates or fats." Instruct students to use text information to support their arguments.

Food Sources of Protein

9. **RT** Review the food groups in MyPyramid and identify which groups provide the most grams of protein per portion.

10. **RF** Show students two food products that are good sources of protein—one an animal source and one a plant source. Give students the price of each product and the number of servings per package. Have students compute cost per serving then cost per gram of protein. Ask students to use their findings to compare relative costs of animal and plant sources of protein.

11. **RF** *Animal vs. Plant Proteins,* Activity C, SAG. Students are to complete a chart contrasting plant and animal proteins.

12. **ER** Guest speaker. Invite a vegetarian who is knowledgeable about nutrition to speak to students about meeting protein needs without meat. Have students prepare questions about the vegetarian lifestyle.

13. **RT** *Health Benefits of a Vegetarian Diet,* color transparency CT-7. Use the transparency to highlight the nutritional advantages and disease prevention benefits of a vegetarian diet. Emphasize that maximum benefits are derived when diet planning follows the MyPyramid system and when lifestyle behaviors include avoiding the use of tobacco and alcohol and other drugs.

14. **EX** Have three students role-play a situation in which a teen shares a decision to become a lacto-ovo vegetarian with his or her mother and sibling. The mother and sibling should express how they feel about this decision. Family members should

also discuss how this decision will affect the family in terms of grocery purchases and nutrition concerns. Following the role-play, invite the class to share their views about vegetarianism.

15. **EX** Have students design a poster illustrating a "Vegetarian MyPyramid." Encourage students to use vegetarian magazines, the Internet, or other resources for ideas of foods to place in the pyramid.

16. **ER** Have students work in pairs to plan a day's menus for a lacto-ovo vegetarian. Menus should follow MyPyramid. Have students use Appendix C or *Personal Best* software to identify which foods in their menus are high in fiber and which are high in fat.

17. **EX** Review the guidelines presented in the text for combining complementary proteins. Then pass out a picture of a plant source of protein to each student. When you give the cue "Go vegetarian," have each student find a partner with a complementary source of protein. Go around the room and ask partners how they would combine their complementary protein sources in a meal. Give the cue again and have students switch partners to come up with different combinations of complementary proteins. Discuss how a diet with a variety of foods is likely to provide higher-quality protein.

18. **ER** *Complementary Proteins—A "Good Match,"* Activity D, SAG. Students are to identify complementary sources of protein in two recipes. Then students are to find a third example of a recipe containing complementary proteins.

How Much Protein Do You Need?

19. **RT** Have students review Appendix A, *Recommended Nutrient Intakes,* to identify the RDAs for protein for various population groups.

20. **ER** *Estimating Your Protein Intake,* reproducible master 7-2. Have students complete the chart identifying their food group sources of protein for one day. Then have students complete calculations to figure the total number of grams of protein they consumed and answer evaluation questions.

21. **ER** Have the class design a survey about protein needs and the use of protein supplements for sports performance. Have each student use the survey to interview an athlete or coach. Have students compile their findings to identify common beliefs and practices related to protein consumption among athletes. Ask students to evaluate these beliefs and practices based on text information.

The Risks of Too Little or Too Much Protein

22. **RT** Discuss how the typical diet in the United States can easily lead people to consume more than the recommended amounts of protein.

23. **RF** *A Look at Protein Supplements,* transparency master 7-3. Introduce the topic of protein supplements by discussing why some people take them. Ask students what stories they heard about the use of protein or amino acid supplements in strategy 21. Then refer to the transparency to reinforce the value of meeting protein needs through nutritious food choices.

24. **ER** Panel discussion. Organize a panel of athletes to talk about the effects of supplements on their athletic performance. Have panel members discuss the pressures they experience, harmful side effects, and the rules and regulations regarding supplement use. (You may wish to invite parents to attend this discussion.)

25. **RF** *Protein Balance,* Activity E, SAG. Students are to complete a true or false exercise to review the concept of protein balance.

26. **RF** *Not Too Little—Not Too Much,* Activity F, SAG. Students are to use clues provided to identify conditions brought on by too little or too much protein in the diet.

Chapter Review

27. **RF** *Building Blocks of Protein,* Activity A, SAG. Students are to complete a multiple choice exercise to review chapter concepts.

28. **RF** Divide students into pairs. Have each pair write seven sentences summarizing chapter information. Each sentence should begin with a different letter in the word *protein.* Have the class vote on the best sentence for each letter. Then have students prepare a poster with the seven best sentences to display in the school cafeteria.

29. **RF** *Backtrack Through Chapter 7,* Activity G, SAG. Students are to provide complete answers to questions and statements that will help them recall, interpret, apply, and practice chapter concepts.

Above and Beyond

30. **ER** Have students prepare research reports on the design of protein structures that form genetic codes, which make each person a unique human being. (You may wish to coordinate this assignment with the science department.) Have students develop posters to use in giving oral presentations on their findings.

31. **ER** Have each student prepare a report on the various sources of protein in the diet of a chosen culture. Encourage students to contact people from their chosen cultures to learn about favorite high-protein recipes. You may wish to plan a lab experience in which students can prepare and sample these recipes. Have students compile their recipes into a brochure titled "World Protein Preferences," which could be distributed at a schoolwide cultural fair.

32. **ER** Have each student prepare a vegetarian meal for his or her family. Ask students to report to the class the types of foods served and the reactions of family members to the meals.

33. **ER** Have students work in groups to conduct Internet research about specific topics related to protein deficiencies in developing nations. Topics of investigation may include environmental, economic, and political factors that contribute to protein deficiencies. Research might also focus on health conditions that result from protein deficiencies. Have each group write a newsletter article summarizing its findings.

34. **EX** Divide students into teams to debate the following statement by animal rights activists: "If Americans reduced their meat consumption by only 10 percent, there would be 12 million more tons of grain to feed humans. This is enough to feed each of the 560 million people who starve to death each year."

35. **EX** Have each student bring in a product, product label, or advertisement for an amino acid or protein supplement. Have students review the ingredient lists and compute how many grams of protein will be consumed if the products are used as directed. Students should compare these protein values to the RDA. Have students write critiques comparing the costs and protein contents of their products to high-protein foods. Have the class assemble their products and findings into a display for the student body to see.

Answer Key

Text

Check Your Knowledge, page 123

1. The presence of nitrogen makes protein different from carbohydrates and fats.

2. The body can synthesize the nonessential amino acids. The body is not able to make the essential amino acids, so they must be provided by the diet.

3. When you eat a protein food, stomach acids denature the proteins. This makes it easier for enzymes in the stomach to begin breaking down large protein molecules into smaller pieces.

4. As the body grows, it uses protein to help make new tissues.

5. If a diet is low in carbohydrates and fats, the body will use proteins as an energy source. This prevents proteins from being used for their other functions, such as cell-building.

6. (List three animal sources:) beef, veal, pork, lamb, poultry, fish, eggs, milk, yogurt, cheese, ice cream (List three plant sources. See table 7-8 on page 117 in the text.)

7. (Describe two. Student response. See pages 115-116 in the text.)
8. Vegans can get the amino acids missing from one incomplete protein source by combining it with another incomplete source. Combining grains, nuts, or seeds with legumes will create a complete source of protein.
9. 10 to 35 percent
10. (List three:) Choose lowfat protein foods often. Trim visible fat from meats. Remove skin from poultry. Use lowfat cooking methods. Avoid adding high-fat cooking oils, sauces, and gravies to protein foods.
11. A healthy teen would be in positive nitrogen balance because he or she is building new tissue. This requires the teen to take in more protein than he or she excretes.
12. kwashiorkor
13. true
14. liver and kidney problems, calcium loss, excess body fat

Student Activity Guide

Building Blocks of Protein, Activity A

1. A
2. M
3. I
4. N
5. O
6. A
7. C
8. I
9. D
10. S

A Billboard for Proteins, Activity B

1. Build and maintain tissues
2. Make important compounds
3. Regulate mineral and fluid balance
4. Maintain acid-base balance
5. Carry vital substances
6. Provide energy

Protein Balance, Activity E

True: 3, 4, 5, 7, 8, 9, 11, 15
False: 1, 2, 6, 10, 12, 13, 14, 16

Not Too Little—Not Too Much, Activity F

1. body fat
2. calcium loss
3. liver and kidneys
4. positive nitrogen balance
5. protein-energy malnutrition
6. negative nitrogen balance

7. kwashiorkor
8. marasmus

Backtrack Through Chapter 7, Activity G

1. carbon, hydrogen, oxygen, nitrogen
2. heat, acids, bases, alcohol
3. 20; 9; 11
4. build and maintain tissues, make important compounds, regulate mineral and fluid balance, maintain acid-base balance, carry vital substances, provide energy
5. enzymes, hormones, antibodies
6. fats, iron, oxygen
7. (List four:) availability, cost, health concerns, food preferences, religious beliefs, environmental factors
8. (List six:) peanuts, black-eyed peas, kidney beans, black beans, lentils, chickpeas, lima beans, soybeans
9. Plant sources of protein contain no cholesterol. Plant sources of protein are generally high in fiber. Plant sources of protein are generally low in saturated fat.
10. age, gender, body size, state of health
11. milk, yogurt, and cheese group; meat, poultry, fish, dry beans, eggs, and nuts group
12. weaned older children in poor countries who no longer receive protein-rich breast milk when their mothers begin breast-feeding newborn siblings
13. About three percent of body protein is broken down each day. Adults need dietary protein to maintain existing tissues.
14. When proteins are used to provide energy, they cannot be used for other purposes, such as building cells.
15. Complete proteins provide all the essential amino acids humans need. Incomplete proteins are missing or short in one or more of the essential amino acids.
16. An extra half glass of milk or a chicken wing will provide the extra protein an athlete needs.
17. Protein is the only energy nutrient that provides nitrogen.
18. (Student response.)
19. males: 52 grams per day; females: 46 grams per day
20. (Student response.)

Teacher's Resources

Testing Foods for Protein, reproducible master 7-1

Food color change results:
    beans—color change
    broccoli—color change
    carrots—no change
    cheese—color change
    egg white—color change
    ground beef—color change

Chapter 7 Test

1.	B	10.	B	19.	T	28.	A
2.	G	11.	B	20.	T	29.	D
3.	C	12.	A	21.	F	30.	C
4.	A	13.	A	22.	F	31.	C
5.	D	14.	B	23.	T	32.	A
6.	H	15.	F	24.	T	33.	C
7.	I	16.	T	25.	C	34.	C
8.	F	17.	F	26.	D	35.	D
9.	B	18.	F	27.	B	36.	C

37. Body cells use amino acids from food proteins to build new proteins. Cells can also convert amino acids to other compounds including other amino acids.

38. (List five:) growth, pregnancy, lactation, male gender, large body size, illness, injury, intense athletic training

39. (List four:) Choose fat free and lowfat dairy products. Choose fish and legumes instead of meat. Trim visible fat from meats. Remove skin from poultry. Use lowfat cooking methods. Avoid adding high-fat cooking oils, sauces, and gravies to protein foods.

Testing Foods for Protein

Name_____ Date _____ Period _____

Objective: To identify the presence of protein in foods.

Supplies:

5   g baked beans, mashed
5   g broccoli, fresh, crushed
5   g carrots, fresh, mashed
5   g cheese, mashed
5   g egg white, cooked
5   g ground beef, raw
6   test tubes
    Biuret solution
    eyedropper

Procedure:

1. Place each of the foods in a separate test tube.
2. Add 10 to 15 drops of the Biuret solution to each test tube.
3. The Biuret solution provides an accurate test for the presence of protein. If protein is present, the Biuret solution will change color from blue to violet pink. Record your results in the chart below. (Since this reaction is reversible, the color may fade.)

Food Item	Change Noted
beans	
broccoli	
carrots	
cheese	
egg white	
ground beef	

Which of the above results did you find surprising? Explain your answer. _____

_____

_____

_____

© Goodheart-Willcox

Reproducible Master 7-2

Estimating Your Protein Intake

Name_____   Date _____   Period _____

Complete the chart below by listing all the foods you ate during one day from each food group. Refer to Chart 4-5 in the text for a reminder of how much food equals a portion. Then write the total number of portions from each group in the space below the chart. Complete each equation to determine the approximate number of grams of protein you consumed from each group. Add the products of all the equations to determine the approximate number of grams of protein you consumed during the day. Then answer the questions at the bottom of the page.

Grains	Vegetables
	Fruits
Milk	**1-Ounce Equivalents of Meat**

	Total Portions		Grams of Protein per Portion		
grains	_____	×	3	=	_____
milk	_____	×	8	=	_____
vegetables	_____	×	2	=	_____
fruits	_____	×	1	=	_____
meat (total ounces)	_____	×	8 (per ounce)	=	_____

Total grams of protein consumed   _____

1. How did your protein intake compare to your protein needs (52 grams per day for teenage males, 46 grams per day for teenage females)? _____

2. If someone said to you, "The more protein, the better," how would you respond? _____
_____

© Goodheart-Willcox

A Look at Protein Supplements

Protein Supplements

- do not increase muscle size or performance
- may promote kidney problems
- may be less digestible than protein-rich foods
- cost more than protein-rich foods

Amino Acid Supplements

- may impair absorption of other amino acids, causing a deficiency
- may have a high risk of toxicity
- perform no nutrient function in the body
- rarely live up to their claims

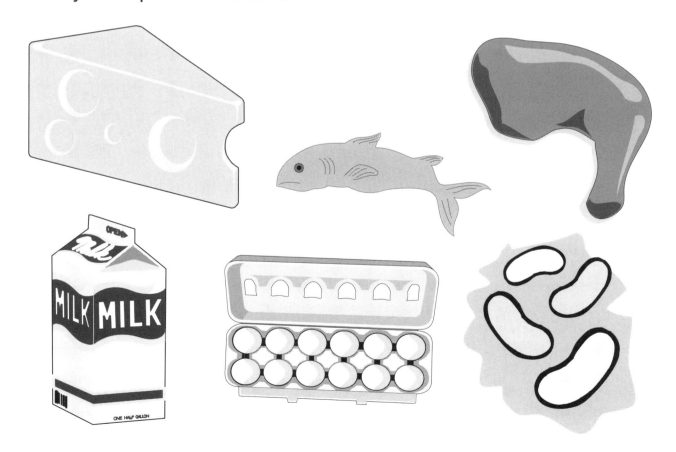

The typical U.S. diet will easily meet your protein needs.

© Goodheart-Willcox

Protein: The Body's Building Blocks

Name_____

Date _____   Period _____   Score _____

Chapter 7 Test

Matching: Match the following terms and identifying phrases.

_____ 1. One of the building blocks of protein molecules.

_____ 2. A change in shape that happens to protein molecules when they are exposed to heat, acids, bases, or alcohol.

_____ 3. A protein made by the immune system to defend the body against infection and disease.

_____ 4. The maintenance of the correct level of acidity of a body fluid.

_____ 5. A compound that can counteract an excess of acid or base in a fluid.

_____ 6. A plant that has a special ability to capture nitrogen from the air and transfer it to protein-rich seeds.

_____ 7. A comparison of the nitrogen a person consumes with the nitrogen he or she excretes.

_____ 8. A sickness caused by a lack of a nutrient.

A. acid-base balance
B. amino acid
C. antibody
D. buffer
E. complementary proteins
F. deficiency disease
G. denaturation
H. legume
I. nitrogen balance

Matching: Match the food characteristics with the sources of protein.

_____ 9. The largest source of dietary protein in the United States.

_____ 10. A source of dietary cholesterol.

_____ 11. Higher costs per serving size.

_____ 12. Soybeans, tofu, seeds.

_____ 13. A source of fiber.

_____ 14. Eggs, milk.

A. plant source of protein
B. animal source of protein

True/False: Circle *T* if the statement is true, and *F* if the statement is false.

T   F   15. The essential amino acids can be synthesized in the body.

T   F   16. Stomach acids denature protein that enters the stomach.

T   F   17. Protein plays a role in only a few specific cells in the body.

T   F   18. A vegetarian diet is fat free.

T   F   19. Corn provides an incomplete source of protein.

T   F   20. Two incomplete protein sources can be combined to provide all the essential amino acids.

T   F   21. Children and teens have a lower proportional need for protein than adults.

T   F   22. A person's protein needs are directly related to his or her level of physical activity.

T   F   23. A diet very high in protein from animal sources may promote calcium loss from the bones.

T   F   24. Excess amino acids in the diet will be stored as body fat.

(Continued)

© Goodheart-Willcox

Name_____

Multiple Choice: Choose the best response. Write the letter in the space provided.

_____25. What chemical element is found in protein that is not found in fats and carbohydrates?
   A. Carbon.
   B. Hydrogen.
   C. Nitrogen.
   D. Oxygen.

_____26. Which of the following functions of protein can also be performed by carbohydrates and fats?
   A. Build and maintain body tissues.
   B. Carry iron and oxygen in the blood.
   C. Form hormones, enzymes, and antibodies.
   D. Provide energy.

_____27. Seiko gets about 10 percent of her daily 2,000-calorie energy needs from protein. About how many grams of protein does Seiko consume each day?
   A. 5 grams.
   B. 50 grams.
   C. 200 grams.
   D. 400 grams.

_____28. Which type of vegetarian consumes dairy products and eggs but no meat, fish, or poultry?
   A. Lacto-ovo vegetarian.
   B. Lacto-vegetarian.
   C. Semivegetarian.
   D. Vegan.

_____29. Which is a common reason for becoming vegetarian?
   A. Concern for animals.
   B. Interest in health.
   C. Religious beliefs.
   D. All the above.

_____30. Which of the following combinations demonstrates two incomplete proteins forming a complete protein?
   A. Oatmeal and toast.
   B. Orange juice and cereal.
   C. Rice and beans.
   D. Steak and milk.

_____31. John is 16 years old. What is his RDA for protein?
   A. 16 grams.
   B. 44 grams.
   C. 52 grams.
   D. 120 grams.

_____32. Most of an athlete's calories should come from _____.
   A. carbohydrates
   B. fats
   C. proteins
   D. water

(Continued)

© Goodheart-Willcox

Name_____

_____33. Negative nitrogen balance is associated with _____.
　　　　　　　　　　A. infant growth
　　　　　　　　　　B. pregnancy
　　　　　　　　　　C. starvation
　　　　　　　　　　D. teen growth

_____34. Kwashiorkor is most often associated with _____.
　　　　　　　　　　A. adults in African nations
　　　　　　　　　　B. athletes
　　　　　　　　　　C. children who are weaned when younger siblings are born
　　　　　　　　　　D. infants

_____35. On the average, protein consumption among men in the United States is _____.
　　　　　　　　　　A. about half the RDA
　　　　　　　　　　B. fairly close to the RDA
　　　　　　　　　　C. one and one-half times the RDA
　　　　　　　　　　D. twice the RDA

_____36. What might happen as a result of consuming a high-protein diet?
　　　　　　　　　　A. Dramatic increase in muscle tissue.
　　　　　　　　　　B. Intense hunger pangs.
　　　　　　　　　　C. Liver and kidney problems.
　　　　　　　　　　D. Loss of appetite.

Essay Questions: Provide complete responses to the following questions or statements.

37. How do body cells use amino acids from food proteins?

38. What are five factors that increase a person's protein needs?

39. What are four tips for limiting fats in the diet when choosing protein sources?

Vitamins: Drivers of Cell Processes

8

Objectives

After studying this chapter, students will be able to
- state the major roles of vitamins in the diet.
- classify vitamins as fat-soluble or water-soluble.
- identify functions and sources of specific vitamins.
- describe symptoms of various vitamin deficiencies and excesses.
- discuss considerations of using vitamin supplements.
- demonstrate how to select, cook, and store foods to preserve vitamin content.

Bulletin Boards

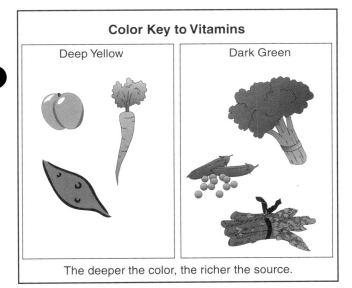

Color Key to Vitamins

Deep Yellow | Dark Green

The deeper the color, the richer the source.

Title: *Color Key to Vitamins*

Group pictures of deep yellow and dark green fruits and vegetables on the bulletin board. For example, you might show deep yellow carrots, apricots, and sweet potatoes and dark green broccoli, spinach, and Brussels sprouts. At the bottom of the board, place a caption stating *The deeper the color, the richer the source.*

Teaching Materials

Text, pages 126–149
  Learn the Language
  Check Your Knowledge
  Put Learning into Action
  Explore Further

Student Activity Guide, pages 57–64
  A. *Vitamin Analogies*
  B. *Vitamin Sources and Functions*
  C. *Cause and Effect*
  D. *Foods vs. Supplements*
  E. *Viva Las Vitamins!*
  F. *Backtrack Through Chapter 8*

Teacher's Resources
  Load Up on Antioxidants, transparency master 8-1
  Meeting Vitamin Needs, reproducible master 8-2
  Testing Foods for Vitamin C, reproducible master 8-3
  Effects of Storage and Cooking on Vitamins, reproducible master 8-4
  Chapter 8 Test

Introducing the Chapter

1. Read the following paragraph aloud to the students one sentence at a time. Ask students to raise their hands as soon as they know what the paragraph is describing. Wait until you have finished reading the paragraph before asking a student to identify the topic.

   The discovery of this minute substance ushered in a new era of nutrition in the early 1900s. The earliest existence of this nutrient came during the search for treatment of diseases. One of these diseases was experienced by sailors who spent long periods at sea. The sailors were cured of this disease, called scurvy, when their diet on the ship started including oranges and lemons.

2. Discuss what people believe about vitamins that often leads them to use vitamin supplements. List student responses on the chalkboard. Keep this list of beliefs to be reviewed after studying the chapter.

3. Supply students with several Nutrition Facts panels from food product labels. Have students identify which vitamins are included on the panel. Ask why they think other vitamins are not listed. Explain that only vitamins A and C are required on Nutrition Facts panels because these vitamins have been determined to be most important to the health of today's consumers. Listing of other vitamins is optional.

4. Display MyPyramid. Ask students which of the food groups they think provides the most abundant sources of vitamins. Explain that each food group provides sources of different vitamins.

5. Review the meaning of the term *nutrient density.* Display several well-liked foods, such as crackers, potato chips, peanuts, apple, soft drink, and taco on a table. Ask students to arrange the foods based on their vitamin density, from most to least. Then have students refer to Appendix C or *Personal Best* software to rearrange the foods if necessary.

6. Review the terms *grams, milligrams, micrograms,* and *international units* with students. Then place 1/8 teaspoon of salt on a piece of black paper to illustrate the minute amount of all vitamins needed for one day. Explain that failing to get enough vitamins can lead to a deficiency disease, whereas getting too much can create a toxicity. Discuss how a person can know if he or she is getting enough of each vitamin.

Strategies to Reteach, Reinforce, Enrich, and Extend Text Concepts

What Are Vitamins?

7. **ER** Guest speaker. Invite a registered dietitian, nutrition educator from the community WIC program, or an extension home economics professional to speak to the class about vitamin deficiencies that are most common among families on very low food budgets.

8. **ER** Guest speaker. Invite a laboratory technician to speak to the class about the tests that are used to identify vitamin deficiencies. Ask the speaker to bring sample lab reports for students to practice interpreting. Discuss how vitamin deficiencies can be treated.

9. **RT** On the chalkboard, make a parallel list of the properties of fat-soluble and water-soluble vitamins. Ask students to name the vitamins that fall into each category.

10. **RF** Place two clear containers filled with water side by side. Drop a vitamin A supplement into one container and a vitamin C supplement into the other. Have students observe and describe the results. Relate this demonstration to the transport of fat-soluble and water-soluble vitamins in the body.

The Fat-Soluble Vitamins at Work

11. **RF** Divide students into groups. Assign each group one of the fat-soluble vitamins and have group members work together to prepare a fact sheet. Fact sheets should discuss functions, deficiency symptoms, food sources, and recommended intake. Encourage students to add interest to their fact sheets with computer graphics or other art. Display the nutrient fact sheets in the classroom.

12. **RF** Supply labels from fortified and enriched food products. Ask students to explain the meanings of the terms *fortified* and *enriched.* Have students look on the labels to determine which nutrients have been added to each product.

13. **ER** Have each student conduct an Internet search on the newest findings related to deficiency diseases associated with one of the fat-soluble vitamins. Have students share their findings in oral reports.

14. **RT** *Load Up on Antioxidants,* transparency master 8-1. Use the transparency to introduce the functions and sources of antioxidants.

15. **ER** Guest speaker. Invite a physician or health educator to explain how free radicals can cause damage to healthy cells. Ask the speaker to share the latest research findings on the role of antioxidants, such as carotenoids and vitamin E, in reducing the risks of cancer due to free radical damage. Ask students to summarize the speaker's talk in an article for the school newspaper.

16. **ER** Have groups of students prepare snacks that include foods high in antioxidants. (Most fruits and vegetables are high in carotenoids and vitamins C and E.) Students should prepare a place card describing the antioxidants in each snack. Serve the snacks and take a poll to see which foods students enjoyed most.

The Water-Soluble Vitamins at Work

17. **ER** Guest speaker. Invite a pediatric nurse to discuss how folate can help prevent neural tube damage in unborn infants. Ask the speaker to identify foods that are good sources of folate.

18. **ER** Have students plan a day's menus for a pregnant woman that meet the DRI of 400 micrograms of folic acid. The menus should also provide the recommended number of servings from the Food Guide Pyramid.

19. **EX** *Meeting Vitamin Needs,* reproducible master 8-2. Have students use Appendix A, *Recommended Nutrient Intakes,* to complete the second column of the first chart on the handout. Tell students to multiply the values in the second column by 0.1 to determine the vitamin requirements of good food sources to list in the third column of the chart. Then have students use Appendix C or *Personal Best* software to find the vitamin values of the food items in the dinner menu shown in the second chart. Students are to use the information in the two charts to answer the questions at the bottom of the page.

20. **ER** *Testing Foods for Vitamin C,* reproducible master 8-3. Have lab groups complete the experiment as directed on the master. Students will be

determining whether vitamin C is present in various foods. Following the experiment, discuss answers to the questions and review learning outcomes. (You should be able to obtain starch solution and iodine solution from the chemistry lab.)

21. **RF** *Vitamin Analogies,* Activity A, SAG. Students are to underline the term in parentheses that best completes each analogy.

22. **RF** *Vitamin Sources and Functions,* Activity B, SAG. Students are to complete a chart by recording food sources, functions, classification, and RDA or AI for listed vitamins.

23. **RF** *Cause and Effect,* Activity C, SAG. Students are to complete a chart with missing information about the causes and effects of various vitamin deficiencies and excesses.

Nonvitamins and Other Nonnutrients

24. **RT** Play a "What Am I?" quiz game. Read the following description of phytochemicals and ask the students to guess what is being discussed.

    I am a plant chemical. Thousands of me exist in fruits, vegetables, and whole grains. I am neither vitamin nor mineral. I supply no calories. I am essential to good health. Researchers think I protect against cancer, heart disease, and other diseases.

25. **ER** Guest speaker. Have each student bring in an advertisement for nonvitamin supplements, such as melatonin or ginseng. Invite a registered dietitian to review the ads and speak to the class about the safety and effectiveness of nonnutrient products. If you are unable to bring in a guest speaker, you might have students use the Internet to see what reliable information they can find about their nonnutrient products.

Are Vitamin Supplements Needed?

26. **RF** Display a bottle of multivitamin tablets and a bowl of fresh fruits and vegetables. Ask students to list as many similarities and differences between supplements and foods as they can.

27. **EX** Provide a selection of modern lifestyle and teen magazines to groups of students. Also encourage students to bring in vitamin literature from health food stores. Have groups go through these materials to find claims about vitamin supplements. Have groups use information from the text to evaluate the validity of the claims.

28. **ER** Have half of the class create a poster advertisement for a vitamin pill that truthfully informs consumers of the benefits of the supplement. Have the other half of the class create an advertisement expounding the benefits of fruits, vegetables, and whole grains. Check for accuracy of information and creativity. Display the posters in the classroom.

29. **RF** *Foods vs. Supplements,* Activity D, SAG. Students are to use the space provided to compare and contrast the benefits of getting vitamins from supplements with the benefits of getting vitamins from food sources.

Preserving Vitamins in Foods

30. **ER** Field trip. Take a field trip to a local supermarket. Ask the produce manager to talk to the students about the qualities to check when selecting fresh and frozen produce.

31. **RF** Leave a bunch of broccoli in a visible area for students to see over several days. Then ask the students what is happening to the nutrient content of the food. Ask how the vitamins could have been preserved more carefully. Ask students what they think should be done with the wilted broccoli.

32. **RF** *Viva Las Vitamins!* Activity E, SAG. Students are to use the boxes provided to design mini-posters about the preservation of vitamins in foods through careful food selection, preparation, and storage.

33. **ER** *Effects of Storage and Cooking on Vitamins,* reproducible master 8-4. Distribute the handout for students to use as a reference when selecting, storing, and preparing foods at home.

34. **RF** Demonstrate the preparation of a fresh food item, such as using apples to make applesauce. As students watch your preparation steps, they should note any techniques you use that help preserve vitamins. Students should also note any techniques that might promote vitamin destruction. Following the demonstration, ask students to share what they observed.

Chapter Review

35. **RF** Refer to the list of beliefs about vitamins compiled in strategy 2. Have students work in small groups to write responses to each of the belief statements. Students' responses should reflect what they learned through study of this chapter. Have groups share their responses with the class.

36. **RF** Have each student use Appendix C or *Personal Best* software to find the vitamin content of one food item. Students should list the functions of all the vitamins for which their chosen foods are good sources.

37. **RF** Have the class develop a vitamin trivia game. Students should write thirty to fifty questions with varying levels of difficulty. Students can write their questions on index cards that are color coded by difficulty level or question category. Answers should be written on the backs of the cards. Identify a monitor to ask the questions and keep score. Individuals or teams accumulate points related to question difficulty by answering questions correctly.

38. **RF** *Backtrack Through Chapter 8,* Activity F, SAG. Students are to provide complete answers to questions and statements that will help them recall, interpret, apply, and practice chapter concepts.

Above and Beyond

39. **ER** Have each student conduct Internet research about a specific phytochemical. Have students write three-page reports identifying the phytochemicals they researched. The reports should also discuss where the phytochemicals are found and how they function to provide health benefits.

40. **EX** Have teams of students videotape public service announcements demonstrating techniques for preserving vitamins in foods through careful selection, storage, or preparation. Show the videotapes at a school health and wellness fair.

Answer Key

Text

Check Your Knowledge, page 148

1. nutrient metabolism, energy production and release, tissue maintenance, normal digestion, infection resistance
2. true
3. insufficient amount of a vitamin in the diet, failure of the body to absorb a vitamin
4. (List three:) Fat-soluble vitamins are soluble in fats; water-soluble vitamins are soluble in water. Excess fat-soluble vitamins are stored in the body; excess water-soluble vitamins are excreted in the urine. Fat-soluble vitamins are more likely to build up to toxic levels in the body than water-soluble vitamins. It is not crucial to consume fat-soluble vitamins every day, water-soluble vitamins should be consumed daily.
5. provitamin carotenes
6. With exposure to sunshine, the body can make all the vitamin D it needs.
7. The main function of vitamin E in the body is as an antioxidant. It protects the membranes of white and red blood cells and the cells of the lungs from harmful effects of oxygen exposure.
8. The main function of vitamin K is to make proteins needed in the coagulation of blood.
9. (List three:) nausea, loss of weight, loss of appetite, severe exhaustion, irritability, depression, forgetfulness, heart problems, skin problems, impaired functioning of the immune system
10. beriberi
11. (List three:) milk and milk products, enriched and whole grain cereals, meats, poultry, fish
12. false

13. Studies on pantothenic acid have not produced enough conclusive data to set an RDA. However, the AI for people ages 14 and over is 5 milligrams per day.
14. Women who have inadequate folate intakes are more likely to give birth to babies with neural tube damage.
15. People exposed to cigarette smoke need extra vitamin C because smoke hinders the use of vitamin C.
16. (List two:) prompting the body to make enzymes, binding harmful substances, acting as antioxidants
17. (List three:) pregnant women, breast-feeding women, infants, older adults, patients who are ill or recovering from surgery
18. Natural vitamins are extracted from foods. Synthetic vitamins are made in a laboratory.
19. (List three. Student response. See page 146 in the text.)
20. (Student response. See pages 146-147 in the text.)

Student Activity Guide

Vitamin Analogies, Activity A

1. vitamin A
2. B-complex and vitamin C
3. large doses of supplements
4. siding
5. night blindness
6. retinol equivalent
7. dairy products
8. osteomalacia
9. vitamin D
10. tissue damage
11. red blood cells
12. clotting
13. coenzymes
14. vitamin C
15. thiamin
16. pellagra
17. collagen
18. skin tingling

Vitamin Sources and Functions, Activity B

(For food sources, see "Meeting Needs" section for each vitamin, pages 130-142.)
(For functions, see "Functions" section for each vitamin, pages 130-142.)
Classification

1. water-soluble
2. water-soluble
3. water-soluble
4. water-soluble
5. water-soluble
6. water-soluble
7. fat-soluble
8. water-soluble
9. water-soluble
10. water-soluble

11. fat-soluble
12. fat-soluble
13. fat-soluble
(For RDA and AI information, see "Meeting Needs" section for each vitamin, pages 130-142.)

Cause and Effect, Activity C
1. vitamin A deficiency
2. thiamin deficiency
3. inflamed tongue, cracked skin in corners of mouth
4. vitamin D deficiency
5. broken red blood cells
6. deficiency of biotin
7. damage to the liver
8. walking difficulty, numbness
9. excess vitamin K
10. tiredness, weakness, diarrhea, infection
11. deficiency of niacin
12. pernicious anemia
13. hardening of the kidneys and soft organs
14. severe vitamin C deficiency
15. painful rash, nausea, diarrhea
16. stomach cramps

Backtrack Through Chapter 8, Activity F
1. 0
2. to regulate body processes
3. They contain carbon.
4. about a month
5. pregnancy, infancy, adolescence
6. Toxicity is a poisonous condition. If a person consumes an excess of a vitamin, it can lead to toxicity.
7. retinol activity equivalent (RAE)
8. vitamin D
9. vitamin K
10. thiamin, riboflavin, niacin, pantothenic acid, biotin, B_6, folate, and B_{12}
11. A coenzyme is a nonprotein compound that combines with an enzyme to form an active enzyme system that can metabolize nutrients.
12. severe vitamin C deficiency
13. They can prevent heart disease and some forms of cancer. People can gain these benefits by consuming fruits, vegetables, herbs, spices, legumes, and grains.
14. Antioxidants help deactivate or transform free radicals, preventing them from generating harmful chain reactions that can damage body tissue. Vitamins C and E are antioxidants.
15. Thiamin—alcohol diminishes the body's ability to absorb and use thiamin.
16. Adequate folate intake can reduce the risk of neural tube damage that can occur during the early stages of pregnancy before many women realize they are pregnant.
17. In most cases, doctors advise getting most of your vitamins from food sources. A nutritious diet can provide all the nutrients most people need. In some cases, however, doctors do advise vitamin supplements to help a person meet his or her vitamin needs.
18. (Student response.)
19. (Student response.)
20. valid—second, fourth, and fifth claims; invalid—first and third claims

Teacher's Resources

Meeting Vitamin Needs, reproducible master 8-2
1. A. 900 µg
   B. 90 µg
2. A. 1.2 mg
   B. 0.12 mg
3. A. 1.3 mg
   B. 0.13 mg
4. A. 16 mg
   B. 1.6 mg
5. A. 90 mg
   B. 9 mg
6. A. 5 µg
   B. 0.06 mg
   C. 0.10 mg
   D. 11.8 mg
   E. 0 mg
7. A. 218 µg
   B. 0.13 mg
   C. 0.32 mg
   D. 1.2 mg
   E. 97 mg
8. A. 0 µg
   B. 0.22 mg
   C. 0.07 mg
   D. 3.3 mg
   E. 26 mg
9. A. Tr
   B. 0.12 mg
   C. 0.08 mg
   D. 1.2 mg
   E. Tr
10. A. 149 µg
    B. 0.09 mg
    C. 0.34 mg
    D. 0.2 mg
    E. 2 mg
11. A. 8 µg
    B. 0.02 mg
    C. 0.12 mg
    D. 0.2 mg
    E. Tr
12. A. broccoli
    B. baked potato
    C. milk
    D. chicken
    E. broccoli

13. thiamin
14. milk chocolate bar
15. (Student response.)

Testing Foods for Vitamin C, reproducible master 8-3

Color change results:

fresh orange juice—color will change after very few drops added

frozen orange juice—color will change

canned orange juice— color will change, but only after many drops are added

gelatin—no color change

lemonade—color will change, but only after many drops are added

orange or lemon-lime soda—no color change

1. Fresh orange juice has the highest amount of vitamin C. It takes very few drops for the iodine to change colors.
2. The gelatin and lemon-lime soda will not change colors. There is little to no vitamin C in these products.
3. Fresh orange juice contains more vitamin C than other forms of orange juice.

Chapter 8 Test

1. D	10. T	19. T	28. A
2. H	11. F	20. T	29. D
3. E	12. T	21. B	30. A
4. B	13. T	22. B	31. A
5. A	14. F	23. B	32. C
6. F	15. F	24. D	33. C
7. G	16. T	25. D	34. D
8. I	17. F	26. C	35. B
9. F	18. F	27. C	

36. (List three:) Fat-soluble vitamins dissolve in fats; water-soluble vitamins dissolve in water. The body stores excess fat-soluble vitamins; excess water-soluble vitamins are normally excreted in the urine. It is not essential to consume fat-soluble vitamins every day; water-soluble vitamins should be consumed every day. Fat-soluble vitamins can build up in the body to toxic levels; water-soluble vitamins do not readily build up to toxic levels.
37. Buying supplements is costly and vitamin tablets do not provide the fiber, energy, or taste offered by food sources of vitamins.
38. (List three:) Choose fresh fruits and vegetables that have bright colors and firm textures. Avoid produce with wilted leaves, mold growth, or bruised spots. Do not buy cans that are dented or bulging. Avoid frozen foods that have a layer of ice on the package. When buying dried foods, look for packages that are securely sealed.

Load Up on Antioxidants

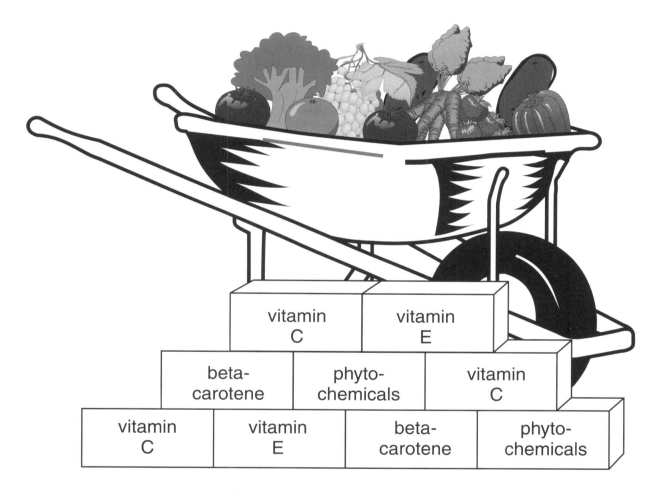

vitamin C	vitamin E

beta-carotene	phyto-chemicals	vitamin C

vitamin C	vitamin E	beta-carotene	phyto-chemicals

Build a Foundation of Risk Reduction

© Goodheart-Willcox

Meeting Vitamin Needs

Name_____ Date _____ Period _____

For a food to be described as a good source of a vitamin, it should provide at least 10 percent of the recommended daily intake for an adult male. Use Appendix A, *Recommended Nutrient Intakes,* to complete the second column of the first chart below. Multiply the values in the second column by 0.1 to determine the vitamin requirements of good food sources to list in the third column of the chart. Then use Appendix C, *Nutritive Values of Foods,* to find the vitamin values of the food items in the dinner menu shown in the second chart. Use the information in the two charts to answer the questions at the bottom of the page.

Vitamin	A. Recommended Daily Intake for Adult Male	B. Vitamin Requirements of Good Food Sources
1. Vitamin A		
2. Thiamin		
3. Riboflavin		
4. Niacin		
5. Vitamin C		

Food Item	A. Vitamin A	B. Thiamin	C. Riboflavin	D. Niacin	E. Vitamin C
6. chicken breast, roasted, flesh only, 3 ounces					
7. broccoli, cooked from raw spears, 1 cup					
8. baked potato with skin					
9. whole wheat bread, 1 slice					
10. fat free milk, 1 cup					
11. milk chocolate bar with almonds, 1 ounce					

12. Which food item was the best source of each vitamin?

    A. vitamin A _____

    B. thiamin _____

    C. riboflavin _____

    D. niacin _____

    E. vitamin C_____

13. For what vitamin is wheat bread a good source? _____

14. Which food item is the poorest source of vitamins overall?_____

15. What could you substitute for the poorest vitamin source to improve the vitamin content of this meal?

    _____

© Goodheart-Willcox

Testing Foods for Vitamin C

Name_____ Date _____ Period _____

Objective: To identify the presence of vitamin C in foods.

Supplies:

6 test tubes	orange juice, frozen reconstituted
100mL graduated cylinder	orange juice, canned
starch solution	gelatin dessert, dissolved but not set
iodine solution	lemonade
eyedropper	lemon-lime soda
orange juice, fresh	

Procedure:

1. Using the graduated cylinder, measure 20 mL of starch solution into each test tube.
2. Add 7 drops of iodine solution to each test tube.
3. Add one of the liquids listed to each test tube, one drop at a time. Stir after each drop is added. Count the number of drops you add.
4. If vitamin C is present, the iodine will change to an orange color. In the chart below, indicate if the color of the iodine changed. If a color change occurred, indicate how many drops of the liquid were added before the change occurred.

Food Item	Change Noted	Number of Drops Added
Fresh orange juice		
Frozen reconstituted orange juice		
Canned orange juice		
Gelatin		
Lemonade		
Lemon-lime soda		

Conclusions

1. Which of the liquids had the highest amount of vitamin C? Explain your answer. _____

_____

2. Which of the liquids had the lowest amount of vitamin C? Explain your answer. _____

_____

3. What can you conclude about the amount of vitamin C in various forms of orange juice?_____

_____

_____

Reproducible Master 8-4

Effects of Storage and Cooking on Vitamins

Name_____   Date _____   Period _____

Vitamins	Storage Considerations	Cooking Considerations
Fat-soluble vitamins—A, D, E, and K	Fat-soluble vitamins are destroyed through long exposure to oxygen and the passing of time. Exposure to air, metals, and light destroys vitamin E.	Use vitamin-dense outer leaves, skins, and peels. Repeated use of oils in deep frying destroys vitamin E.
B Vitamins	B vitamins are relatively stable in oxygen. Riboflavin is sensitive to light. Store milk in cardboard or opaque container. Warm temperatures destroy B-vitamins. Always chill food immediately. The faster a food loses moisture, the greater the vitamin losses. Store foods in airtight containers.	Soaking foods leaches vitamins. Use small amounts of water to cook foods. Heat destroys vitamins; cook food only until tender. Use a pan with a tight-fitting lid to speed cooking time. Boil or bake potatoes in skins where vitamins are dense. Use liquids from cooking in soups, casseroles, sauces, or gravies.
Vitamin C	The higher the storage temperatures, the greater the vitamin loss. Keep fruits and vegetables chilled. Because of sensitivity to air, consume immediately after harvesting or opening canned products.	Vitamin C dissolves in water when food is washed, boiled, or canned. Reuse liquids. Cut foods in large pieces with a sharp blade so little surface is exposed to oxygen. Prepare salads and fruits as close to serving time as possible. Avoid high temperatures and long cooking times. Reheating foods adds to vitamin loss. Acid foods protect vitamin C; tomatoes, citrus foods, and orange juice can be kept in the refrigerator for several days. Vitamin C is unstable when in contact with iron and copper.

© Goodheart-Willcox

Vitamins: Drivers of Cell Processes

Name_____

Date _____   Period _____   Score _____

Chapter 8 Test

Matching: Match the following conditions related to vitamin deficiencies with the vitamins that cause them.

_____ 1. A vitamin A deficiency condition in which the cells in the eyes adjust slowly to dim light, causing night vision to become poor.

_____ 2. A deficiency disease in children caused by a lack of vitamin D and characterized by soft, misshapen bones.

_____ 3. A vitamin D deficiency disease in adults that causes the bones to become misshapen.

_____ 4. A vitamin E deficiency condition that is sometimes seen in premature babies and is characterized by broken red blood cells, resulting in weakness and listlessness.

_____ 5. The thiamin deficiency disease, which is characterized by weakness, loss of appetite, irritability, poor arm and leg coordination, and a tingling throughout the body.

_____ 6. The niacin deficiency disease, which is characterized by diarrhea and dermatitis and can lead to dementia and death.

_____ 7. A deficiency disease caused by an inability to absorb vitamin B_{12}, which is characterized by fatigue; weakness; a red, painful tongue; and a tingling or burning in the skin.

_____ 8. The vitamin C deficiency disease, characterized by tiredness, swollen and bleeding gums, slow healing of wounds, and tiny bruises on the skin.

A. beriberi
B. erythrocyte hemolysis
C. neural tube damage
D. night blindness
E. osteomalacia
F. pellagra
G. pernicious anemia
H. rickets
I. scurvy

True/False: Circle *T* if the statement is true or *F* if the statement is false.

T   F   9. Vitamins are considered to be nonessential nutrients.

T   F   10. Provitamins are compounds the body can convert into active forms of vitamins.

T   F   11. Vitamin toxicity occurs when daily vitamin needs are not met over an extended period.

T   F   12. With exposure to sunlight, the body can make vitamin D.

T   F   13. Milk and milk products are good sources of riboflavin.

T   F   14. Because pantothenic acid and biotin are found in only a limited number of food sources, deficiencies are fairly common.

T   F   15. Vitamin B_6 helps the body make essential amino acids.

T   F   16. Cigarette smoke hinders the body's use of vitamin C.

T   F   17. Research provides evidence that extra vitamin C in the diet will prevent people from getting the common cold.

T   F   18. Natural vitamins are more effective in the body than synthetic vitamins.

T   F   19. Canned green beans are likely to have a higher vitamin content than fresh green beans that are not stored properly.

T   F   20. Cutting foods into smaller pieces increases their exposure to vitamin losses.

(Continued)

© Goodheart-Willcox

Name_____

Multiple Choice: Choose the best response. Write the letter in the space provided.

_____ 21. What will eventually happen if a vitamin is missing from the diet?
   A. A craving for rich food sources of the vitamin will develop.
   B. Deficiency symptoms will appear.
   C. The body will adapt to getting along without the vitamin.
   D. The body will produce the missing vitamin.

_____ 22. Which of the following factors can interfere with vitamin absorption?
   A. An active lifestyle.
   B. Diarrhea.
   C. High blood pressure.
   D. All the above.

_____ 23. Which of the following is *not* a water-soluble vitamin?
   A. Riboflavin.
   B. Vitamin A.
   C. Vitamin B_6.
   D. Vitamin C.

_____ 24. What is indicated by a milk carton labeled *fortified with vitamins A and D?*
   A. The daily requirements for vitamin A and D will be met by drinking one serving.
   B. The food has passed all safety tests.
   C. The food is a perfect food.
   D. Two nutrients have been added during processing.

_____ 25. Which of the following vitamins are antioxidants?
   A. Niacin and folate.
   B. Thiamin and riboflavin.
   C. Vitamins B_6 and B_{12}.
   D. Vitamins C and E.

_____ 26. Which of the following best describes a free radical?
   A. A cell that lines the passages of the lungs, intestines, and reproductive tract.
   B. A compound in plant foods that is active in the body.
   C. A highly reactive, unstable single oxygen molecule that can generate a harmful chain reaction.
   D. A substance that reacts with unstable single oxygen molecules to protect other substances.

_____ 27. What is the main function of vitamin K?
   A. Assists in the formation of collagen.
   B. Helps form healthy epithelial tissue.
   C. Promotes blood coagulation.
   D. Regulates levels of calcium in the bloodstream.

_____ 28. The B-vitamin coenzymes _____.
   A. combine with inactive enzymes to form active enzyme systems
   B. help release energy from carbohydrates, proteins, and minerals
   C. include thiamin, riboflavin, and ascorbic acid
   D. All the above.

_____ 29. Common symptoms of B vitamin deficiencies include _____.
   A. depression and exhaustion
   B. loss of weight and appetite
   C. nausea and irritability
   D. All the above.

(Continued)

© Goodheart-Willcox

Name_____

_____ 30. Why is flour enriched?
   A. To add back nutrients that were lost in processing.
   B. To give it a better flavor.
   C. To help it stay fresh longer.
   D. To restore its natural color.

_____ 31. Women of childbearing age should strive to fully meet folate requirements _____.
   A. before becoming pregnant
   B. during the sixth month of pregnancy
   C. just prior to giving birth
   D. during lactation

_____ 32. Which vitamin poses the greatest deficiency risk for people who eat no foods from animal sources?
   A. Vitamin A.
   B. Vitamin B_6.
   C. Vitamin B_{12}.
   D. Vitamin C.

_____ 33. Which of the following is a good source of vitamin C?
   A. Enriched breads and cereals.
   B. Fortified margarine.
   C. Grapefruit.
   D. Milk.

_____ 34. How do phytochemicals protect the body?
   A. They act as antioxidants.
   B. They bind harmful substances.
   C. They help the body make enzymes.
   D. All the above.

_____ 35. Which foods are a good source of phytochemicals?
   A. Fats and oils.
   B. Fruits and vegetables.
   C. Poultry and fish.
   D. Red meats.

Essay Questions: Provide complete responses to the following questions or statements.

36. Describe three major differences between fat-soluble and water-soluble vitamins.

37. Explain why foods are a better source of vitamins than vitamin supplements.

38. List three tips for selecting foods high in vitamins.

Minerals: Regulators of Body Functions

Objectives

After studying this chapter, students will be able to
- list the major roles of minerals in the diet.
- identify functions and sources of specific macrominerals and microminerals.
- describe symptoms of various mineral deficiencies and excesses.
- write guidelines for maximizing mineral absorption and availability in the body.

Bulletin Board

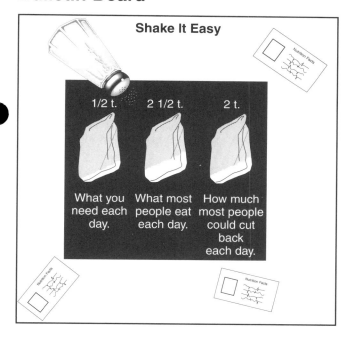

Title: *Shake It Easy*

　　Place a large cutout of a salt shaker under the title. Tack food labels around the board from products with a high sodium content. In the center of the board, place a large sheet of colored construction paper. Tape three small, sealed, clear plastic bags to the construction paper. In the first bag, place ½ teaspoon of salt with a label underneath reading *What you need each day*. In the second bag, place 2½ teaspoons of salt with a label underneath reading *What most people eat each day*. In the third bag, place 2 teaspoons of salt with a label underneath reading *How much most people could cut back each day*.

Teaching Materials

Text, pages 150–171
> *Learn the Language*
> *Check Your Knowledge*
> *Put Learning into Action*
> *Explore Further*

Student Activity Guide, pages 65–70
> A. *Mineral Match*
> B. *Go to the Source*
> C. *Mineral Mysteries*
> D. *Minerals, More or Less*
> E. *Backtrack Through Chapter 9*

Teacher's Resources
> *Bone-Up on Calcium,* color transparency CT-9
> *Risk Factors for Osteoporosis,* transparency master 9-1
> *Where's the Sodium in Your Diet?* reproducible master 9-2
> *Testing Beverages for Iron,* reproducible master 9-3
> Chapter 9 Test

Introducing the Chapter

1. Hold up an iron pan for the class to see. Ask students what an iron pan might have to do with nutrition. Mention that foods cooked in iron pans can provide a dietary source of iron, which is just one of many minerals students will study in this chapter.
2. Have students look at a Nutrition Facts panel from a food product label. Ask them to identify which minerals are listed. Ask students if they are aware of any health issues related to these minerals, which would indicate why they are required to be listed on food labels.

Strategies to Reteach, Reinforce, Enrich, and Extend Text Concepts

How Minerals Are Classified

3. **RT** Ask students to describe the differences between minerals and vitamins.
4. **RF** Use a metric scale to show students what 100 milligrams of salt looks like. Explain that minerals needed in amounts less than this are called microminerals and minerals needed in

amounts equal to or greater than this are called macrominerals. Have students refer again to the elements they highlighted on handouts of reproducible master 3-1, *Periodic Table of the Elements.* Ask students to label the macrominerals *MAC* and the microminerals *MIC.*

The Macrominerals at Work

5. **RT** Ask students to estimate how much calcium is in their bodies by multiplying their weights by 0.02. Use a 3-pound bag of flour to represent the approximate weight of calcium in a 150-pound adult.

6. **RT** *Bone-Up on Calcium,* color transparency CT-9. Use the transparency as you discuss steps teens can take to help build bone mass.

7. **ER** Have groups of students place washed chicken bones in jars and add vinegar to cover the bones. Have groups cover their jars and let them stand for a few days. Then have groups examine the bones, which should be rubbery because the calcium in the bones dissolved in the vinegar. Explain that in humans, calcium losses from the bones also result in weakened bones.

8. **ER** Guest speaker. Invite a health care professional to explain how bone mass is analyzed. Ask the speaker to show sample X rays to illustrate the difference between dense and porous bones.

9. **RT** Display 4 glasses of milk, explaining that this amount of milk would provide the calcium AI of 1,300 mg for 14- to 18-year-olds. Gradually substitute pictures of other foods that would provide the 300 mg of calcium in each glass of milk. Substitutions might include 1½ ounces Cheddar cheese, 2¼ cups cottage cheese, 1¾ cups ice cream, 1 cup yogurt, 1 cup calcium-fortified orange juice, 5 ounces salmon, 2½ ounces sardines, 1¾ cups broccoli, 2 cups cream of tomato soup, 1 cup cooked spinach, and 1 cup almonds.

10. **RT** *Risk Factors for Osteoporosis,* transparency master 9-1. Use the transparency to identify factors that increase the risk of developing osteoporosis.

11. **ER** Guest speaker. Invite a registered dietitian who works with senior citizens to speak to the class. Ask the speaker to describe the effects and treatment of osteoporosis he or she has observed among clients. Also have the speaker describe who is likely to develop osteoporosis and what can be done to prevent bone deterioration over a lifetime.

12. **ER** Have students interview parents, grandparents, or older adults to learn of their current health practices to prevent osteoporosis. Ask students to share their findings in class.

13. **ER** Have students place various calcium supplements in glasses of white vinegar for half an hour, stirring frequently. Have students record the amount of time required for the supplements to dissolve. Relate the supplements' solubility in vinegar to their absorption in the body.

14. **ER** Have each student survey three teens about their daily consumption of carbonated soft drinks and milk. Have students compile their findings and calculate the percentage of the teen population that may be at risk of reduced calcium absorption due to high phosphorus intake. Have the class formulate a recommendation in an article for the school newspaper.

15. **RT** Discuss the role of magnesium in enzymatic reactions and in the activation of ATP for the release of energy.

16. **RF** Burn a sample of hair so students can smell the sulfur content. Discuss the role of sulfur as a part of the protein tissue in the body.

17. **RF** Demonstrate the process of osmosis by slicing a cucumber and dividing the slices into two bowls. Salt the slices in one bowl. Leave the slices in the other bowl unsalted. After 30 minutes, have students compare the contents of the two bowls. Students should notice that a larger pool of water formed in the bowl of salted cucumbers. Explain this occurred because the salt drew the water out of the cucumber slices. Relate this demonstration to the way sodium draws water out of body cells to equalize mineral concentrations in the body.

18. **EX** Have students use litmus paper to identify the pH of a variety of common substances.

19. **RF** Using an overhead projector, list the day's menu in the school cafeteria. Have students identify which of the food items are good sources of potassium. Discuss menu alternatives that would improve potassium content. Review the functions of potassium in transmitting nerve impulses and maintaining a normal heartbeat.

20. **ER** Survey the class to find an average of how often students salt foods at the table. Cut three circles from dark construction paper, each 5 inches in diameter. Place each circle under a sheet of waxed paper. Tell three student volunteers to imagine the circles represent servings of French fries. Give the volunteers salt shakers and ask them to shake on the amount of salt they would add to their fries. Measure the salt collected on the waxed paper and figure an average amount added per serving. Knowing that 1/8 teaspoon of salt provides about 250 mg of sodium, have students calculate how many milligrams of sodium an average person might add to foods at the table each day. Discuss how reducing sodium in the diet can begin by limiting salt use at the table.

21. **RF** *Where's the Sodium in Your Diet?* reproducible master 9-2. Have students answer the questions to evaluate their sodium consumption and assess their understanding of sodium needs, deficiencies, and excesses.

22. **EX** Collect and distribute menus from local family and fast-food restaurants to small groups of students. Have students identify menu items that are high in sodium as well as low-sodium alternatives. Place the high- and low-sodium food lists on the board.

23. **RF** Have students use Nutrition Facts panels to determine the sodium content of three processed food products. Discuss how quickly sodium intake can add up when a person's diet includes a number of processed foods. Inform students a food providing 140 mg or less sodium per serving is considered a low-sodium food. Discuss why this is important information for people with high blood pressure.

24. **RF** Have each student read the ingredients list from a different processed food label. Help students identify ingredients that are sources of sodium, such as onion, celery, and garlic salts; monosodium glutamate; baking soda; baking powder; bouillon; meat tenderizer; sodium caseinate; sodium nitrate; and sodium saccharin.

The Microminerals at Work

25. **RT** Review iron functions, dietary needs, deficiencies, and excesses.

26. **ER** *Testing Beverages for Iron,* reproducible master 9-3. Have lab groups complete the experiment as directed on the master. Students will be identifying beverage sources of iron. Following the experiment, discuss answers to the questions and review learning outcomes. (You may wish to brew the tea ahead of time. Steep two teabags in two cups of water for five minutes.)

27. **RF** Have students check the Nutrition Facts panels from a variety of foods to identify those that are good sources of iron. Have students also check the ingredients lists to determine whether foods are naturally rich in iron or fortified with iron.

28. **EX** Review the sources of iron in the diet, emphasizing the difference between heme and nonheme iron. Then have students plan a snack that takes advantage of the partnership between vitamin C and iron.

29. **RT** Review the functions of zinc. Then survey students to find out how many have taken zinc lozenges to reduce the symptoms and duration of a cold. Find out if students found this treatment to be effective. Also ask whether students experienced any side effects, such as nausea or aftertastes.

30. **ER** Have students compose letters or e-mail to the Thyroid Foundation of America (TFA) asking for information about the prevalence of thyroid problems due to iodine deficiencies and excesses in the United States and throughout the world. Students should also request information about symptoms of thyroid disorders and how they are diagnosed.

31. **ER** Have each student conduct an Internet search for the latest findings on the role of one of the trace minerals in nutrition. Encourage some students to select minerals not discussed in the text, such as boron, cobalt, nickel, silicon, arsenic, barium, cadmium, lead, lithium, mercury, silver, tin, and vanadium. Have students share their findings in oral reports.

32. **RF** *Go to the Source,* Activity B, SAG. Students are to complete a chart by filling in functions and food sources of listed minerals.

33. **RF** *Mineral Mysteries,* Activity C, SAG. Students are to choose the best responses to complete statements about mineral deficiencies and excesses.

Minerals and Healthful Food Choices

34. **ER** Guest speaker. Invite an agriculture agent from the county extension office to speak to your class about the mineral content of the soil in your area. Ask the speaker to explain how soil is analyzed and discuss the impact mineral content has on locally grown food products.

35. **RT** *Minerals, More or Less,* Activity D, SAG. Students are to complete statements about minerals and healthful food choices with the words *more* or *less.*

Chapter Review

36. **RF** Play the game "What Mineral Am I?" Have each student write information about functions, deficiencies, or excesses of a mineral on one side of an index card. Have students write the names of the appropriate minerals on the backs of the cards. Pass the cards around the room for pairs of students to use in quizzing each other.

37. **RF** *Mineral Match,* Activity A, SAG. Students are to match terms from the chapter with identifying phrases.

38. **RF** *Backtrack Through Chapter 9,* Activity E, SAG. Students are to provide complete answers to questions and statements that will help them recall, interpret, apply, and practice chapter concepts.

Above and Beyond

39. **EX** Have students prepare a fun, interactive presentation on "Minerals for Life" for a middle school or elementary class. Students could

develop role-plays or puppet shows about the sources and functions of minerals. Students could also make up quiz games, crossword puzzles, and other strategies to assess the comprehension of the young members of their audience.

40. **EX** Have students debate the statement "Salt is bad for teens." Have students contact the American Heart Association or the National Heart, Lung, and Blood Institute for information about sodium, hypertension, and heart health to include in their arguments.

41. **EX** Have teams of students write children's stories about the role of one or more minerals on health. Have students illustrate the stories with pictures or cartoons.

Answer Key

Text

Check Your Knowledge, page 170

1. false
2. in the bones
3. milk group
4. (List two:) smaller bones, longer life expectancy, drop in estrogen levels after menopause or due to amenorrhea
5. (List three:) works with calcium to help form strong bones and teeth, helps maintain an acid-base balance in the blood, plays vital roles in key metabolic processes, functions as part of some enzymes, forms part of every cell
6. (List five:) leafy green vegetables, legumes, seafood, nuts, milk, whole grain products, hard water
7. hair, nails, skin
8. osmosis
9. 7
10. sodium and chloride; processed foods
11. heart
12. iron
13. (List two:) iron needs increase during the teenage growth spurt, teenage females are beginning their menstrual cycles and losing iron supplies that must be replaced, teenage females have trouble eating enough to get an adequate amount of iron in their diets
14. supplements
15. the thyroid gland
16. from fluoridated water
17. Selenium works with vitamin E in an antioxidant capacity. It assists an enzyme that helps reduce damage to cell membranes due to exposure to oxygen.
18. (List two:) copper, chromium, manganese, molybdenum (Functions are student response. See pages 167-168 in the text.)
19. soil, water, and fertilizers used to grow them
20. true

Student Activity Guide

Mineral Match, Activity A

1. M
2. J
3. L
4. P
5. K
6. B
7. O
8. A
9. Q
10. H
11. I
12. D
13. R
14. G
15. E
16. F

Mineral Mysteries, Activity C

1. A
2. B
3. A
4. C
5. D
6. B
7. B
8. C
9. A
10. C
11. C
12. B

Minerals, More or Less, Activity D

1. more
2. less
3. more
4. more
5. less
6. less
7. less
8. more
9. less
10. more
11. more
12. less
13. more
14. more
15. more
16. more
17. less
18. less
19. more
20. more

Backtrack Through Chapter 9, Activity E

1. major minerals; 100 or more milligrams per day
2. helps muscles contract, assists blood-clotting processes, transmits nerve impulses
3. teenage and young adult women who develop amenorrhea
4. It hinders calcium absorption and absorption of other minerals.
5. A. (List three:) weakness, heart irregularities, disorientation, seizures
   B. weakness, nausea
6. sulfur
7. sodium, potassium, chloride
8. (List three:) heart malfunctions, muscle cramps, loss of appetite, constipation, confusion
9. heme and nonheme; heme
10. during periods of rapid growth and sexual development
11. either an iodine deficiency or excess
12. heart disease
13. (List three:) bone breakage, tooth loss, spinal compression, height reduction
14. They combine with other elements to form alkaline compounds that neutralize acid-forming elements in the body.
15. Females in this age group lose iron through the monthly blood loss of menstruation.
16. Excess zinc will reduce the body's ability to absorb iron and copper.
17. Fluoride from fluoridated drinking water helps strengthen bones and teeth, reduce the incidence of dental caries, and may help prevent the onset or decrease the severity of osteoporosis.
18. (Student response. See Chart 9-12 on page 162 in the text.)
19. potassium deficiency; Discuss symptoms with a doctor. If he or she diagnoses a deficiency, consult with a registered dietitian to evaluate my diet for good potassium sources.
20. (Student response. See pages 168-169 in the text.)

Teacher's Resources

Where's the Sodium in Your Diet? reproducible master 9-2

(Questions 1-9 are student response.)
10. 500 mg
11. 2,400 mg
12. processed foods
13. fluid losses

14. people who are sodium sensitive
15. (List three. Student response. See Chart 9-12 on page 162 in the text.)

Testing Beverages for Iron, reproducible master 9-3

Precipitate results:
  Apricot nectar—precipitate forms
  Cola—no precipitate
  Milk—no precipitate
  Orange juice—small amount of precipitate
  Pineapple juice—small amount of precipitate
  Prune juice—large amount of precipitate

1. (Student response. Approximate order should be: prune juice, apricot juice, orange juice, pineapple juice, cola, and milk.)
2. A. 1.0 mg
   B. 0.2 mg
   C. 0.1 mg
   D. 0.5 mg
   E. 0.7 mg
   F. 3.0 mg
3. (Student response.)
4. Typically, beverages are not good sources of iron.
5. (List three:) red meat, clams, oysters, duck, goose, legumes, dark green leafy vegetables, whole grains, enriched bread and cereal products (Students may justify other responses.)

Chapter 9 Test

1. I	10. E	19. F	28. B
2. J	11. F	20. T	29. C
3. A	12. F	21. T	30. C
4. G	13. T	22. T	31. C
5. H	14. T	23. T	32. D
6. C	15. F	24. F	33. B
7. K	16. F	25. T	34. A
8. F	17. T	26. A	35. C
9. D	18. T	27. B	

36. (List four:) help enzymes complete chemical reactions, become part of body components, aid normal nerve functioning and muscle contraction, promote growth, regulate acid-base balance in the body, maintain body fluid balance
37. Discuss suspected deficiency symptoms with a physician. If he or she diagnoses a deficiency, a registered dietitian can help evaluate your diet for good mineral sources.
38. (List three. Student response. See pages 168-169 in the text.)

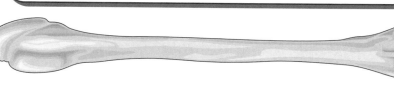

Risk Factors for Osteoporosis

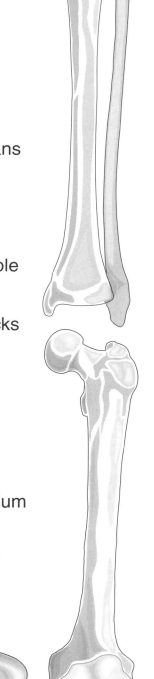

Which factors are controllable, which are not?

- Age—risks of osteoporosis increase with age.

- Sex—women are at greater risk than men.

- Race—Caucasians and Asians are more prone to developing osteoporosis than African Americans and Hispanics.

- Inactivity—bones are less dense among people who do not engage in weight-bearing exercise.

- Body size and weight—risks are greater for people with small body frame and low weight.

- Calcium intake—risks increase when the diet lacks balance or is chronically low in calcium.

- Family history—risks increase if family members have developed osteoporosis.

- Eating disorders—nutrient imbalances and amenorrhea increase risks.

- Cigarette smoking—smokers do not absorb calcium efficiently from food.

A larger number of risk factors means an increased chance of developing osteoporosis later in life.

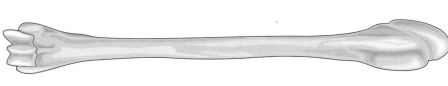
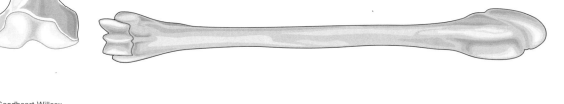

© Goodheart-Willcox

Reproducible Master 9-2

Where's the Sodium in Your Diet?

Name_____   Date _____   Period _____

Answer questions 1 through 8 by checking the column that best describes you. Then write your responses to the remaining questions in the space provided.

Once a week or less	3-4 times a week	Daily	
_____	_____	_____	1. How often do you eat ham, bacon, sausage, hot dogs, and other processed or cured meats?
_____	_____	_____	2. How often do you eat canned vegetables or frozen vegetables with sauce?
_____	_____	_____	3. How often do you eat frozen dinners or canned or dehydrated soups?
_____	_____	_____	4. How often do you eat processed cheeses and cottage cheese?
_____	_____	_____	5. How often do you eat salty snacks, such as nuts, popcorn, pretzels, and chips?
_____	_____	_____	6. How often do you add salt to foods while cooking?
_____	_____	_____	7. How often do you use soy sauce, catsup, mustard, pickles, and other condiments that are high in sodium?
_____	_____	_____	8. How often do you salt food on the plate before tasting it?

9. What do your answers tell you about your diet? (The more checks you have in the second and third columns, the higher your diet is likely to be in sodium.) _____

_____

10. What is the daily safe and adequate intake of sodium for adolescents and adults? _____

11. What daily limit for sodium appears on Nutrition Facts panels on food labels?_____

12. What is the source of the majority of sodium in the typical U.S. diet?_____

13. What is the most frequent cause of a drop in the body's sodium level? _____

14. Who is most at risk of health problems due to excess sodium in the diet?_____

15. Suggest three ways to help people "shake the salt habit."

_____

_____

_____

Testing Beverages for Iron

Name_____   Date _____   Period _____

Objective: To identify the presence of iron in beverages.

Supplies:

10   mL apricot nectar
10   mL cola
10   mL milk
10   mL orange juice
10   mL pineapple juice
10   mL prune juice
 6   test tubes
60   mL brewed tea

Procedure:

1. Pour apricot nectar, cola, milk, orange juice, pineapple juice, and prune juice into separate test tubes.
2. Add 10 mL of brewed tea to each test tube.
3. Tannic acid in the tea reacts with iron to form a brown precipitate. Indicate in the chart below whether a precipitate formed in each beverage.

Beverage	Appearance of Precipitate
Apricot nectar	
Cola	
Milk	
Orange juice	
Pineapple juice	
Prune juice	

Conclusions:

1. List the beverages in order from largest amount of precipitate to smallest amount of precipitate. _____
   _____

2. Using Appendix B, *Nutritive Values of Foods,* look up the amount of iron present in 1 cup of each beverage.

   _____ A. Apricot nectar   _____ D. Orange juice

   _____ B. Cola   _____ E. Pineapple juice

   _____ C. Milk   _____ F. Prune juice

3. Did the results of the experiment agree with the amounts of iron listed in the appendix? _____

4. How would you evaluate beverages as a source of iron? _____
   _____

5. Name three foods that would be good sources of iron. _____
   _____

© Goodheart-Willcox

Minerals: Regulators of Body Functions

Name_____

Date _____   Period _____   Score _____

Chapter 9 Test

Matching: Match the following minerals with the functions and deficiencies.

_____ 1. The movement of water across a semipermeable membrane to equalize the concentrations of solution on each side of the membrane.

_____ 2. A term used to express a substance's acidity or alkalinity.

_____ 3. A compound that has a pH lower than 7.

_____ 4. An iron-containing protein that helps red blood cells carry oxygen from the lungs to cells throughout the body.

_____ 5. An iron-containing protein that carries oxygen and carbon dioxide in muscle tissue.

_____ 6. A substance that acts with enzymes to increase enzyme activity.

_____ 7. A hormone produced by the thyroid gland that helps control metabolism.

_____ 8. An enlargement of the thyroid gland.

_____ 9. Severe mental retardation and dwarfed physical features of an infant caused by the mother's iodine deficiency during pregnancy.

_____ 10. A spotty discoloration of teeth caused by high fluoride intake.

A. acid
B. base
C. cofactor
D. cretinism
E. fluorosis
F. goiter
G. hemoglobin
H. myoglobin
I. osmosis
J. pH
K. thyroxine

True/False: Circle *T* if the statement is true or *F* if the statement is false.

T   F   11. Minerals are considered organic compounds.

T   F   12. The macrominerals are more important to good health than the microminerals.

T   F   13. Teens have greater calcium needs than adults in their 30s and 40s.

T   F   14. Women are affected by osteoporosis more than men.

T   F   15. Most nutrition experts recommend supplements over food sources for meeting calcium needs and reducing the risks of osteoporosis.

T   F   16. Because alcohol increases magnesium absorption, alcoholics are at increased risk of magnesium toxicity.

T   F   17. Sulfur is part of protein tissues and is concentrated in hair, nails, and skin.

T   F   18. The pH of body fluids must remain within a narrow range for life processes to be maintained.

T   F   19. Most people in the United States have difficulty meeting their recommended daily sodium needs.

T   F   20. Iron is needed to make new cells and release energy from macronutrients.

T   F   21. Zinc is often associated with periods of rapid growth and sexual development.

T   F   22. Seafood is a rich source of iodine.

T   F   23. Selenium functions as an antioxidant.

T   F   24. Chromium helps the body make hemoglobin and collagen.

T   F   25. The body tends to absorb a greater percentage of minerals from foods during times of increased mineral needs.

(Continued)

© Goodheart-Willcox

Name_____

Multiple Choice: Choose the best response. Write the letter in the space provided.

_____26. Which of the following is an example of a macromineral?
A. Chlorine.
B. Fluoride.
C. Iron.
D. Selenium.

_____27. Which of the following best describes bone tissue affected by osteoporosis?
A. A small-celled sponge with a hard shell layer.
B. A large-celled sponge with a brittle outer layer.
C. A rubbery core with a flaky covering.
D. Osteoporosis affects blood calcium levels but not bone tissue.

_____28. If Sasha cannot tolerate milk in her diet, what options does she have for food sources of calcium?
A. Deep yellow vegetables.
B. Legumes.
C. Tuna.
D. All the above are dietary calcium sources.

_____29. The condition called amenorrhea, common among young women with eating disorders, causes _____.
A. excess calcium in the bones
B. excess estrogen in the body
C. monthly menstrual periods to stop
D. vomiting and diarrhea

_____30. Which of the following is an effect of excess phosphorus in the diet?
A. Kidney stones.
B. Liver damage.
C. Reduced calcium absorption.
D. Weakness and nausea.

_____31. Which of the following is a disorder associated with sodium retention?
A. Anemia.
B. Goiter.
C. Hypertension.
D. Menopause.

_____32. Which of the following is a source of heme iron?
A. Broccoli.
B. Brown rice.
C. Navy beans.
D. Round steak.

_____33. Which of the following is a symptom of iron-deficiency anemia?
A. Blurred vision.
B. Fatigue.
C. Heart malfunction.
D. Muscle cramps.

(Continued)

© Goodheart-Willcox

Name_____

_____34. Which of the following minerals may be added to water to reduce the risks of tooth decay?
   A. Fluoride.
   B. Iodine.
   C. Iron.
   D. Zinc.

_____35. The longer a food is soaked in water, the greater the chances for _____.
   A. decreased absorption rate
   B. increased absorption rate
   C. mineral losses
   D. toxic effects

Essay Questions: Provide complete responses to the following questions or statements.

36. List four major roles of minerals in the diet.

37. What should you do if you have symptoms you suspect are due to a mineral deficiency?

38. What are three guidelines for maximizing mineral absorption and availability in the body?

Water: The Forgotten Nutrient

10

Objectives

After studying this chapter, students will be able to
- identify four main functions of water in the body.
- list sources of the body's water supply.
- describe effects of water loss on the body.
- determine whether their water intake is adequate.

Bulletin Board

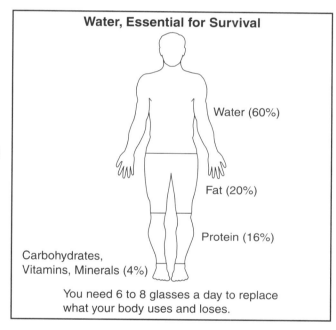

Water, Essential for Survival

Water (60%)

Fat (20%)

Protein (16%)

Carbohydrates, Vitamins, Minerals (4%)

You need 6 to 8 glasses a day to replace what your body uses and loses.

Title: *Water, Essential for Survival*

From construction paper, make an outline of the human body. Draw lines through the body at the hip, knee, and ankle levels. Label the section from head to hip *Water (60%),* from hip to knee *Fat (20%),* from knee to ankle *Protein (16 %).* Label the feet *Carbohydrates, Vitamins, Minerals (4%).* Under the silhouette, place the sentence "You need 6 to 8 glasses a day to replace what your body uses and loses."

Teaching Materials

Text, pages 172–182
Learn the Language
Check Your Knowledge
Put Learning into Action
Explore Further

Student Activity Guide, pages 71–76
   A. *Water Crossword*
   B. *Drinking Water—The Undiluted Truth*
   C. *Examining Your Water Needs*
   D. *"Water Under the Bridge"*
   E. *Backtrack Through Chapter 10*

Teacher's Resources
Water Works: The Functions of H_2O, color transparency CT-10
Water Experiment: A Solvent for Nutrients, reproducible master 10-1
Dehydration and Water Losses: The Body Signals, transparency master 10-2
Chapter 10 Test

Introducing the Chapter

1. Ask students to describe what it feels like to be very thirsty. List on the board all the adjectives they can identify. Relate the constant need to replenish fluids with the good feeling of a quenched thirst.
2. Explain that water is the most essential nutrient because a person can only live a few days without it. Ask which situations seem to require drinking more fluids than usual.
3. Hold up a glass of tap water and a purchased bottle of water. Ask students to vote on which is better for health. Record the number of votes for each choice. Repeat the survey at the end of the chapter to see if there is a change of opinion.

Strategies to Reteach, Reinforce, Enrich, and Extend Text Concepts

The Vital Functions of Water

4. **RT** *Water Works: The Functions of H_2O,* color transparency CT-10. Use the transparency to highlight the important functions of water. Review the concepts and provide examples for each.
5. **ER** Give each student a soda cracker to slowly chew and swallow. As the students are eating the crackers, ask them to write a one-paragraph description of what is happening to the crackers in their mouths. Students should describe the role of saliva in the chewing and swallowing process as the cracker softens and dissolves. Relate this to the lubrication role of water in other parts of the digestive system.

6. **ER** *Water Experiment: A Solvent for Nutrients,* reproducible master 10-1. Have students form teams of two. Each team should complete the experiment to demonstrate the function of water as a solvent. Discuss with students how water aids digestion and the role of water in the transport of nutrients.

7. **RF** Show three quarts of water to the students. Tell students this is the quantity of water lost every day by the human body. Ask students why the recommended amount of water intake is only two quarts a day. They should explain that the other quart comes from food sources.

8. **ER** Guest speaker. Invite a paramedic to describe what happens to someone who has suffered extreme temperature exposure to cold or heat for an extended period of time. Ask about first aid procedures for the victims.

Keeping Fluids in Balance

9. **RF** Place glasses equally full of water on each side of a balance scale. One glass represents the daily water intake; the other represents daily water output. When the amount of water is equal, fluid balance is present. Then remove water from the output glass to demonstrate a need for more fluids. Use water from the input glass to refill the output glass. Repeat the process until the input glass is empty, and the output glass is near empty. Discuss the meaning of *dehydration.*

10. **ER** Have students dehydrate slices of a juicy fruit, such as an apple or cherry. Compare the amount of water in the fresh fruit with that of the dehydrated fruit by weighing the food before and after dehydration. Discuss that water is a part of foods (1-94% by weight), much as water is a part of the human body (approximately 60%).

11. **RF** Discuss the relationship of a food's water content to the number of calories in the food. Refer students to Appendix C or *Personal Best* software. Fruits and vegetables are usually higher in water than fats and oils, which are higher in calories. Also, the higher the water content of the solid food, the more fluid is provided to a person's daily diet.

12. **ER** Have students prepare a bar graph illustrating where water is located in the body and the percentages for each of these tissue areas. Students might use the following information: bones—25% water; brain—74% water; muscles—75% water; blood—83% water; body fat—20-35% water.

13. **RF** Ask students why people may choose to buy water instead of using tap water. Discuss why each reason may or may not be valid.

14. **RF** *Drinking Water—The Undiluted Truth,* Activity B, SAG. Students are to identify true and false statements and answer questions about bottled versus tap water. After students have completed their worksheets, discuss their answers and identify common myths associated with the booming sales of bottled water.

15. **RF** *Dehydration and Water Losses: The Body Signals,* transparency master 10-2. Discuss percentages of water weight loss and their effects on state of wellness. Discuss situations in which people may experience serious water weight loss.

16. **EX** Have students determine how many pounds of water a 150-pound person could lose before his or her athletic performance would decrease. Then ask students to determine their own maximum water weight loss.

17. **ER** Guest speaker. Invite one of the school's sports coaches to discuss the effects of dehydration. Also discuss how a student can become aware of dehydration and how it can be prevented.

18. **RF** Demonstrate the effects of a diuretic by showing what happens when a water-filled sponge is squeezed. What are the implications for fluid intake?

19. **RF** Ask students to explain why a fever tends to increase the need for fluids.

20. **ER** Have students form small groups to discuss ways a heat wave can cause people to become ill. Have students develop a pamphlet on increasing fluid intake during hot weather.

21. **ER** *Examining Your Water Needs,* Activity C, SAG. Students are to keep a beverage diary for 24 hours. Then, using Appendix C or *Personal Best* software, they should determine what percentage of each beverage is water and answer the questions that follow.

22. **EX** *"Water Under the Bridge,"* Activity D, SAG. Students are to read each case situation and explain how the teen in each case could avoid similar situations in the future.

Chapter Review

23. **RF** *Water Crossword,* Activity A, SAG. Students are to complete a crossword puzzle using terms from the chapter.

24. **RF** *Backtrack Through Chapter 10,* Activity E, SAG. Students are to provide complete answers to questions and statements that will help them recall, interpret, apply, and practice chapter concepts.

Above and Beyond

25. **EX** Have students create a "Fluid Thought for the Day" poster to hang in the school cafeteria. Students should place a new water-related fact on the poster each day. Students may decorate the

poster with pictures of water or people drinking water.

26. **EX** Have teams of students choose a topic to research and write a report for the school newspaper. Topics might include the special water/health connections for people with diabetes, athletes, and people trying to lose weight.

27. **EX** Have students contact the local public health department to learn the process for testing the quality of the home water supply. If a water testing program is available, have the students submit a sample of their water supply for purity testing.

Answer Key

Text

Check Your Knowledge, page 182

1. (List five:) saliva, blood, lymph, digestive juices, urine, perspiration
2. Amino acids from proteins, glucose from carbohydrates, minerals, and water-soluble vitamins are dissolved in the water of digestive fluids. Then these nutrients are absorbed from the small intestine and transported through the water-based blood to all the cells of the body.
3. The water in blood and perspiration helps the body release excess heat. When the body becomes warm, the blood vessels near the skin surface expand. The expanded blood vessels allow more blood to flow near the skin surface, releasing excess body heat into the air. Perspiration also transmits heat from the body through pores in the skin surface.
4. sodium, potassium, chlorine
5. (Student response. See Chart 10-4 on page 177 in the text.)
6. false
7. Diarrhea and vomiting pull electrolytes as well as water from an infant's body. When fluid losses are excessive, electrolytes as well as fluids must be replaced.
8. Caffeine is a diuretic.
9. Fluids make up a high percentage of body weight. Therefore, when you lose water, you lose weight.
10. (List three:) infants, older adults, pregnant women, lactating women, people on high-protein diets

Student Activity Guide

Water Crossword, Activity A

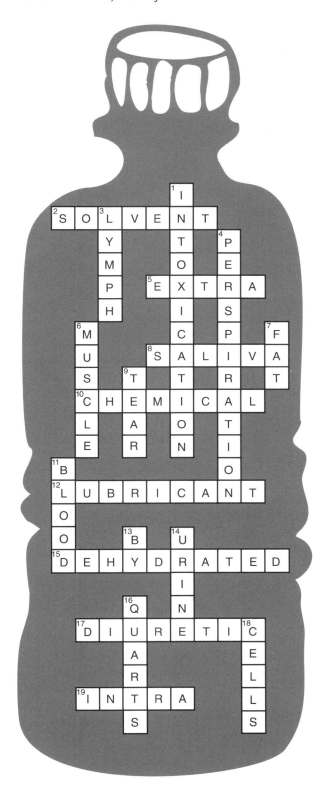

Drinking Water—The Undiluted Truth, Activity B

1. F
2. T
3. T
4. F
5. T
6. F
7. T
8. F
9. F
10. T
11. (Student response.)
12. (Student response.)
13. (Student response.)
14. (Student response.)
15. (Student response.)

Backtrack Through Chapter 10, Activity E

1. about 10 to 12 gallons
2. 50 to 70 percent
3. facilitates chemical reactions, transports nutrients and waste products, lubricates surfaces, regulates body temperature, keeps fluids in balance
4. (Student response. See Figure 10-4 on page 177 in the text.)
5. (List three:) they think bottled water contains minerals that promote health; they think it tastes better; they fear tap water may be contaminated; they like the convenience of bottled water
6. 2 to 3 quarts
7. through breath, perspiration, urine, and bowel wastes
8. An electrolyte is a mineral that helps in fluid balance. It regulates water movement both inside and outside cells.
9. A diuretic is a substance that increases urine production. (List two examples:) coffee, soft drinks, some prescription medicines
10. serious organ malfunction can occur
11. 6 to 8
12. 1 to 2 quarts daily
13. Water is an essential nutrient that must be replaced every day. The body cannot live without it. Water makes up 50 to 70 percent of body weight and serves many other important functions.
14. Water dissolves substances for digestion. Blood is made up mostly of water, and many substances dissolve in blood to be transported through the body.
15. Water aids in regulating body temperature in cold weather by conserving heat. The body restricts the amount of blood (a water-containing substance) flowing near the skin surface. In warm weather conditions, the body allows more blood to flow close to the surface and release heat into the air.

The body also perspires, using the released water to cool itself down.

16. Water moves across cell membranes to keep the proper level of fluids inside the cell and surrounding it. Minerals called electrolytes help move the water into and out of the cells as needed to keep the proper balance.
17. Women who are pregnant have extra fluid needs because they have an increased volume of body fluids to support their developing babies. Lactating women need extra fluids to produce breast milk.
18. (Student response.)
19. (Student response.)
20. (Student response.)

Teacher's Resources

Water Experiment: A Solvent for Nutrients, reproducible master 10-1

1. The candy should be almost completely dissolved in the water.
2. There should be no change in the color or size of the candy.
3. Water is an excellent solvent for sugars.
4. Oil is not a very effective solvent for sugars.
5. Water acts as a solvent for glucose in carbohydrates during digestion. Water is also a solvent for amino acids, minerals, and water-soluble vitamins.

Chapter 10 Test

1. D	9. D	17. F	25. D
2. F	10. A	18. T	26. C
3. C	11. T	19. F	27. C
4. E	12. F	20. T	28. D
5. B	13. F	21. T	29. A
6. E	14. F	22. T	30. D
7. F	15. T	23. C	31. C
8. B	16. T	24. B	32. A

33. (List three:) urine, perspiration, breathing moisture losses, bowel waste
34. It is better to lose fat than water weight; water weight is quickly regained when body fluids are replenished; loss of more than two percent of water weight can make a person ill.
35. (List three:) infants—immature kidneys are not as efficient at filtering waste from the bloodstream, older adults—lose some water-conserving abilities, pregnant women—have increased volume of body fluids to support the developing babies, lactating women—need fluid to produce breast milk, people on high-protein diets—require extra water to rid their bodies of the waste products of protein metabolism

Water Experiment: A Solvent for Nutrients

Name_____ Date _____ Period _____

Objective: To understand the function of water as a solvent.

Supplies:

    2   150-mL beakers
         masking tape
  125   mL water (room temperature)
  125   mL canola oil
    2   pieces of hard peppermint candy
    2   stirring rods

Procedure:

1. Label the beakers *A* and *B* with the masking tape.
2. Pour the water into beaker A. Pour the canola oil into beaker B.
3. Put one peppermint candy in each beaker.
4. Stir the contents of each beaker continuously for 5 minutes. At the end of 5 minutes, examine the candies and answer the questions below.

Questions:

1. What happened to the candy in beaker A? _____

   _____

2. What happened to the candy in beaker B? _____

   _____

3. Based on your findings, what conclusion would you draw about the effectiveness of water as a solvent for sugars?_____

   _____

   _____

4. What conclusion would you draw about the effectiveness of oil as a solvent for sugars?_____

   _____

   _____

5. How does this information relate to the importance of water as a solvent during digestion? _____

   _____

   _____

   _____

© Goodheart-Willcox

Dehydration and Water Losses: The Body Signals

Percentage of Body Weight Loss	Effects on the Body
0-1% weight loss	Experience of thirst
2% weight loss	Feelings of discomfort, lack of appetite
3% weight loss	Nausea, irritability, fatigue
6% weight loss	Increased pulse and breathing rate
7% weight loss	Rise in body temperature
8% weight loss	Dizziness, weakness, confusion
9% weight loss	Difficulty breathing
10% weight loss	Decreased blood volume, muscle spasms, collapse of the circulatory system
11% weight loss	Kidney failure
20% weight loss	Coma, death

© Goodheart-Willcox

Water: The Forgotten Nutrient

Name_____

Date _____ **Period** _____ **Score** _____

Chapter 10 Test

Matching: Match the following functions of water with their descriptions.

_____ 1. Helps maintain body temperature.

_____ 2. Carries nutrients through the bloodstream.

_____ 3. Splits the bonds in a starch chain and becomes part of the separate glucose molecules.

_____ 4. Dissolves amino acids and glucose.

_____ 5. Mixes with foods to soften and moisten.

A. diuretic
B. lubricant
C. reactant
D. regulator
E. solvent
F. transporter

Matching: Match the following terms and identifying phrases.

_____ 6. Water inside the cells.

_____ 7. A condition that results from drinking too much water.

_____ 8. Substances that increase urine production.

_____ 9. Water outside of cells.

_____ 10. State in which the body contains a lower-than-normal amount of body fluids.

A. dehydration
B. diuretics
C. electrolyte
D. extracellular
E. intracellular
F. water intoxication

True/False: Circle *T* if the statement is true and *F* if the statement is false.

T   F   11. Most people can survive a longer period without food than they can without water.

T   F   12. Fat tissue contains proportionally more water than muscle tissue.

T   F   13. The liver filters waste from blood and forms urine.

T   F   14. More heat can be lost when the blood vessels near the surface of the skin constrict.

T   F   15. Electrolytes help water move freely inside and outside the cells.

T   F   16. Foods as well as beverages are a source of water.

T   F   17. Bottled water is a better source of minerals than tap water.

T   F   18. It is possible to drink too much water, but this rarely happens.

T   F   19. The use of diuretics decreases urine production.

T   F   20. Exercise causes increased water losses.

T   F   21. Athletic performance decreases with losses of water weight.

T   F   22. Dark yellow urine can be an indication that fluid intake is low.

(Continued)

© Goodheart-Willcox

Name_____

Multiple Choice: Choose the best response. Write the letter in the space provided.

_____23. For most adults, water is approximately _____ percent of body weight.
  A. 5-20
  B. 30-35
  C. 50-70
  D. 85-90

_____24. About how many gallons of water does the adult body contain?
  A. 2.
  B. 12.
  C. 24.
  D. 50.

_____25. Curin is 35 years old. He exercises regularly and maintains a healthy body weight. His total water weight is likely to be less than that of _____.
  A. Anne, Curin's 35-year-old wife
  B. Tim, Curin's 60-year-old father
  C. Curin's twin brother, who is inactive and overweight
  D. Dan, Curin's 15-year-old son, who is on the track team

_____26. Water is the main component in which of the following?
  A. Bones.
  B. Hair.
  C. Blood.
  D. All the above.

_____27. What keeps cells from bursting with excess fluids?
  A. Extracellular water pressure is greater than intracellular water pressure.
  B. Intracellular water pressure is greater than extracellular water pressure.
  C. Electrolytes keep the water in and out of the cells in balance.
  D. Most cells do not have fluids in them.

_____28. Which one is the most reasonable motive for buying bottled water rather than using tap water?
  A. Bottled water is cheaper than tap water.
  B. Bottled water has been proven to be safer, cleaner, and purer than tap water.
  C. Bottled water contains miracle minerals.
  D. Bottled water is convenient to buy and use when other water sources are not available.

_____29. Through what means can body water be lost?
  A. The skin.
  B. Hair follicles.
  C. Blood circulation.
  D. Enzyme activity.

_____30. Why might more fluids be needed during illness?
  A. Fluids help flush drug metabolism products from the system.
  B. A sick person may not feel like drinking enough fluids.
  C. Vomiting and diarrhea cause fluid loss.
  D. All the above.

(Continued)

© Goodheart-Willcox

Name_____

_____31. How many 8-ounce glasses of water should most people consume each day?
   A.   2-4.
   B.   4-6.
   C.   6-8.
   D.   10-12.

_____32. Who is most likely to suffer the quickest from dehydration?
   A.   Infants.
   B.   Young adults.
   C.   Teens.
   D.   Male athletes.

Essay Questions: Provide complete responses to the following questions or statements.

33. List three ways water leaves the body.

34. Why is it not a good idea for a person to lose weight by losing water weight?

35. Name three groups of people who have above-average needs for water and explain why.

Nutrition for All Ages

11

Objectives

After studying this chapter, students will be able to
- list the five stages of the life cycle.
- describe factors that affect nutritional needs at each stage of the life cycle.
- discuss nutritional problems associated with each stage of the life cycle.
- use nutrient recommendation tables to find the suggested daily intake of specific nutrients for a given person.

Bulletin Boards

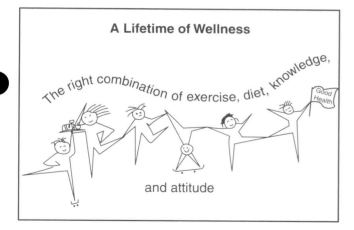

A Lifetime of Wellness

The right combination of exercise, diet, knowledge, and attitude

Good Health

Title: *A Lifetime of Wellness*

Sketch a row of dancing people. The first figure could carry a tray of fruits and vegetables. The last figure could hold a flag labeled *good health*. Place the words *The right combination of exercise, diet, knowledge, and attitude* around the dancing figures.

Title: *Healthy Snacks for Young and Old*

Divide the bulletin board into four quadrants using colorful crepe paper or wide ribbon. Label the quadrants *Refrigerator, Cupboard, Easy Recipes,* and *Prepackaged Snacks.* Use students' suggestions for favorite nutritious foods in each category. Individual food wrappers and/or pictures can be attached to the appropriate square. Refrigerator snacks may include pictures of fresh fruits and vegetables; cupboard snacks might include peanut butter, whole grain breads, cereals, popcorn, and raisins; and prepackaged snacks may include small cans of fruit juices, granola bars, and dried

fruits. Attach simple snack recipes to the recipes section. Include lowfat snack recipes.

Teaching Materials

Text, pages 184-210
> *Learn the Language*
> *Check Your Knowledge*
> *Put Learning into Action*
> *Explore Further*

Student Activity Guide, pages 77-84
> A. *The Life Cycle*
> B. *Nutrition During Pregnancy*
> C. *Feeding an Infant*
> D. *Sticky Situations*
> E. *Ticket to Teen Nutrition*
> F. *Advice for Adults*
> G. *Backtrack Through Chapter 11*

Teacher's Resources
> *Breast Milk vs. Formula,* reproducible master 11-1
> *Food Label for Children,* transparency master 11-2
> *MyPyramid Guidelines for a Six-Year-Old,* color transparency CT-11
> *Rise and Shine for Breakfast,* transparency master 11-3
> Chapter 11 Test

Introducing the Chapter

1. Draw a timeline on the board and list the stages of the life cycle along the line. Discuss with students where they currently fall on the timeline. Also discuss health and nutritional variations of each stage as students have observed them.
2. Refer to Appendix B, *Recommended Nutrient Intakes,* to review where nutrient needs vary depending on age, gender, pregnancy, or lactation. Discuss which nutrient recommendations increase and which decrease. Reasons for nutrient changes will be discussed throughout the chapter.
3. *The Life Cycle,* Activity A, SAG. Students are to list the names and age ranges of each life cycle stage. They should then answer the questions about the life cycle that follow.
4. Have students identify foods commonly associated with infants, teens, and older adults. Ask students why they think the associations exist and if they are valid.

Strategies to Reteach, Reinforce, Enrich, and Extend Text Concepts

Changing Nutritional Needs

5. **ER** Assign students to interview a person in a particular age group about his or her eating patterns. Assign each student to different age groups to cover each of the five stages. Use parents of infants to get responses about infancy. With the assistance of the students, develop several questions to ask. When interview data is collected, have students form groups of five. Every group should have interviews from people in each of the five stages. The groups should compare interviews and discuss what they discovered about changing nutritional needs over the life span.

6. **ER** Guest speaker. Invite an older man and woman to discuss how their food patterns have changed over their life spans. Highlight how and why changes occurred for them. Ask students to think of reasons their food behaviors might change in the future.

7. **ER** Have students complete an Internet search on food pattern changes over the life span. Have each student identify one Internet resource. Combine all the resources to create a directory. This compilation of resources can be used for research throughout the chapter. Distribute the list to students.

Pregnancy and Lactation

8. **ER** Guest speaker. Invite a registered nurse or obstetrician to discuss the importance of good nutrition during pregnancy. Find out how special needs can be met for women who experience morning sickness, allergies, anemia, diabetes, or other health complications.

9. **RF** *Nutrition During Pregnancy,* Activity B, SAG. Students are to complete a fill-in-the-blank activity about nutritional needs during pregnancy.

10. **RF** Have students use Appendix B, *Recommended Nutrient Intakes,* to see the different recommendations for teen women, pregnant women, and lactating women. Discuss why it is important for women to be aware of increased nutrient needs, and review how each of the extra nutrient needs can be met.

11. **ER** Have students plan one week's menus for a pregnant woman. Make sure they take the increased nutrient needs into account.

12. **RT** Have students list on the board factors that reduce health risks in pregnancy and factors that increase health risks in pregnancy.

13. **ER** Guest speaker. Invite a nurse or certified exercise trainer to discuss the role of exercise in pregnancy. Discuss which exercises are safe and which exercises might be restricted during pregnancy.

14. **ER** Guest speaker. Invite a breast-feeding mother and a bottle-feeding mother to talk to the class about the pros and cons of nursing and bottle feeding a baby. Have each relate her goals, satisfactions, and disappointments with her choice.

Infancy and Toddlerhood

15. **RT** *Breast Milk vs. Formula,* reproducible master 11-1. Students are to complete the chart by listing their opinions of the advantages and disadvantages of breast-feeding and bottle-feeding. Discuss with students the nutritional, social, and emotional factors related to the decision to breast- or bottle-feed.

16. **ER** Use the Internet to locate support groups for breast- and bottle-feeding. Gather the name of professional organizations that provide accurate information, such as the LaLeche League.

17. **RF** *Feeding an Infant,* Activity C, SAG. Students are to complete statements about feeding schedules for infants. They will also rank a list of foods in the order they are introduced to an infant's diet. Finally, students will complete sentences about tips for feeding infants.

18. **EX** Provide samples of types of formulas available to consumers. Have students compare ingredients and costs of two prepared formulas to that of two powdered formulas. Have students sample the formulas to decide if there are differences in taste. Discuss why infants do not drink cow's milk their first year of life.

19. **RF** *Food Label for Children,* transparency master 11-2. Review the information on the children's food label. Stress that Dietary Guidelines for Americans and the Adult Nutrition Fact Panel do not apply to children under the age of two.

20. **RF** Have students bring in infant food labels to compare nutrient contents, serving sizes, and costs per serving.

21. **EX** Have students work in groups to investigate how to make homemade baby food. Have students compare homemade baby food to commercial baby food and discuss advantages and disadvantages of each.

22. **ER** Using an infant doll, demonstrate what to do if an infant is choking. Holding the doll upside down, give five blows to the back and five thrusts to the chest. This procedure would be repeated until the object came out.

23. **RF** Discuss foods to avoid giving to very young children. Foods should include small hard foods (nuts, seeds, popcorn, hard candy) and

slippery foods (whole grapes, hot dogs, chicken, cough drops).

24. **RF** Discuss some of the eating problems common in the toddler years. Have students suggest possible strategies for helping toddlers overcome the problems.

Childhood

25. **ER** *MyPyramid Guidelines for a Six-Year-Old,* color transparency CT-11. Use the color transparency to compare and contrast the daily guide recommendations for a 6-year-old with an adult's MyPyramid plan.

26. **ER** Have students interview a preschooler about what snacks he or she likes. Have students list the snacks and indicate the nutritional value of each. Discuss the contribution snacks make to a healthful diet.

27. **EX** *Sticky Situations,* Activity D, SAG. Students are to indicate the eating problem in each example. Students should then state how they would advise each child's caregiver to correct the eating problem.

28. **EX** Discuss the effects television and computer games have on children's activity levels. Brainstorm activities children could do that would be less sedentary, such as jumping rope, dancing, hiking, playing outdoor games, and walking pets.

29. **RF** Have students break into small groups to discuss common health concerns and eating problems of children. Groups should discuss why the problems exist and what preventative measures are possible. Ask each group to create a list of 20 health-promoting guidelines for children.

30. **ER** Ask students to interview parents of small children. Students should ask parents to keep a food diary for their child for three days. Have students use the MyPyramid system to rate the diet. Recommend adjustments that may help to improve the diet.

Adolescence

31. **ER** Have students cut out food ads from popular magazines. Analyze the message given in each ad. Discuss the social and psychological implications of the advertising media on teen nutrition.

32. **RT** *Ticket to Teen Nutrition,* Activity E, SAG. Students are to complete statements about teen nutrition.

33. **RF** *Rise and Shine for Breakfast,* transparency master 11-3. Use the transparency to discuss ways to fit breakfast into a busy lifestyle. Remind students that breakfast offers valuable nutrients to a day's diet and provides the energy to think creatively and perform productively.

34. **ER** Guest speaker. Invite a registered dietitian to discuss the nutritional problems common in the teen years. Have students prepare questions for the dietitian ahead of time.

Adulthood

35. **EX** *Advice for Adults,* Activity F, SAG. Students are to read the case situations and explain whether the advice given was good or bad and why. In instances they have marked as bad advice, students should offer better suggestions.

36. **ER** Guest speaker. Invite a nutritionist who coordinates meals for the elderly to discuss the nutritional concerns of older people. Health concerns should focus on osteoporosis, constipation, diabetes, chewing difficulties, high blood pressure, and obesity. Discuss how diets can be modified to meet the needs of older adults.

Chapter Review

37. **RF** Assign each student a letter of the alphabet. Go around the room and have students give facts or statements that begin with their letter about nutrition in the life span.

38. **RF** *Backtrack Through Chapter 11,* Activity G, SAG. Students are to provide complete answers to questions and statements that will help them recall, interpret, apply, and practice chapter concepts.

Above and Beyond

39. **EX** Ask students to find out the medical histories of family members. Have students identify their own inherited tendencies. If there is a history of family illness, have students identify preventative actions they can take throughout the life span. (Note: Students who do not have access to this information may want to complete the research for a friend.)

40. **EX** Have students visit local agencies that promote wellness to children, teens, and older adults. Prepare a directory of agency names, locations, services, and costs. Make the directory available to students, school staff, and parents to use as a referral source.

Answer Key

Text

Check Your Knowledge, pages 209-210

1. infancy, toddlerhood, childhood, adolescence, adulthood
2. body size and composition, age, gender, activity level, state of health

3. She will build reserves of some nutrients that will help her avoid deficiencies during pregnancy. She will know which foods to select to increase her nutrient intake during pregnancy.

4. true

5. (List two:) Many adolescent women fail to get enough calories, iron, and calcium to fully support their growth. Teens with poor nutritional status do not have the nutrient reserves needed to meet the demands of a developing fetus. Inactive teens are not at an optimum level of physical fitness.

6. (List three:) brain damage and below average intelligence, slowed physical growth, facial disfigurement, short attention span, irritability, heart problems

7. Children require more of each nutrient per pound of body weight than adults do.

8. Introducing only one food at a time to an infant's diet helps caregivers identify food allergies and sensitivities.

9. (Describe two:) lack of teeth, messy eating habits, developing independence, short attention span, picky eating (Suggestions are student response. See pages 199-200 in the text.)

10. (List four:) fruits, yogurt, raisins, carrot sticks, fat free milk (Students may justify other responses.)

11. overweight, dental caries

12. Males generally have a higher percentage of lean body mass than females.

13. (List two:) An adolescent diet that is low in calcium may increase the risk of osteoporosis in adulthood. An adolescent diet high in sugar may increase the risk of gum disease and tooth loss in adulthood. A high-fat diet in adolescence raises the chances of developing heart disease and some forms of cancer in adulthood.

14. (List two:) Many adults have a decrease in basal metabolic rate. Older adults require fewer calories to maintain their body weight. Some older people become less active.

15. (List four:) diminished sense of taste, tooth loss, digestive problems, isolation, limited income, lack of mobility

Student Activity Guide

The Life Cycle, Activity A

1. Infancy—0 to 12 months
2. Toddlerhood—1 to 3 years
3. Childhood—4 to 8 years
4. Adolescence—9 to 18 years
5. Adulthood—19 years and over
6. (Student response.)
7. For the most part, all people in one stage of the life cycle have similar nutritional needs related to age. However, within a stage of the life cycle, persons of different ages may have differing nutritional needs. Subdividing the stages allows people to focus on one particular life-stage group.

8. 9 through 13 years and 14 through 18 years
   (Line should be drawn and area including 14 through 18 should be shaded.)

9. Nutrient needs for adults decrease to a maintenance level; 19 through 30 years, 31 to 50 years, 50 to 70 years, and over 70 years
   (Lines should be drawn to subdivide adulthood at the appropriate ages.)

10. (Student response. See pages 184-186 in the text.)

Nutrition During Pregnancy, Activity B

1. lactation
2. prenatal care
3. low-birthweight
4. premature
5. trimester
6. protein
7. folate
8. B_{12}
9. calcium
10. zinc, iron, magnesium, iodine
11. calories
12. 25; 35
13. fats/sugars
14. morning sickness
15. smoking
16. placenta
17. congenital
18. fetal alcohol syndrome (FAS)

Feeding an Infant, Activity C

1. six
2. four
3. two
4. seven to eight
5. 2
6. 4
7. 1
8. 5
9. 6
10. 3
11. food allergies and sensitivities
12. development of excess fat tissue
13. hold spoons
14. they have small stomachs
15. independence
16. reject that particular food

Ticket to Teen Nutrition, Activity E

1. adolescence
2. puberty
3. growth spurt
4. composition
5. higher

6. 2,300
7. lean body mass
8. 800
9. regular
10. irregular
11. one-fourth
12. moderation
13. anemia
14. menstruation
15. disorders
16. density
17. caries
18. heart

***Backtrack Through Chapter 11,** Activity G*

1. infancy, toddlerhood, and childhood
2. Gender determines body composition, which in turn influences nutrient needs.
3. The woman must provide enough nutrients for her growing baby and adjust to physical changes within her own body during pregnancy.
4. vitamins, minerals, protein, fluids, and calories
5. (Student response. See page 193 in the text.)
6. infancy
7. breast milk (Reasons are student response. See page 195 in the text.)
8. (Student response. See Figure 11-12 on page 198 in the text.)
9. ages four through eight years
10. (List four. Student response. See page 201 in the text.)
11. poor eating habits and lack of exercise
12. The body needs more energy to build new tissue as it grows. A growing body will also contain more cells, which need more nutrients.
13. early adulthood—19-30; early middle adulthood—31 to 50; late middle adulthood—51 to 70; late adulthood—over 70 years
14. (Student response. See pages 184-186 in the text.)
15. When a pregnant woman takes a drug, it enters her bloodstream, then passes through the placenta into the bloodstream of her child. When a lactating mother uses drugs, drugs pass into the milk.

16. Added stress on the teen's body of nourishing the growth of the fetus as well as her own continuing growth; poor nutritional status, lack of nutrient reserves, and inactive lifestyles of many teens
17. (Student response. See page 203 in the text.)
18. (Describe three. See pages 205-206 in the text.)
19. (Student response.)
20. (Student response.)

Teacher's Resources

Chapter 11 Test

1. F	11. I	21. T	31. C
2. A	12. D	22. T	32. A
3. C	13. F	23. F	33. C
4. D	14. A	24. T	34. B
5. B	15. E	25. F	35. D
6. H	16. F	26. T	36. A
7. B	17. F	27. T	37. C
8. K	18. T	28. T	38. C
9. J	19. F	29. F	39. B
10. C	20. T	30. T	40. D

41. (List four:) Breast milk is perfectly designed to meet the nutritional needs of a baby. Babies who are breast-fed develop fewer allergies and infections than formula-fed babies. Mothers who breast-feed lose their pregnancy weight faster. Mothers who breast-feed have a reduced risk of some forms of cancer. Breast-feeding promotes family bonding. Breast-feeding saves the expense of formula and the environmental waste created by formula bottles and cans.
42. (List two:) Before four months of age, infants have trouble swallowing solid foods. Their immature GI tracts can absorb whole proteins instead of amino acids, which increases risks of developing allergies. Infants' kidneys are immature and cannot handle the increased load of excreting wastes generated by solid foods, which can lead to dehydration.
43. (Describe two:) lack of teeth, messy eating habits, developing independence, short attention span, picky eating (Suggestions are student response. See pages 199-200 in the text.)

Breast Milk vs. Formula

Name_____ **Date** _____ **Period** _____

Complete the chart below by listing your opinions of the advantages and disadvantages of breast-feeding and bottle-feeding.

Breast-Feeding	Bottle-Feeding
Advantages	**Advantages**
Disadvantages	**Disadvantages**

© Goodheart-Willcox

Food Label for Children

Serving size: based on the average amount children usually eat at one time.

Total fat: listed only as total fat. Parents and caregivers should not try to limit fat, saturated fat, or cholesterol.

Daily Values: Daily Values for protein and some vitamins and minerals are listed on the food label. Fat, cholesterol, sodium, and fiber have no Daily Values because they have not been set for children under the age of four.

Nutrition Facts

Serving Size 1/4 cup (15g)
Servings Per Container   About 30

Amount Per Serving

Calories 60

Total Fat	1g
Sodium	0mg
Potassium	50mg
Total Carbohydrate	10g
Fiber	1g
Sugars	0g
Protein	2g

	Infants	Children
% Daily Value	**0-1**	**1-4**
Protein	7%	6%
Vitamin A	0%	0%
Vitamin C	0%	0%
Calcium	15%	10%
Iron	45%	60%
Vitamin E	15%	8%
Thiamin	45%	30%
Riboflavin	45%	30%
Niacin	25%	20%
Phosphorus	15%	10%

© Goodheart-Willcox

Rise and Shine for Breakfast

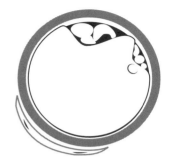

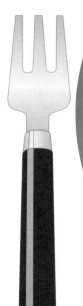

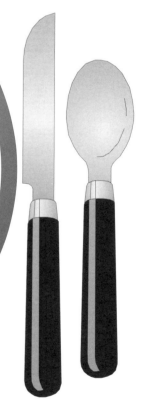

- Get breakfast ready the night before and refrigerate it.

- Eat leftovers from last night's dinner.

- Grab fresh fruit and yogurt.

- Top toast with scrambled egg, cheese, or peanut butter.

- Use a microwave oven to cook single servings— cooked cereal takes three minutes.

© Goodheart-Willcox

Nutrition for All Ages

Name_____

Date _____ Period _____ Score _____

Chapter 11 Test

Matching: Match the following stages with the needs associated with that stage.

_____ 1. Being allowed to choose between two nutritious snacks may help develop a sense of independence.

_____ 2. Body composition changes to include lean muscle development and added weight.

_____ 3. Caregivers need to be concerned about healthy snacks to maintain healthy weight and prevent tooth decay.

_____ 4. Digestive track is immature requiring frequent feedings.

_____ 5. Healthy weight management becomes a challenge as energy needs decrease.

A. adolescence
B. adulthood
C. childhood
D. infancy
E. pregnancy
F. toddlerhood

Matching: Match the following terms and definitions.

_____ 6. An organ inside the uterus through which materials are transferred between the mother and fetus.

_____ 7. A condition existing from birth that limits a person's ability to use his or her body or mind.

_____ 8. One-third of a pregnancy period.

_____ 9. A child that is one to three years old.

_____ 10. The name for a developing human from eight weeks after conception until birth.

_____ 11. A baby born before 35 weeks of pregnancy.

_____ 12. A period of rapid physical growth.

_____ 13. A series of five main stages through which people pass between birth and death.

_____ 14. The period of life between childhood and adulthood.

_____ 15. A child in the first year of life.

A. adolescence
B. congenital disability
C. fetus
D. growth spurt
E. infant
F. life cycle
G. low-birthweight baby
H. placenta
I. premature
J. toddler
K. trimester

True/False: Circle *T* if the statement is true or *F* if the statement is false.

T   F   16. Jack, an 80-year-old male, has the same specific nutritional needs as Jill, an 18-year-old female.

T   F   17. The best time for a woman to attain a healthy weight is after becoming pregnant.

T   F   18. Women who are above or below healthy weight are more likely to experience problems during pregnancy.

T   F   19. When a woman finds out she is pregnant, she should stop her physical fitness program.

(Continued)

© Goodheart-Willcox

● **Name**_____

T   F   20. The negative effects of drug use last longer in the fetus than in the pregnant mother.

T   F   21. Fetal alcohol syndrome can occur in newborns whose mothers drink alcohol while pregnant.

T   F   22. Growth is more rapid during infancy than at any other time in the life cycle.

T   F   23. Proportionately, infants have about the same nutritional needs as those of adults.

T   F   24. The best way to avoid overfeeding a baby is to stop feeding when the infant shows lack of interest in eating.

T   F   25. It is not important to give toddlers snacks because their stomachs are so small.

T   F   26. Children today are more likely to be overweight than their ancestors.

T   F   27. Teens who skip meals tend to have more difficulty concentrating in school.

T   F   28. Eating a healthful diet during the teen years can help prevent health problems during adulthood.

T   F   29. A person's calorie needs increase during adulthood, especially after age 50.

T   F   30. As people age, their ability to absorb some nutrients decreases.

Multiple Choice: Choose the best response. Write the letter in the space provided.

_____ 31. A recommended weight gain for a healthy pregnancy is _____.
     A.   10 to 12 pounds
     B.   15 to 20 pounds
     C.   25 to 35 pounds
     D.   40 to 50 pounds

● _____ 32. A major concern with a teen pregnancy is best represented in which statement?
     A.   Teens with poor nutritional diets do not have the nutrient reserves to meet the needs of a developing fetus.
     B.   Teens are not capable of following a doctor's advice.
     C.   Teens are not able to give adequate love to a newborn.
     D.   All the above.

_____ 33. The serious problem with drug use during pregnancy is drugs can _____.
     A.   increase chances of morning sickness
     B.   affect the mother's appetite
     C.   be passed from the mother's bloodstream through the placenta to the baby
     D.   cause the fetus to stir and move

_____ 34. A pregnant woman may be advised to add which of the following to her diet?
     A.   Caffeine.
     B.   Vitamin and mineral supplements.
     C.   Alcohol.
     D.   Nicotine.

_____ 35. What is usually offered as the first solid food?
     A.   Strained fruits.
     B.   Strained vegetables.
     C.   Strained meats.
     D.   Infant cereals.

● _____ 36. Why are solid foods introduced one at a time?
     A.   To identify allergies.
     B.   To avoid confusing the baby.
     C.   To keep baby's weight normal.
     D.   To cut costs for family.

(Continued)

© Goodheart-Willcox

Name_____

_____37. Which of the following guidelines are used to describe a toddler's daily needs?
   A. Two servings of milk; one serving of meat and beans; one serving of fruits; two servings of vegetables; four servings of cereal or bread.
   B. Four servings of milk; two servings of meat and beans; two servings of fruits; one serving of vegetables; one serving of cereal or bread.
   C. Four servings of milk; two servings of meat and beans; two servings of fruits; three servings of vegetables; six servings of cereal or bread.
   D. Two servings of milk; four servings of meat and beans; four servings of fruits; four servings of vegetables; two servings of cereal or bread.

_____38. A caregiver is planning a snack for her toddler classroom. Which will fit the developing needs of a growing 3-year-old?
   A. Two chocolate chip cookies and a grape drink.
   B. Orange soda and corn chips.
   C. Apple slices and graham crackers.
   D. Milk and a small candy bar.

_____39. A diet lacking in _____ could increase the risk of osteoporosis later in life.
   A. vitamin K
   B. calcium
   C. vitamin A
   D. folate

_____40. Which factor is likely to affect an older adult's ability to maintain healthy nutritional status?
   A. Lack of mobility.
   B. Health of teeth.
   C. Digestive ailments.
   D. All the above.

Essay Questions: Provide complete responses to the following questions or statements.

41. What are four advantages of breast-feeding?

42. What are two reasons caregivers should not add solid foods to infants' diets until they are four to six months of age?

43. Describe two factors that can lead to eating problems during the toddler years and give a suggestion for dealing with each.

© Goodheart-Willcox

The Energy Balancing Act

12

Objectives

After studying this chapter, students will be able to
- describe how the amount of energy in food is measured.
- calculate the three components of their energy expenditure.
- identify the outcomes of energy deficiency and energy excesses.
- use various tools to determine their healthy weight.

Bulletin Board

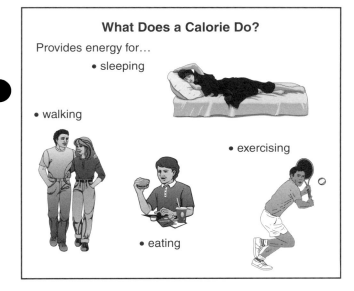

What Does a Calorie Do?

Provides energy for…
- sleeping
- walking
- exercising
- eating

Title: *What Does a Calorie Do?*

Place the title *What Does a Calorie Do?* on the bulletin board. Under the title, place the words *Provides energy for…* followed by a vertical bulleted list using the following words: *sleeping, eating, walking,* and *exercising.* You may also wish to use words for other physical activities. Have students locate magazine pictures that illustrate each of the energy-consuming activities. Attach pictures under the appropriate spaces on the bulletin board.

Title: *Balancing Energy—The Big Picture*

Below the title, place a balance scale made from poster board. Place the words *why, what, when, where,* and *how much you eat* on one side of the balance scale.

On the other side, place the words *BMR, physical activity,* and *thermic effect of food.* Explain to students that this balance indicates weight maintenance.

Teaching Materials

Text, pages 211-224
  Learn the Language
  Check Your Knowledge
  Put Learning into Action
  Explore Further
Student Activity Guide, pages 85-90
  A. *In Balance*
  B. *Calorie Calculations*
  C. *Health Hangs in the Balance*
  D. *Evaluate Your Weight*
  E. *Backtrack Through Chapter 12*
Teacher's Resources
  Everyone Needs Calories! transparency master 12-1
  The Body's #1 Energy Need, transparency master 12-2
  Calories Used for Activities, reproducible master 12-3
  Energy Imbalance, transparency master 12-4
  What Is Healthy Weight, Anyway? transparency master 12-5
  Shape Makes a Difference, color transparency CT-12
  Chapter 12 Test

Introducing the Chapter

1. Write physical activity words (*bicycling, baseball, football*) and food items (*toast, ice cream, corn*) on individual pieces of paper. Put all the papers in a bag. Make sure you have one word for each student. Tell students one side of the room is the "energy in" area and the other side is the "energy out" area. After a student draws a paper out of the bag, have them move to the appropriate side of the room. To represent imbalance, there should either be more food items or activity words in the bag. Ask students what happens when an imbalance occurs and how a balance can be established.
2. Discuss the difference between the "ideal image" defined by the media and society and healthy weight. Healthy weight is a lifetime goal associated with wellness.

3. Show pictures cut from magazines or catalogs of five people of various physical shapes and heights. Number each picture one to five. Include both genders and various physiques. Ask students to silently vote on which person they think is the healthiest. Discuss the reasons for their answers.

Strategies to Reteach, Reinforce, Enrich, and Extend Text Concepts

Energy Input

4. **RT** *Everyone Needs Calories!* transparency master 12-1. Use the transparency to discuss with students the need for calories and the three nutrient groups that provide food energy. As a review, have students suggest foods from each nutrient group.
5. **ER** Have students estimate their recommended calorie intake level. Students should multiply their recommended weight, which can be found in Figure 12-12 in the text, by the following factors: 10 for inactive women and inactive people over the age of 55; 13 for moderately active women, inactive men, and active adults over 55; 15 for moderately active men and active women; or 18 for active men. Tell students these calorie recommendations apply to adults, and people who are still growing will need additional calories.
6. **RF** Discuss with students how the breaking down of food in the body is similar to burning food in a laboratory. Energy is neither created nor destroyed during chemical or physical processes. Food is broken down into simple sugars, which are used to release energy. In the burning process, carbon is left over. In the body, CO_2 and H_2O are left over. Burning of proteins also leaves urea and NH_4 salts.

Energy Output

7. **RF** *The Body's #1 Energy Need,* transparency master 12-2. Use the transparency master to emphasize what BMR is and what factors influence a person's metabolic rate. For each factor, have students provide an example of what makes the BMR faster or slower. Discuss how BMR affects the calorie needs of people.
8. **RF** Discuss how body structure and composition affect how much food a person can eat. Ask students why it is important to accept some unchangeable factors, such as height.
9. **ER** Have several students bring jump ropes to class. Ask volunteer students to jump rope for three minutes. Discuss why they are burning more calories than the students sitting in their seats. Of the rope jumpers, decide who might be burning the most calories.

10. **ER** *Calories Used for Activities,* reproducible master 12-3. Have the students complete an activity diary for one day. Students can record each half hour of activities on the chart and determine the calories used from Chart 12-6 on page 216 of the text. (Remind students that on the chart, calories used are listed *per hour,* so numbers must be divided by 2 to get half-hour totals.) Students should then answer the questions that follow the chart.
11. **RF** *Calorie Calculations,* Activity B, SAG. Students are to complete the worksheet by showing the calculations used to solve problems about energy input and output.

Energy Imbalance

12. **RF** Ask students to describe what happens when they are feeling hungry. Have them visualize the drop in blood glucose and the effects of the body drawing on glycogen stores. When a person is hungry, an energy deficit is occurring. Encourage students to be aware of body needs, a factor often overlooked in weight management.
13. **RT** *Energy Imbalance,* transparency master 12-4. Use the transparency master to explain the consequences of imbalance in calorie intake and expenditure. Remind students that one day's tip of the scale is not the same as a lifestyle of behaviors. Ask students what happens when there is a lifestyle pattern of imbalances over long periods of time. Discuss why lifestyle patterns of imbalance are difficult to reverse.
14. **RF** *Health Hangs in the Balance,* Activity C, SAG. Students are to review concepts about energy imbalance by identifying true and false statements.

Determining Healthy Weight

15. **RF** *What Is Healthy Weight, Anyway?* transparency master 12-5. Discuss why healthy weight, ideal weight, and perfect weight have different definitions. Ask students how weight affects quality of life.
16. **ER** Guest speaker. Invite a health care provider to demonstrate the use of calipers to measure body fat through skin fold tests. Have several students volunteer to undergo the test. Discuss the ranges of body fat percents and what is determined as excess.
17. **RF** *Evaluate Your Weight,* Activity D, SAG. Students are to calculate their BMIs. They are to then answer questions about the status of their weight based on BMI, height-weight tables, and body fat measurement.
18. **ER** Have students look in the Yellow Pages to identify community resources available to assist people who desire to improve their weight.

19. **RF** *Shape Makes a Difference,* color transparency CT-12. Use the transparency to discuss locations where excess fat is stored. Relate body shape to the hereditary tendency to store fat.

Chapter Review

20. **RF** Have each student select one new word they learned in the chapter. Have them write that word on a card. Students can gather in groups of three and play a game. The other two group members must ask the cardholder questions that can be answered with yes or no until they have enough clues to guess the word.
21. **RF** *Backtrack Through Chapter 12,* Activity E, SAG. Students are to provide complete answers to questions and statements that will help them recall, interpret, apply, and practice chapter concepts.
22. **RF** *In Balance,* Activity A, SAG. Students are to fill in the letters that correspond with the described terms. Then they are to arrange the letters to describe the energy balance formula.

Above and Beyond

23. **EX** Have students create posters explaining why energy balance is important and what it takes to maintain an energy balance. Posters can be placed in a community fitness center or nutrition program center.
24. **EX** Have students write a short article for the school newspaper on the role of exercise and calories in maintaining energy balance.

Answer Key

Text

Check Your Knowledge, page 223

1. false
2. One gram of pure carbohydrate or protein yields 4 calories. One gram of pure fat yields 9 calories.
3. secreting hormones, maintaining body temperature, making new cells
4. (List six:) body structure, body composition, gender, internal temperature, external temperature, thyroxine secretion, age, diet, growth
5. (List three. Student response. See page 215 in the text.)
6. Keep an accurate record of all your activities for one typical 24-hour period. Note the amount of time spent on each activity. Multiply the calories used per hour by the number of hours spent doing each activity. Total the number of calories burned for all activities.
7. thermic effect of food
8. because of the potential danger of ketone formation, which changes the acid-base balance of the blood

9. 3,500 calories
10. body mass index (BMI)
11. For men, over 25 percent body fat is considered excessive. For women, over 30 percent body fat is excessive.
12. Fat stored in the abdomen increases the liver's production of low-density lipoproteins, which is a risk factor for heart disease.

Student Activity Guide

In Balance, Activity A

1. calorie density
2. underweight
3. thermic effect of food
4. basal metabolic rate
5. energy
6. sedentary activity
7. basal metabolism
8. bioelectrical impedance
9. ketone bodies
10. skinfold test
11. obese
12. overweight
13. healthy weight
14. body mass index
15. body composition
16. subcutaneous fat
17. ketosis

The Energy Balance Equation: energy in = energy out

Calorie Calculations, Activity B

1. 9 grams × 4 calories per gram = 36 calories from protein
   26 grams × 4 calories per gram = 104 calories from carbohydrate
2. 260 grams × 4 calories per gram = 1040 calories from carbohydrates
   75 grams × 9 calories per gram = 675 calories from fat
   60 grams × 4 calories per gram = 240 calories from protein
   1040 + 675 + 240 = 1,955 total calories
   675 calories from fat ÷ 1,955 total calories = 0.345
       No, you are not following your doctor's advice because about 35 percent of your calories are coming from fat.
3. chicken sandwich: 540 calories ÷ 248 grams = 2.18 calories per gram
   bacon cheeseburger: 460 calories ÷ 159 grams = 2.89 calories per gram
   The double bacon cheeseburger is more calorie dense.
4. 175 pounds × 0.5 calories per pound = 87.5 calories per hour
   87.5 calories per hour × 24 hours = 2,100 calories per day for basal energy needs

5. strenuous activity—running: 1 hour × 350 calories per hour = 350 calories

   sedentary activities—eating, reading: 1 hour × 90 calories per hour = 90 calories

   light activities—doing dishes, grooming: 1 hour × 135 calories per hour = 135 calories

   vigorous activities—yard work: 2 hours × 300 calories per hour = 600 calories

   350 + 90 + 135 + 600 = 1,175 total calories

6. basal metabolism: 2,400 total calories × .60 = 1,440; 2,400 total calories × .65 = 1,560 calories

   physical activity: 2,400 total calories × .25 = 600 calories; 2,400 total calories × .35 = 840 calorie

   thermic effect of food: 2,400 total calories × .05 = 120 calories; 2,400 total calories × .10 = 240 calories

   Stephanie burns approximately 1,440 to 1,560 calories per day for basal metabolism. She burns 600 to 840 calories per day for physical activity. She burns 120 to 240 calories per day for the thermic effect of food.

Health Hangs in the Balance, Activity C

1.	T	12.	T
2.	F	13.	F
3.	T	14.	T
4.	F	15.	F
5.	T	16.	T
6.	F	17.	T
7.	T	18.	T
8.	F	19.	F
9.	F	20.	T
10.	F	21.	T
11.	T	22.	T

Backtrack Through Chapter 12, Activity E

1. chemical
2. carbohydrates, fats, proteins
3. basal metabolism, physical activity, thermic effect of food
4. digestive system
5. thyroxine
6. muscle movement, breathing harder, pumping more blood
7. (List five:) watching television, studying, working in an office, driving, using a computer, reading, eating, sewing, playing cards, other sitting activities
8. thermic effect of food
9. The body draws on liver glycogen stores.
10. Healthy body weight is the weight at which a person's body fat is in an appropriate proportion to his or her lean tissue.
11. (List one:) They are not precise. They are not designed for people under age 19. They do not take into account body composition or individual health risks.

12. about 50 percent
13. Water yields no energy, whereas fats are a concentrated source of energy. Therefore, when a large percentage of a food's weight is due to water content, the food will have a low calorie density. However, when a large percentage of a food's weight is due to fat content, the food will have a high calorie density.
14. The larger the body size, the greater the amount of energy needed to make the muscles work.
15. to lose or gain weight
16. Consuming just a few excess calories each day can result in pounds of excess weight over a period of years. Excess weight due to body fat increases the risks of a number of health problems.
17. Fat around the waist increases the liver's production of low-density lipoproteins, which is a risk factor for heart disease. Thus, fat stored in the abdomen seems to pose a greater risk than fat stored in the buttocks, hips, and thighs.
18. (Student response.)
19. (Student response.)
20. The Swansons have a BMI of 24. This puts Mrs. Swanson within the healthy weight range for adults. However, recommended BMI cutoffs for children and adolescents vary according to age and sex. Therefore, although a BMI of 24 is within the healthy range for Janet, this BMI puts Jake in the at-risk category.

Teacher's Resources

Chapter 12 Test

1.	C	9.	F	17.	F	25.	T
2.	A	10.	F	18.	T	26.	D
3.	G	11.	F	19.	T	27.	B
4.	D	12.	T	20.	F	28.	A
5.	E	13.	F	21.	T	29.	B
6.	I	14.	T	22.	F	30.	A
7.	B	15.	F	23.	T	31.	D
8.	F	16.	T	24.	F	32.	A

33. (List four:) Take stairs instead of riding in an elevator. Swing your arms when walking. Stand rather than sit when waiting for someone. Walk or ride a bicycle instead of riding in a car. Park the car away from your destination and walk the last few blocks. (Students may justify other responses.)
34. A. $(170 \div 65^2) \times 705 = 28$

    B. overweight
35. (List three:) height-weight charts, BMI, calipers for skinfold test, bioelectrical impedance to measure current flow through lean and fat tissues

Everyone Needs Calories!

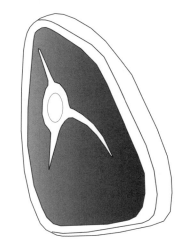

**Protein =
4 calories per gram**

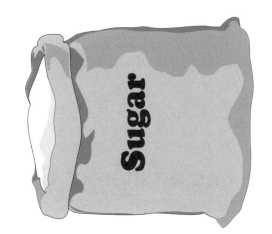

**Carbohydrates =
4 calories per gram**

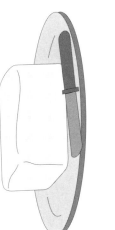

**Fat =
9 calories per gram**

© Goodheart-Willcox

The Body's #1 Energy Need

Basal metabolism is the amount of energy required to support the operation of all internal body systems except digestion.

BMR is the rate at which the body uses energy for basal metabolism. It depends on
- body structure
- body composition
- gender
- temperature (internal and external)
- thyroid
- age
- diet
- growth

Everyone has a different BMR!

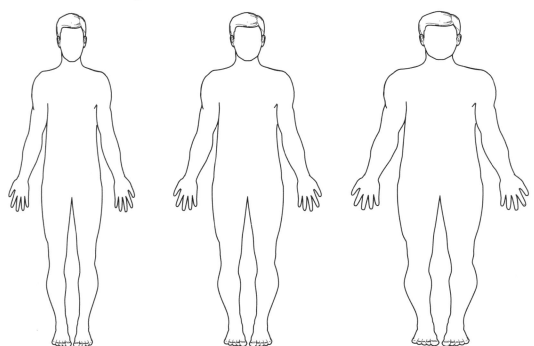

© Goodheart-Willcox

Calories Used for Activities

Name_____ Date _____ Period _____

Record your activities for one day in one-half hour blocks of time. Use Chart 12-6 on page 216 of the text to determine calories used for each activity. (Use the higher figures in the range for large body frames and lower figure in the range for small body frames.) Determine total number of activity calories burned. Then answer the questions that follow.

Time	Activity	Calories	Time	Activity	Calories
12:00 AM			12:00 PM		
12:30			12:30		
1:00			1:00		
1:30			1:30		
2:00			2:00		
2:30			2:30		
3:00			3:00		
3:30			3:30		
4:00			4:00		
4:30			4:30		
5:00			5:00		
5:30			5:30		
6:00			6:00		
6:30			6:30		
7:00			7:00		
7:30			7:30		
8:00			8:00		
8:30			8:30		
9:00			9:00		
9:30			9:30		
10:00			10:00		
10:30			10:30		
11:00			11:00		
11:30			11:30		
Total Calories Used					

1. Were the majority of your activities for the day sedentary, light, moderate, vigorous, or strenuous? _____

2. Were there times when you could have chosen activities that would burn more calories? When? _____
_____

3. What activities could you work into your schedule that would burn more calories? _____
_____

4. How does this day's analysis influence your activity goals for the future? _____
_____
_____

© Goodheart-Willcox

Energy Imbalance

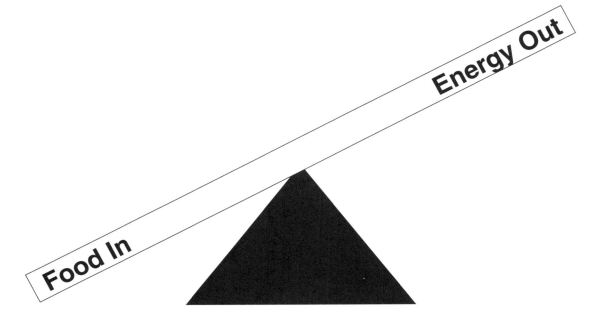

Calorie Excess

Energy in is greater than energy need. Weight will be gained.

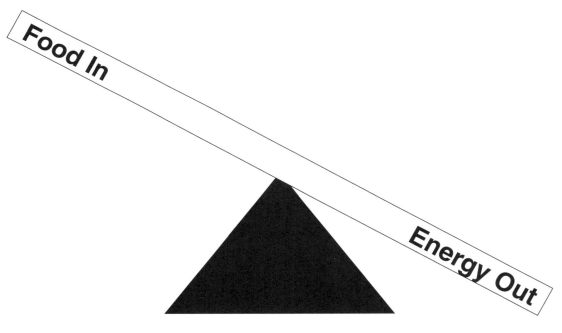

Calorie Deficit

Energy in is less than energy need. Weight will be lost.

© Goodheart-Willcox

What Is Healthy Weight, Anyway?

- the weight that is best for the person
- a range that is statistically related to good health
- a weight in which risk of diseases is reduced
- an appropriate proportion of body fat to lean mass
- a weight at which a person feels healthy and can function effectively to achieve life goals

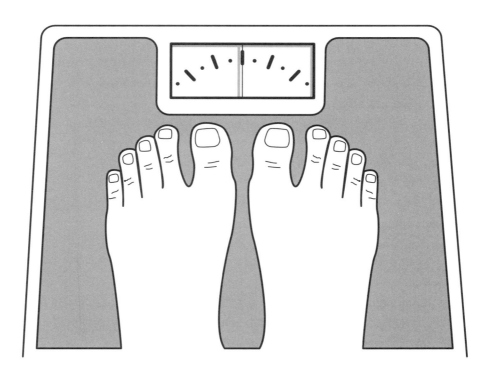

The Energy Balancing Act

Name_____

Date _____ Period _____ Score _____

Chapter 12 Test

Matching: Match the following terms and identifying phrases.

_____ 1. A calculation of body weight and height used to evaluate weight.

_____ 2. Energy required for the operation of all internal systems except digestion.

_____ 3. Activities that require much sitting.

_____ 4. The ability to do work.

_____ 5. A BMI of 18.5 to 24.9.

_____ 6. Fat that lies underneath the skin.

_____ 7. Method for measuring body fat using the body's resistance to a low-energy electrical current.

_____ 8. A BMI of 25 to 29.9.

A. basal metabolism
B. bioelectrical impedance
C. body mass index
D. energy
E. healthy weight
F. overweight
G. sedentary
H. skinfold test
I. subcutaneous

True/False: Circle *T* if the statement is true or *F* if the statement is false.

T   F   9. When energy supplied in foods is greater than the energy needs of the body, a person loses weight.

T   F   10. For most people in the United States, the majority of daily calories comes from proteins.

T   F   11. The bomb calorimeter is used to measure the weight of a food after it is cooked.

T   F   12. Foods high in fat are also calorie dense.

T   F   13. Women need more calories per pound of body weight per hour to support basal metabolism than men do.

T   F   14. Jim, who is tall, has a higher BMR than Jane, who is short.

T   F   15. The less active a person is, the more calories he or she expends.

T   F   16. Basal metabolism keeps your body alive when it is at rest.

T   F   17. All the factors that impact BMR can be changed.

T   F   18. Energy output varies depending on body size.

T   F   19. Calories burned during an activity can be measured by comparing oxygen intake and carbon dioxide output.

T   F   20. For most people, approximately 75 percent of energy output is for physical activity.

T   F   21. People who are trying to lose weight intentionally create an energy imbalance.

T   F   22. The nervous system can use fat as a fuel source.

T   F   23. Ketosis can be harmful because it changes the acid-base balance of the blood.

T   F   24. Height-weight tables take body composition and individual health risks into account.

T   F   25. Excess fat stored around the abdomen poses a greater health risk than excess fat stored around the hip area.

(Continued)

© Goodheart-Willcox

Name_____

Multiple Choice: Choose the best response. Write the letter in the space provided.

_____26. How is the number of calories in a food measured?
  A. By weighing the food before and after dehydration.
  B. By measuring the density of the food.
  C. By adding chemicals to the food to measure change.
  D. By measuring the amount of heat produced when the food is burned.

_____27. The hormone thyroxine affects _____.
  A. calorimetric measures
  B. BMR
  C. BMI
  D. ketone stores

_____28. Which factor increases BMR?
  A. Pregnancy.
  B. Personality.
  C. Intake of B-vitamins.
  D. Food likes and dislikes.

_____29. If Carmen's basal energy needs and physical activity needs amount to 2,000 daily calories, what are her needs for thermic effect of food?
  A. 2,000 calories.
  B. 200 calories.
  C. 20 calories.
  D. None of the above.

_____30. When carbohydrates are not available to the body, what will happen?
  A. The body will slowly begin to convert fatty acids into ketone bodies for energy needs.
  B. The body will obtain glucose from fat.
  C. An energy excess will occur.
  D. Muscles will expand and become stronger.

_____31. Measuring thickness of skinfolds of subcutaneous fat is done with a device called _____.
  A. bioelectrical impedance
  B. indirect calorimetry
  C. a bomb calorimeter
  D. a caliper

_____32. Which of the following is most likely to have a "pear-shaped" body?
  A. Young women.
  B. Young men.
  C. Older women.
  D. Older men.

Essay Questions: Provide complete responses to the following questions or statements.

33. List four examples of how someone might complete daily tasks in more energy-intensive ways.

34. A. Compute body mass index for Ben, who weighs 170 pounds and is 65 inches tall. The formula for BMI is (weight ÷ height^2) × 705.

   B. In what range is Ben's BMI?

35. List three methods that can be used to determine if a person is within a healthy weight range.

© Goodheart-Willcox

Healthy Weight Management

13

Objectives

After studying this chapter, students will be able to
- describe health risks of obesity and underweight.
- recognize factors that influence a person's weight status.
- estimate their daily calorie needs and their daily calorie intake.
- state why some rapid weight-loss plans are dangerous and ineffective.
- explain guidelines for safe loss of body fat.
- list tips for safe weight gain.

Bulletin Board

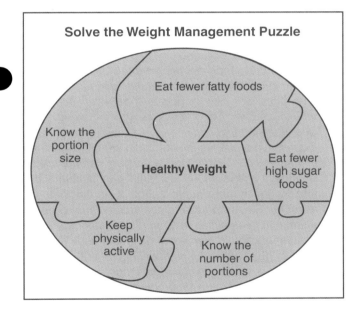

Solve the Weight Management Puzzle

Eat fewer fatty foods

Know the portion size

Healthy Weight

Eat fewer high sugar foods

Keep physically active

Know the number of portions

Title: *Solve the Weight Management Puzzle*

Cut a circle out of posterboard. Cut the circle into six "puzzle pieces." Place in the center the words *healthy weight.* In the outer puzzle pieces, place words that contribute to healthy weight maintenance: *eat fewer fatty foods, know the number of portions; know the portion size; keep physically active;* and *eat fewer high sugar foods.*

Title: *Health Comes in Different Shapes and Sizes*

Cut pictures from magazines of people with various body shapes and sizes and hang them on the bulletin board. Discuss with students which of the people seem to be at a healthy weight.

Teaching Materials

Text, pages 225-242
> *Learn the Language*
> *Check Your Knowledge*
> *Put Learning into Action*
> *Explore Further*

Student Activity Guide, pages 91-98
> A. *Weigh the Risks*
> B. *Facts and Factors*
> C. *The Math of Weight Loss*
> D. *Believe It or Not?*
> E. *In the Driver's Seat*
> F. *Backtrack Through Chapter 13*

Teacher's Resources
> *Health Risks of Obesity,* transparency master 13-1
> *Questions to Ask About Weight Management Programs,* reproducible master 13-2
> *Lowfat May Not Mean Low Calorie,* color transparency CT-13
> *Food Diary,* reproducible master 13-3
> Chapter 13 Test

Introducing the Chapter

1. Ask students why society places so much emphasis on the tall, thin body build as the ideal. Does an ideal type really exist? How does the image of "ideal type" affect people who can never fit that image? What makes a person healthy?
2. Ask a student to walk around the room several times carrying a 10-pound sack of sand or flour. The sack represents excess body fat. Ask the student to describe what seems to be happening to his or her body while carrying the extra weight. Discuss how excess fat can affect heart health.
3. Refer to The Dietary Guidelines for Americans. Read the guideline that states "Balance the food you eat with physical activity—maintain or improve your weight." Discuss why this guideline is necessary for Americans today.
4. Have students brainstorm reasons so many Americans have difficulty maintaining weight over the life span. List the ideas on the board and discuss.

Strategies to Reteach, Reinforce, Enrich, and Extend Text Concepts

Healthy People Need a Healthy Weight

5. **RT** Have each student write a definition of *healthy weight*. Have students read their definitions to the class. Discuss any misconceptions.

6. **RF** Review the conflicting influences in society that encourage people to overeat, yet place value on being thin. One example would be the media, which advertises high-calorie food with underweight models. Another might be family members who offer people dessert while complimenting them on losing weight. Ask students how this dilemma affects individuals who struggle with poor body image.

7. **RF** *Health Risks of Obesity,* transparency master 13-1. Use the transparency master to highlight the potential for health risks related to overweight. Refer students to Figure 12-10 to review the BMIs for defining overweight and obesity.

8. **EX** Have students debate the pros and cons of the expression "A person can never be too thin or too rich." Review the health risks associated with underweight.

9. **RF** *Weigh the Risks,* Activity A, SAG. Students are to determine if listed health risks are risks of being underweight, overweight, or both. Then students are to write a paragraph about the risk of most interest to them.

Factors Affecting Your Weight Status

10. **RF** *Facts and Factors,* Activity B, SAG. Students are to determine which statements are true and which are false. Students should change the underlined word in false statements to make them true.

11. **ER** Guest speakers. Invite a panel of guests who have successfully lost weight to discuss the factors that related to their gaining excess weight. What methods were successful in helping them achieve a healthier weight?

12. **EX** Have students debate which is easier for most people: reducing calorie intake or increasing activity levels. Have students justify their responses.

Losing Excess Body Fat

13. **ER** *The Math of Weight Loss,* Activity C, SAG. Students are to use mathematical formulas presented in the chapter to solve the problems in each situation.

14. **ER** Guest speaker. Invite a dietitian or medical professional to discuss treatment for obese patients. Discuss the dangers of rapid weight loss, weight loss gimmicks, and fad diets. Discuss the successful methods for safe weight loss.

15. **RF** *Believe It or Not?* Activity D, SAG. Students are to evaluate each of the weight-loss claims in the activity. Students will indicate if they believe each claim and write statements to support their responses.

16. **RF** Discuss why people want to believe in fad diets. What effects does advertising have on people's wellness choices? What clues are available to indicate the claims are not reliable? What agencies are responsible for regulating misinformation?

17. **EX** *Questions to Ask About Weight Management Programs,* reproducible master 13-2. Students are to evaluate a weight management program by answering given questions.

18. **RF** *Lowfat May Not Mean Low Calorie,* CT-13. Use the transparency to discuss how to watch calorie intake in addition to fat intake. Discuss which foods are naturally low in fats and which foods are higher in calories.

19. **ER** Ask students to make two lists. See how many foods they can name that are less than 80 calories per serving and how many foods they can name that are more than 120 calories per serving.

20. **RF** *Food Diary,* reproducible master 13-3. Give each student three copies of the handout so they can complete food diaries for three days. Students are to record the foods they ate, amounts eaten, time, location, people present, activity, and mood while eating. They should then answer the questions that follow.

21. **ER** Have students list common snack foods they regularly include in their diets. Have sample snack wrappers available so students can evaluate the snacks for nutrient content. Focus on calories per serving, fats, saturated fats, calcium, iron, protein, vitamin A, vitamin C, and sodium. Have students determine how many servings of the food would it take to get 100% of a vitamin or mineral. Discuss alternative snacks that will add more nutrients and fewer calories to the food choice.

22. **ER** Collect take-out menus from several restaurants. Have students study the menus and select items that are lower in calories and fat. Then have students prepare a list of recommendations for anyone planning to dine out while trying to lose weight.

Gaining Weight

23. **RF** Discuss why some people may want to gain weight. What factors contribute to underweight? What are the social and health issues faced by teens who think they are too thin? Have students think of ways to add extra calories needed to build body mass.

24. **ER** Bring in a sample of health food products that are intended to increase body size. Read the ingredients label. Have students prepare a research report on the safety and effectiveness of the product. Students may want to write to the company to ask for data that supports the product.

Chapter Review

25. **RF** *In the Driver's Seat,* Activity E, SAG. Students are to determine if given statements are good or bad advice about weight loss and explain why.
26. **RF** *Backtrack Through Chapter 13,* Activity F, SAG. Students are to provide complete answers to questions and statements that will help them recall, interpret, apply, and practice chapter concepts.
27. **EX** Have each student write a question related to healthy weight management. Collect all the questions and put them in a box. Have students draw questions from the box at random and research responses for the questions.

Above and Beyond

28. **EX** Have students plan a workshop for healthy weight management. Invite other classes to attend the event. The workshop could include student handouts, an audio-visual corner, consultants such as dietitians, and samples of low-fat snacks.
29. **EX** Divide students into groups. Have each group prepare a poster that focuses on the evaluation of popular fad diets and products. Have students identify clues that indicate the diet or product is unreliable. Place the posters around the school.

Answer Key

Text

Check Your Knowledge, page 241

1. true
2. (List five:) high blood pressure, coronary heart disease, stroke, diabetes, arthritis, respiratory problems, certain types of cancer, accidents, problems during surgery, problems during pregnancy
3. (List two:) problems during pregnancy, problems after surgery, feelings of fatigue, difficulty staying warm, cessation of menstruation
4. The size of bones and the location of fat stores in the body are inherited traits. Heredity also affects basal metabolic rate.
5. parents or guardians
6. 1,440 + (7.3 × 160) = 2,608 calories
7. In a food diary, list all foods and beverages consumed. Use food composition tables or diet analysis software to find the calorie values of each food listed. Add the totals for each day. Then add the daily totals and divide by the number of days to find the average.
8. During a fast, the body will slowly begin to break down lean tissues, including muscles and organs, to produce energy. The body can also go into ketosis, which affects the acid-base balance of the blood.
9. (List two:) Very low calorie diets trigger the body to lower BMR, which makes it harder to lose weight. Fad diets give people no control over their food choices. Fad diets require eating patterns that are radically different from most people's normal eating habits. Fad diets teach people nothing about better eating behaviors to help them maintain their new weight.
10. maintain weight while continuing to grow
11. time of day, where you eat, who you are with, what you are doing, how you are feeling
12. (List five. Student response. See pages 233-238 in the text.)
13. 700 to 1,000 extra calories
14. (List three. Student response. See pages 239-240 in the text.)

Student Activity Guide

Weigh the Risks, Activity A

Underweight: F, G, I, J, K, M, O
Overweight: A, B, C, D, E, H, L, M, N, O
(Summary is student response.)

Facts and Factors, Activity B

1. status
2. true
3. true
4. true
5. does not
6. harder
7. true
8. true
9. true
10. high
11. true
12. true
13. on the go
14. true
15. environmental
16. is
17. emotional
18. true
19. out
20. inactive

The Math of Weight Loss, Activity C

1. Answer: 2,462 calories.
   Explanation: 1,440 + (7.3 × 140) = 2,462

2. Answer: Salena.
   Explanation: (Serena) $960 + (3.8 \times 125) = 1,435$
   (Salena) $1,120 + (4.5 \times 145) = 1,772.5$
3. Answer: 10 days. Explanation: $3,500 \div 350 = 10$
4. Answer: deficit of 375 calories.
   Explanation: $3,500 \times 3 = 10,500 \div 28 = 375$.
       Yes, that is a safe goal because 375 calories is within the recommended range of 250 to 500.
5. Answer: greater. Explanation: $1,120 + (4.5 \times 135) = 1,727.5; 2,100 > 1,727.5$.

Believe It or Not? Activity D

1. NOT: unrealistic promises of rapid weight loss, fad diet lacking in variety, no control over food choices, radically different eating pattern
2. BELIEVE IT: promotes lifestyle changes rather than miracle cures; uses dietitians and fitness experts; emphasizes planning and health
3. NOT: unrealistic promise; pills can have harmful side effects
4. NOT: fad diet lacking in variety; no control over food choices; unsupported claims; radically different eating pattern
5. NOT: weight-loss gimmick, it is doubtful anyone could achieve the advertised results
6. BELIEVE IT: if claims are true that doctors have tested, may be worth investigating; use of term *management* instead of *loss* implies self-control in learning new eating patterns; offers encouragement; offers education; features exercise
       (Note: For each question, there are other acceptable reasons for responses.)

In the Driver's Seat, Activity E

1. BA
2. GA
3. GA
4. GA
5. BA
6. GA
7. BA
8. GA
9. GA
10. BA
11. BA
12. GA
13. GA
14. GA
15. BA
16. BA
17. GA
18. GA
19. GA
20. BA
21. GA
22. BA
23. GA
24. GA
25. GA

(Reasons are student response.)

Backtrack Through Chapter 13, Activity F

1. attaining healthy weight and keeping it throughout life
2. over 50 percent
3. because of the health risks associated with obesity
4. (List three. See page 226 in the text.)
5. heredity, eating habits, activity level
6. (List three:) sight, smell, and taste of foods; time of day, and social settings
7. 3,500
8. 250 to 500
9. increase

10. A fad diet is an eating plan that is popular for a short time because it promises rapid weight loss. A crash diet is a weight-loss plan that provides fewer than 1,200 calories per day.
11. a lifelong pattern of weight gain and loss; also called yo-yo diet syndrome
12. 1 to 2 pounds
13. The extra fluids might make the person feel full, causing him or her to consume fewer calories at the meal.
14. (List two:) fatigue, irritability, nausea, digestive upsets, problems with digestion, problems with heartbeat rhythm, problems with the acid level of the blood, lack of needed calories and nutrients
15. burning fewer calories than you consume
16. The FDA takes action only when false claims are made about particular products or foods. Many misleading weight-loss schemes do not fit into that category.
17. body breakdown of lean tissues, muscles, and organs to produce energy; conversion of fatty acids from body fat into ketone bodies, producing an abnormal buildup of ketone bodies; abnormal acid-base balance of the blood
18. (Suggest five. See pages 239 and 240 in the text.)
19. (Student response.)
20. (Student response.)

Teacher's Resources

Chapter 13 Test

1. G
2. E
3. B
4. C
5. F
6. D
7. F
8. F
9. T
10. T
11. F
12. T
13. T
14. T
15. F
16. T
17. F
18. T
19. C
20. A
21. C
22. D
23. C
24. B
25. B
26. D
27. A
28. A

29. Sonja wants to lose five pounds. For each pound, she must create an energy deficit of 3,500 calories. Her total calorie deficit will be 17,500 calories. She will be losing the weight gradually over a period of four weeks, or 28 days. Sonja will have to cut her daily calorie consumption by 625 calories to reach her goal.
30. Crash diets usually involve eating patterns that are radically different from normal eating patterns. This eventually leads to people giving up the diet because they miss the foods they are used to eating. Following the diet, people eat more than before because they feel starved and deprived of food. Some people gain more weight than they lost by dieting. Discouragement over the lack of success in maintaining weight loss causes them to try another crash diet.
31. (List six. Student response. See pages 237-238 in the text.)

Health Risks of Obesity

- High blood pressure

- Coronary heart disease and stroke

- Type II diabetes

- Pressure on the joints—arthritis and gout

- Breathing complications

- Some forms of cancer

- More accidents due to loss of agility

- Increased health risks during pregnancy

- Hernia

- Gallbladder disease

Reproducible Master 13-2

Questions to Ask About Weight Management Programs

Name_____   Date _____   Period _____

Find a weight management program advertised in a magazine. Evaluate it by checking *yes* or *no* to the following criteria. Then answer the questions that follow.

Name of program: _____

Yes   No

_____ _____   1. Does the program provide all the nutrients needed by the body?

_____ _____   2. Are a variety of food choices offered?

_____ _____   3. Would the diet keep you from being hungry or unusually tired?

_____ _____   4. Would you be able to order food in a restaurant comfortably while following this program?

_____ _____   5. Does the program include foods from all the groups of the MyPyramid system?

_____ _____   6. Does the program promote weight loss without the use of diet pills?

_____ _____   7. Does the program promote losing weight slowly?

_____ _____   8. Does the program include physical activity?

_____ _____   9. Will the program help you change your eating habits?

_____ _____ 10. Will the program help you succeed in losing weight without jeopardizing your health?

Questions:

1. Based on your answers above, do you believe the program would be effective? Why or why not? _____
   _____

2. Do you think the program is safe? Why or why not? _____
   _____

3. Would you recommend this program to a friend who wants to lose weight? Why or why not? _____
   _____

4. How could the program be improved? _____
   _____
   _____
   _____
   _____
   _____
   _____
   _____
   _____
   _____

© Goodheart-Willcox

Food Diary

Name_____ **Date** _____ **Period** _____

Keep a food diary for three days. Evaluate your eating habits by answering the questions.

Meal	Amount	Food	Time	Location	People Present	Activity	Mood

1. Analyze your food diary. When, if ever, did you eat more than you really wanted or needed? _____
   _____

2. Why do you think you might have eaten more at those particular times? _____
   _____

3. How many times did you snack? _____
   From which food group did most of your snacks come? _____

4. In what ways might you want to change your eating habits?_____
   _____
   _____
   _____
   _____

© Goodheart-Willcox

Healthy Weight Management

Name_____

Date _____ Period _____ Score _____

Chapter 13 Test

Matching: Match the following terms and identifying phrases.

_____ 1. Attaining healthy weight and keeping it throughout life.

_____ 2. A routine behavior that is often difficult to break.

_____ 3. An event or situation that triggers a person to eat.

_____ 4. Eating plan promising rapid weight loss that is popular for a short time.

_____ 5. A lifelong pattern of weight gain and loss.

_____ 6. Refraining from consuming most or all sources of calories.

A. crash diet

B. environmental cue

C. fad diet

D. fasting

E. habit

F. weight cycling

G. weight management

True/False: Circle *T* if the statement is true and *F* if the statement is false.

T F   7. All people who are overweight have excess body fat.

T F   8. There are no associated health risks with underweight.

T F   9. The more excess fat a person carries, the greater the health risks.

T F   10. Obesity can be a source of social and emotional problems as well as physical ones.

T F   11. A family history of obesity means a person is destined to be obese.

T F   12. Children who develop eating behaviors based on good nutrition are more likely to practice healthful eating habits throughout life.

T F   13. A certain time of day can be an environmental cue.

T F   14. Eating habits can be responses to psychological factors.

T F   15. The less active you are, the more calories you need for energy.

T F   16. People who are most likely to succeed in a weight management plan are those who receive encouragement.

T F   17. A person should attempt to lose no more than 8 to 10 pounds a week.

T F   18. Like weight loss, weight gain requires a management plan.

Multiple Choice: Choose the best response. Write the letter in the space provided.

_____19. Which of the following is *not* an example of an environmental cue?
   A. Sampling food from a buffet table at a party.
   B. Buying a hot dog from a vendor at a baseball game.
   C. Eating when you are hungry.
   D. Eating a snack every day after school.

Name_____

_____20. The main goal of weight management is _____.
   A. good health
   B. a slim appearance
   C. to become popular
   D. to achieve a sports goal

_____21. How many calories must be burned before one pound (0.45 kg) of body fat is lost?
   A. 35.
   B. 350.
   C. 3,500.
   D. 35,000.

_____22. An ad claims, "This pill taken with our diet supplement plan will help you lose 30 pounds in one month." This is an example of _____.
   A. an effective diet plan
   B. a pill that can help burn off body fat
   C. a diet approved by the American Dietetic Association
   D. a fad diet

_____23. Of the following factors, which is the best explanation for poor results of a fad diet?
   A. Lack of support from friends.
   B. A weight loss plan is too expensive to maintain after weight is lost.
   C. After weight is lost, a return to former eating patterns results in weight gain.
   D. Genetic factors cause people to regain weight that was lost.

_____24. People who lose weight slowly _____.
   A. are not going to lose enough to reach a healthy weight
   B. are more likely to maintain a healthy weight once they reach it
   C. don't really care about losing weight
   D. aren't following the MyPyramid system

_____25. A habit change should _____.
   A. punish you for failing to maintain a healthy weight
   B. help you plan permanent actions to change eating and activity habits
   C. be a temporary change that will help you lose a few pounds
   D. make you feel guilty for making poor lifestyle choices

_____26. Which eating habit change is likely to help you lose weight?
   A. Watching more TV talk shows on how to lose weight.
   B. Eating high-fat foods only when emotionally upset.
   C. Skipping meals to reduce calorie intake.
   D. Recognizing moods that cause you to overeat.

_____27. Which of the following groups should focus on increased physical activity without reducing calorie intake from nutritious foods when trying to lose weight?
   A. Teens.
   B. Young adults.
   C. Older adults.
   D. None of the above.

(Continued)

© Goodheart-Willcox

Name_____

_____28. A healthful tip for someone trying to gain weight is to _____.
   A.   eat bigger, more frequent meals
   B.   eat more bulky low-calorie foods such as salads
   C.   eat snacks high in saturated fats
   D.   drink extra fluids with meals

Essay Questions: Provide complete responses to the following questions or statements.

29. Sonja wants to lose five pounds in four weeks. Assuming she is not changing her activity level, how many calories must Sonja cut out of her daily diet to reach her goal?

30. Explain how crash diets can lead to weight cycling.

31. List six tips that would help a person lose weight.

© Goodheart-Willcox

Eating Disorders 14

Objectives

After studying this chapter, students will be able to
- identify characteristics and health risks associated with three common eating disorders.
- analyze possible causes of eating disorders.
- describe sources of help for people with eating disorders.

Bulletin Board

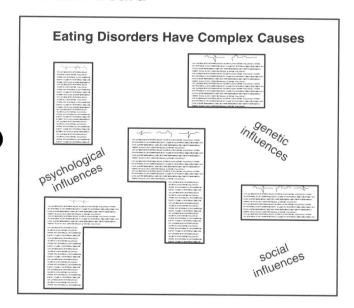

Eating Disorders Have Complex Causes

Title: *Eating Disorders Have Complex Causes*

Cut out newspaper articles about people who have eating disorders. Attach the articles to the bulletin board. Around the articles, randomly arrange the words *social influences, psychological influences,* and *genetic influences.* Relate these to the multiple causes of eating disorders.

Title: *Is Good Health in Style?*

Cut out pictures from magazines of people with healthy body weights. Place them on one side of the bulletin board. Then cut out pictures featuring very thin popular models. Place them on the other side of the bulletin board. Have students compare the appearance of the people in all the pictures. Discuss with students how the media promotes popularity of the models and how this popularity reflects on adolescents.

Teaching Materials

Text, pages 243-254
Learn the Language
Check Your Knowledge
Put Learning into Action
Explore Further

Student Activity Guide, pages 99-104
A. *Read the Warning Signs*
B. *Help for Eating Disorders*
C. *Evaluating Theories*
D. *Backtrack Through Chapter 14*

Teacher's Resources
Symptoms of Anorexia Nervosa, transparency master 14-1
Positive Reflections—Steps to Accepting Your Body, transparency master 14-2
Words of Self-Affirmation, color transparency CT-14
Thoughts About My Eating Behaviors, reproducible master 14-3
Chapter 14 Test

Introducing the Chapter

1. Have students privately pick a number between one and ten that indicates their degree of satisfaction with their body image. (One represents low body image and ten represents high body image.) Do not ask students to share their responses. Discuss with students why they think many people are not completely satisfied with their body image.
2. Have students look at pictures of models for several minutes. Use images of heavily muscled male models for males and very thin female models for the females. Ask students to privately write feelings they have about themselves in relation to the models. Then ask students to again score their satisfaction with body image. Ask for volunteers to share their thoughts. Determine how many students scored themselves lower after seeing the pictures of models.
3. Review the difference between an eating disorder and an eating problem. Stress that a person with an eating disorder has a condition they cannot change without the help of medical and psychological counseling. A person with an eating problem has a temporary difficulty, usually due to unusual circumstances, with maintaining a healthy eating pattern.

Strategies to Reteach, Reinforce, Enrich, and Extend Text Concepts

Characteristics of Eating Disorders

4. **RT** *Symptoms of Anorexia Nervosa,* transparency master 14-1. Use the transparency master to discuss the dangers of anorexia nervosa.

5. **RF** Have students develop a chart describing the similarities and differences of characteristics associated with anorexia nervosa, bulimia nervosa, and binge eating disorder.

6. **ER** Guest speaker. Ask a professional counselor from a local clinic to speak to the class about symptoms of eating disorders.

7. **RF** *Read the Warning Signs,* Activity A, SAG. Students are to determine if given characteristics are associated with bulimia nervosa, anorexia nervosa, or binge eating disorder.

Probable Causes of Eating Disorders

8. **ER** Have students form small groups. Ask them to discuss factors that decrease self-image. Ask how these factors affect school performance, relationships, and personal satisfaction with life. Have each group determine one method they could use to help a person build a positive self-image.

9. **RT** *Positive Reflections—Steps to Accepting Your Body,* transparency master 14-2. Use the transparency to encourage students to appreciate their uniqueness.

10. **ER** Have students role-play situations in which feelings of guilt, low self-esteem, depression, and anxiety affect eating patterns. Discuss how long-term effects of emotions on eating behaviors might lead to eating disorders.

11. **EX** *Evaluating Theories,* Activity C, SAG. Students are to evaluate three theories about the causes of eating disorders. They will then write conclusions they have drawn from their evaluations.

12. **RF** Have students think of experiences when they felt pressure to look thinner. Discuss how people react to pressure from society. Discuss examples of how people get the message that "thin is in."

13. **ER** Guest speaker. Invite a sports coach to discuss how students with eating disorders are identified. Discuss how sports goals can affect ideas about healthy weight.

What Help Is Available?

14. **ER** Guest speaker. Ask a professional counselor from a local eating disorder clinic to speak to the class. Ask the counselor to describe symptoms, causes, and treatment of eating disorders.

15. **ER** Have students use library resources or the Internet to learn about programs available for the treatment of eating disorders. Ask students to write a report on the results of the search and present it to the class.

16. **ER** Guest speaker. Invite a physician or counselor to talk about treatment of eating disorders. Have the speaker discuss why some people have difficulty accepting healthy eating behaviors. Summarize the criteria a person can use to evaluate treatment programs.

17. **ER** Have students identify community agencies, services, or support groups that counsel people with eating disorders. Prepare a complete list of the community resources to use in Activities 23 and 24.

18. **RF** *Help for Eating Disorders,* Activity B, SAG. Students are to describe the roles various people play in the treatment of someone with an eating disorder.

19. **EX** Have students role-play a supportive friend who is reaching out to someone they suspect has an eating disorder.

20. **ER** *Words of Self-Affirmation,* color transparency CT-14. Use the transparency master to discuss how eating disorders are related to psychological difficulties. Have students explain how finding affirming words to describe the self is a step toward building positive self-esteem. Have each student draw his or her own affirmation flower.

Chapter Review

21. **ER** *Thoughts About My Eating Behaviors,* reproducible master 14-3. Students are to complete the activity by evaluating their eating behaviors. They will then answer questions about whether some of their eating behaviors need improvement. This activity should be done privately and should not be collected or graded.

22. **RF** *Backtrack Through Chapter 14,* Activity A, SAG. Students are to provide complete answers to questions and statements that will help them recall, interpret, apply, and practice chapter concepts.

Above and Beyond

23. **EX** Have students create a display on eating disorders to put up in the school cafeteria. Students might contact the organizations listed in the text on page 249 to request resources. They should include handouts about different eating disorders and a list of community contacts for students who may have questions.

24. **EX** Organize an eating disorder awareness day for the school. Have students prepare pamphlets to pass out and posters to hang around the school. Ask counselors to be available to answer students' questions. You might wish to invite a panel of nutritionists, physicians, and counselors to discuss topics related to eating disorders at an assembly.

Answer Key

Text

Check Your Knowledge, page 253

1. (List five:) a large drop in weight; amenorrhea (for females); restlessness; irritability; feeling cold; a covering of fine hair over the body; rough, dry skin; hair loss
2. true
3. Unlike bulimics, binge eaters do not engage in a follow-up behavior after bingeing to prevent weight gain.
4. (Student response. See Chart 14-4 on page 247 of the text.)
5. Many coaches focus on body weight during training. Constantly trying to achieve and maintain weight goals for their sports leads some athletes to develop eating disorders.
6. early treatment
7. attending to the physical health problems the disorder has caused
8. stress and change
9. (List three. Student response. See page 251 in the text.)
10. Be careful when encouraging someone to lose weight. Emphasize acceptance of the person regardless of his or her weight. Show concern for the person's health and well-being.

Student Activity Guide

Read the Warning Signs, Activity A

1. BN
2. AN
3. AN
4. AN
5. BN
6. AN
7. AN
8. BN
9. AN, BN
10. AN
11. AN
12. BED
13. BN
14. BED
15. BN, BED
16. BED
17. AN
18. BN
19. BN
20. BED

Backtrack Through Chapter 14, Activity D

1. anorexia nervosa, bulimia nervosa, binge eating disorder
2. teenage women, young adult women
3. psychological
4. forced vomiting, abuse of laxatives, abuse of diuretics, abuse of enemas
5. guilt, frustration, rejection
6. media
7. concern with appearances and high achievement, lack of communication skills, tendency to avoid conflicts
8. disordered eating, amenorrhea, osteoporosis
9. about 20 percent remain underweight and struggle with low self-esteem and weight distortion throughout life
10. medical care that does not require a hospital stay
11. to give clients the emotional tools to take control of their eating behaviors
12. helping the patient form healthful eating habits
13. their sense of pride in reaching weight goals and the compliments they receive from others
14. Anorexics typically have a large drop in body weight. Bulimics, on the other hand, may maintain a fairly average body size. This may keep others from identifying the bulimics' problem for a long time.
15. (Student response. See page 247 in the text.)
16. Verbal skills can help anorexics relate better to their family members and friends. Stress management techniques can help anorexics respond appropriately to their emotions.
17. Counseling can help bulimics prepare for and manage stressful events and thus avoid a relapse.
18. (Student response.)
19. (Student response.)
20. (Student response.)

Teacher's Resources

Chapter 14 Test

1. D	11. T	20. F
2. A	12. T	21. C
3. B	13. T	22. B
4. F	14. F	23. A
5. H	15. F	24. C
6. C	16. T	25. D
7. I	17. T	26. A
8. E	18. T	27. A
9. F	19. F	28. D
10. F		

29. (List five:) skipping meals; a large drop in weight; eating little food or bingeing; exercising excessively; wearing baggy clothes; restlessness or irritability; withdrawal from social events; feeling cold; complaining of feeling fat; secrecy about food

30. (List three:) Teens are especially vulnerable to feelings of rejection, worthlessness, and guilt. Their lives are in a state of physical, social, and emotional change. Facing the challenges of growing up creates stress. Some teens feel powerless over their lives. Some teens feel they cannot live up to society's ideal of body image.

31. (List four:) medical doctor—treatment for the effects on physical health; psychologist—help deal with emotional issues at the root of the disorder; registered dietitian—help the patient form healthful eating habits; exercise specialist—help plan a moderate exercise program

Symptoms of Anorexia Nervosa

- Large drop in weight

- Stress, restlessness, or irritability

- Coldness caused by loss of insulation

- Growth of fine hair on body to trap heat

- Nutrient deficiencies, which cause rough, dry skin and hair loss

- Low blood pressure

- Depression

- Decrease in bone density; risk of osteoporosis

- Slowdown in growth and development

- Amenorrhea in females

© Goodheart-Willcox

Positive Reflections—Steps to Accepting Your Body

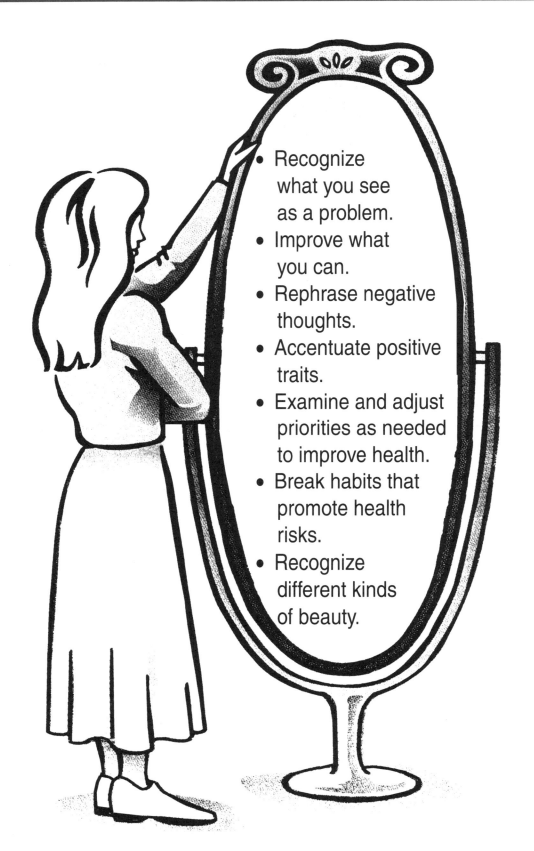

- Recognize what you see as a problem.
- Improve what you can.
- Rephrase negative thoughts.
- Accentuate positive traits.
- Examine and adjust priorities as needed to improve health.
- Break habits that promote health risks.
- Recognize different kinds of beauty.

© Goodheart-Willcox

Thoughts About My Eating Behaviors

Name_____ **Date** _____ **Period** _____

Answer the multiple choice questions by checking one option or filling in the "other" blank. Then answer the questions that follow. (This activity will not be graded or collected.)

1. How often do you think about food and your weight?

    _____ All the time.   _____ Daily.   _____ Rarely.   _____ I don't think about it.   Other: _____

2. How do you feel about the possibility of becoming overweight?

    _____ Afraid.   _____ Anxious.   _____ Depressed.   _____ I'm not concerned.   Other: _____

3. What emotion do you most often feel when you are eating?

    _____ Guilt.   _____ Pleasure.   _____ Fulfillment.   _____ None.   Other: _____

4. Which best describes your weight status?

    _____ I'm always trying to lose weight.   _____ I sometimes need to lose a few pounds.

    _____ I pretty much maintain my healthy weight.   _____ I'm trying to gain some weight.   Other: _____

5. How often do you lose control and overeat?

    _____ I often continue to eat after I'm full.   _____ I sometimes overeat at special functions.

    _____ I always stop eating when I'm full.   _____ I stop eating before I'm really full.   Other: _____

6. Why might you hide your eating behaviors?

    _____ I don't want people to know how much I eat.   _____ I don't want people to bother me about how little

    I eat.   _____ I never hide my eating behaviors.   Other: _____

7. How often do you weigh yourself?

    _____ More than once a day.   _____ Every day.   Once a week.   _____ Seldom.   Other: _____

8. Which of the following do you think is most important?

    _____ Being as thin as possible.   _____ Losing weight.   _____ Maintaining a healthy weight.

    _____ Gaining weight.   Other: _____

9. What are some of your healthy eating behaviors?_____

    _____

    _____

10. Which eating habits would you like to improve? How might you improve them?_____

    _____

    _____

11. Which of your eating habits could lead to health risks?_____

    _____

12. Which of your eating habits influence weight management?_____

    _____

    _____

© Goodheart-Willcox

Eating Disorders

Name_____

Date _____   Period _____   Score _____

Chapter 14 Test

Matching: Match each of the following eating disorders with the characteristic that describes it.

_____ 1. Uncontrollable eating of huge amounts of food.

_____ 2. Eating disorder typified by an intense fear of weight gain.

_____ 3. A drug that alters the nervous system and relieves depression.

_____ 4. An abnormal eating pattern that endangers physical and mental health.

_____ 5. Medical care that does not require a hospital stay.

_____ 6. An eating disorder that involves repeatedly eating very large amounts of food without a follow-up behavior to prevent weight gain.

_____ 7. Clearing the food from the digestive system.

_____ 8. An eating disorder that involves uncontrollable eating of huge amounts of food followed by an inappropriate behavior to prevent weight gain.

A. anorexia nervosa
B. antidepressant
C. binge eating disorder
D. bingeing
E. bulimia nervosa
F. eating disorder
G. female athlete triad
H. outpatient treatment
I. purging

True/False: Circle *T* if the statement is true or *F* if the statement is false.

T F   9. Overstuffing yourself at a holiday dinner is a sign that you have an eating disorder.

T F   10. Eating disorders are most common among teenage and young adult men.

T F   11. Anorexics often skip meals.

T F   12. Some people alternate between bulimic and anorexic behaviors.

T F   13. Thinking constantly about food is a common symptom of both anorexia nervosa and bulimia nervosa.

T F   14. Bulimia nervosa does not cause as much damage to the body as anorexia nervosa does.

T F   15. The only cause of eating disorders is the media's emphasis on thinness as the ideal.

T F   16. A female athlete may develop an eating disorder because she wants to achieve certain weight goals to be more competitive.

T F   17. As part of treatment, patients with eating disorders are taught how to set realistic weight management goals.

T F   18. Many professionals advise family therapy as part of treatment for anorexics.

T F   19. Once people with eating disorders have received treatment, they are completely cured.

T F   20. If you suspect a friend has an eating disorder, it is best to keep your suspicions to yourself.

(Continued)

© Goodheart-Willcox

Name_____

Multiple Choice: Choose the best response. Write the letter in the space provided.

_____21. Which of the following characteristics is most descriptive of a person with anorexia nervosa?
   A.   Thinks of self as extremely thin.
   B.   Exercises moderately once or twice a week.
   C.   Will eat only small amounts of food.
   D.   Thinks little about body size and shape.

_____22. Which of the following is a physical effect of anorexia nervosa on the body?
   A.   Blood pressure and pulse rate rise.
   B.   Bone density decreases and symptoms of osteoporosis occur.
   C.   Body fat builds up.
   D.   Rate of growth and development increases.

_____23. Which of the following is a characteristic of someone with bulimia nervosa?
   A.   May consume thousands of calories in a few hours.
   B.   Often binges on foods low in fats and carbohydrates.
   C.   Usually possesses high self-esteem.
   D.   Does not engage in follow-up behavior to prevent weight gain.

_____24. A person with _____ is likely to be overweight.
   A.   anorexia nervosa
   B.   bulimia nervosa
   C.   binge eating disorder
   D.   All the above.

_____25. Which of the following views of food could be harmful?
   A.   I enjoy food.
   B.   I like sharing food with friends.
   C.   I eat when I'm hungry.
   D.   I'm emotionally dependent on food.

_____26. What is the set of problems associated with the female athlete triad?
   A.   Eating disorder, amenorrhea, osteoporosis.
   B.   Binge eating, vitamin D deficiency, low self-esteem.
   C.   Depression, emotional dependency, weight image distortion.
   D.   Powerlessness, psychological distress, physical change.

_____27. Which of the following would most likely be used for treatment of a person diagnosed with anorexia nervosa?
   A.   Counseling.
   B.   A weight-reduction diet.
   C.   Increased use of diuretics.
   D.   A more rigorous exercise plan.

_____28. The function of a support group in an eating disorder recovery program is to _____.
   A.   assist with nutrition counseling
   B.   recommend a drug treatment plan
   C.   replace the need for professional therapy
   D.   share information and give encouragement

(Continued)

© Goodheart-Willcox

Name_____

Essay Questions: Provide complete responses to the following questions or statements.

29. List five signals that might cause a person to suspect a friend has an eating disorder.

30. List three reasons teens are especially vulnerable to the development of eating disorders.

31. List four professionals involved in the treatment of a person with an eating disorder. Briefly explain each professional's role in treatment.

Staying Physically Active: A Way of Life

Objectives

After studying this chapter, students will be able to
- choose their goals for physical activity.
- describe the benefits of physical activity.
- list the health and skill components of physical fitness.
- determine their target heart rate zone.
- identify four keys to a successful exercise program.
- plan a personal exercise program.

Bulletin Board

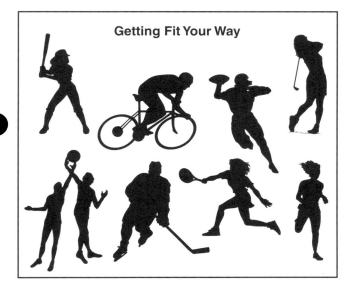

Getting Fit Your Way

Title: *Getting Fit Your Way*

Prepare silhouette outlines of people in various sports activities to display the many choices available for becoming physically active.

Title: *Staying Fit to Meet Life's Adventures*

Collect magazine pictures of active people throughout the life span. Arrange the pictures on the bulletin board from youngest to oldest. Have students create a caption for each photo.

Teaching Materials

Text, pages 256-273
Learn the Language
Check Your Knowledge
Put Learning into Action
Explore Further

Student Activity Guide, pages 105-110
A. *Assessing Activity Goals*
B. *Physical Activity Crossword*
C. *The Physical Activity Runaround*
D. *Backtrack Through Chapter 15*

Teacher's Resources
What Can Physical Activity Do for You? transparency master 15-1
Skill Components of Physical Fitness, color transparency CT-15
Health- and Skill-Related Benefits of Exercise, reproducible master 15-2
What Makes an Exercise Right for You? reproducible master 15-3
Warm Up to Exercise, reproducible master 15-4
Chapter 15 Test

Introducing the Chapter

1. Discuss what students have heard about the need to exercise and how it relates to fitness. Use the feedback as an indication of students' level of knowledge and a measure of their attitude toward exercise. Summarize the interest areas and share results with the class.
2. Ask students how they think a person becomes physically fit. Ask students if they think it is important to become physically fit and why.
3. Ask students how they feel after they have exercised or participated in a sports activity. Discuss why it is important to exercise on a regular basis and make physical activity a lifestyle behavior.

Strategies to Reteach, Reinforce, Enrich, and Extend Text Concepts

Goals for Physical Activity

4. **RF** Have each student list three goals for becoming more physically active. Then ask students to classify each goal into one of three categories: good health outcomes (H), total fitness outcomes (F), or peak athletic performance outcomes (P). Tally the results to learn the primary interests of the class. Discuss how goals for improved fitness might change over the life span.
5. **ER** *Assessing Activity Goals,* Activity A, SAG. Students are to answer questions that help them assess their activity goals. Ask students to

compare their answers with the goals they listed in Activity 5.

6. **ER**   Guest speakers. Invite a fitness trainer, physical education director, and physical therapist to speak on the common goals of people who enter their programs. Discuss how activities could be added to sedentary lifestyles. Have students prepare questions beforehand.

7. **ER**   Use the Internet to locate statistics about physical activity and related effects on the health of young people. You can find these at the U.S. Centers for Disease Control and Prevention's Web site, www.cdc.gov. Locate and list the physical activity goals for people by the year 2010. In small group discussions, determine what individuals, parents, teachers, schools, and communities can do to help achieve these goals.

The Benefits of Physical Activity

8. **RF**   *What Can Physical Activity Do for You?* transparency master 15-1. Use the transparency master to discuss with students the benefits of physical activity.

9. **RF**   Ask students to give examples of how physical activity can help improve a person's mental outlook.

10. **EX**   Have students use the Internet or library resources to research the connections between physical activity and health and longevity. Have students write a summary to publish in the school newspaper.

What Is Total Fitness?

11. **RT**   Have students discuss how life choices impact fitness. Make sure the discussion includes eating a nutritious diet, avoiding harmful substances, maintaining a healthy weight, and getting enough exercise.

12. **ER**   Contact the President's Council on Physical Fitness and Sports to identify the fitness norms recommended. Refer to the *Using Other Resources* section in the front of this product for contact information.

13. **ER**   Ask students to suggest exercises that promote cardiovascular endurance, muscular endurance, strength, and flexibility. Write students' examples on the board. Discuss how these different exercises will affect body composition.

14. **RF**   *Skill Components of Physical Fitness,* color transparency CT-15. Use the transparency to discuss the skill components of physical fitness. Have students give examples of exercises that promote each skill component.

15. **RF**   *Health- and Skill-Related Benefits of Exercise,* reproducible master 15-2. Use the handout to discuss with students how various

forms of exercise may be beneficial for some health or skill components of physical fitness, but not for others.

Exercise and Heart Health

16. **RT**   Demonstrate how to take a pulse rate. Have students practice taking pulse rates for themselves and a partner.

17. **RF**   Have each student determine his or her maximum heart rate and individual target heart rate zone.

18. **ER**   Rent a beginners' exercise videotape with music that appeals to teens. Make the tape available for students to take home for use.

19. **ER**   Ask for student volunteers who exercise regularly or those who have just begun an exercise program. Have the volunteers record their pulse rates before and after they exercise for several days. Ask the volunteers if they notice a difference in their pulse rates as fitness levels improve.

Keys to a Successful Exercise Program

20. **RF**   Discuss with students the benefits of balancing exercise choices, much as food choices should be balanced. Have students draw their own "activity pyramid" and place the names of activities they do at each level. Have them evaluate the balance in their daily activities.

21. **EX**   Have students brainstorm a list of tips they would suggest to someone trying to lose weight by exercising. Compile the list of ideas to create a pamphlet.

22. **ER**   *What Makes an Exercise Right for You?* reproducible master 15-3. Students are to evaluate exercise activities that best match their lifestyle and interests. Then, based on their responses, students should choose exercises that would be best for them.

Planning an Exercise Program

23. **ER**   Have each student research a community exercise program. Ask students to find out the purpose, history, cost, difficulty level, and health benefits of each program. Have students report their findings to the class.

24. **ER**   Guest speaker. Invite a certified personal trainer to talk to the class about types and benefits of warm-ups, workouts, and cooldowns. Discuss safety precautions to take when exercising indoors or outdoors.

25. **RF**   *Warm Up to Exercise,* reproducible master 15-4. Use the handout to discuss some methods of warm-up exercises with students.

Chapter Review

26. **RF** *Backtrack Through Chapter 15,* Activity D, SAG, Students are to provide complete answers to questions and statements that will help them recall, interpret, apply, and practice chapter concepts.

27. **RF** *Physical Activity Crossword,* Activity B, SAG. Students are to complete the crossword puzzle using vocabulary from the chapter.

28. **RF** *The Physical Activity Runaround,* Activity C, SAG. Use the game to review concepts from the chapter with students.

29. **RF** Ask students if they have modified their exercise levels or programs since beginning the chapter. Have students name or demonstrate particular exercises they use to meet their exercise goals.

Above and Beyond

30. **EX** Have students create bookmarks from heavy paper. On the bookmarks, they should write motivational information about the benefits of daily exercise. Pictures may be sketched to add interest. Distribute bookmarks to other classes.

31. **EX** Have students plan an exercise session for elementary students. Research the age group exercise capabilities before planning activities.

32. **EX** Have students organize an exercise laboratory after school. Ask students to create posters and handouts to advertise the session and its benefits. Students may act as leaders of the activities.

Answer Key

Text

Check Your Knowledge, page 272

1. Accumulate at least 60 minutes of moderate activity daily nearly every day.
2. developing better posture, making more graceful movements, maintaining healthy weight
3. aerobic activities
4. muscular endurance
5. (List four:) power, agility, balance, coordination, speed, reaction time (Examples are student response. See pages 261-263 in the text.)
6. The heart beats slower because it is able to work more efficiently, pumping more blood with each beat.
7. the wrist or the neck
8. 190
9. 60 to 90 percent
10. You will be less likely to skip an exercise session if you know it will show up on a written record. You will also feel good about yourself when you see how faithfully you are following your exercise plan.

11. Doing different types of activities can keep you from getting bored. Different activities also help develop different components of fitness.
12. frequency, intensity, duration
13. false
14. The warm-up period prepares the heart and other muscles for work.
15. (Student response. See page 271 in the text.)

Student Activity Guide

Physical Activity Crossword, Activity B

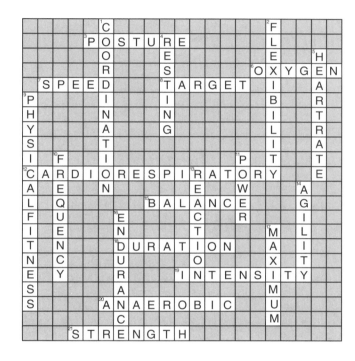

Backtrack Through Chapter 15, Activity D

1. good health, total fitness, peak athletic performance
2. at least 60 minutes
3. Exercise can strengthen the muscles of the abdomen and back, allowing people to stand and sit with erect posture.
4. (List four:) osteoporosis, coronary heart disease (CHD), some cancers, diabetes mellitus, and stroke
5. cardiorespiratory fitness, muscular endurance, strength, flexibility, and body composition
6. (List three:) walking, bicycling, swimming (Other correct answers may be accepted.)
7. (List three:) sprinting, football, tennis (Other correct answers may be accepted.)
8. (List three:) hiking, rowing, gymnastics (Other correct answers may be accepted.)
9. Body composition is the percentage of different types of tissues in the body.
10. (Student response.)
11. written goals, enjoyable activities, a convenient exercise schedule, and knowledge of personal fitness level

12. burning muscles, out of breath
13. warm-up period, workout period, cool-down period
14. to help keep weight at a healthy level throughout life
15. Anaerobic activities cannot be sustained long enough to develop cardiorespiratory fitness.
16. When the heart beats more slowly, this means it is working more efficiently. The heart is under less strain and does not have to work so hard. This is a sign of increased cardiorespiratory fitness.
17. Exercise can lower LDL and increase HDL. This increases blood flow and allows the heart to work more efficiently.
18. (Student response.)
19. (Student response.)
20. (Student response. See pages 264 and 265 in the text for formulas.)

Teacher's Resources

Chapter 15 Test

1. A	9. D	17. F	25. F
2. K	10. C	18. F	26. B
3. G	11. T	19. T	27. A
4. H	12. F	20. F	28. C
5. B	13. T	21. T	29. C
6. F	14. T	22. F	30. D
7. E	15. T	23. T	31. B
8. J	16. F	24. F	32. A

33. improved appearance, disease prevention, improved mental outlook
34. power, agility, balance, coordination, speed, reaction time (Exercise examples are student response. See pages 262-263 in the text.)
35. Tony's maximum heart rate is 199 beats per minute (220 – 21 = 199). His target heart rate zone is 119 to 179 beats per minute (199 × 0.6 = 119; 199 × 0.9 = 179).

What Can Physical Activity Do for You?

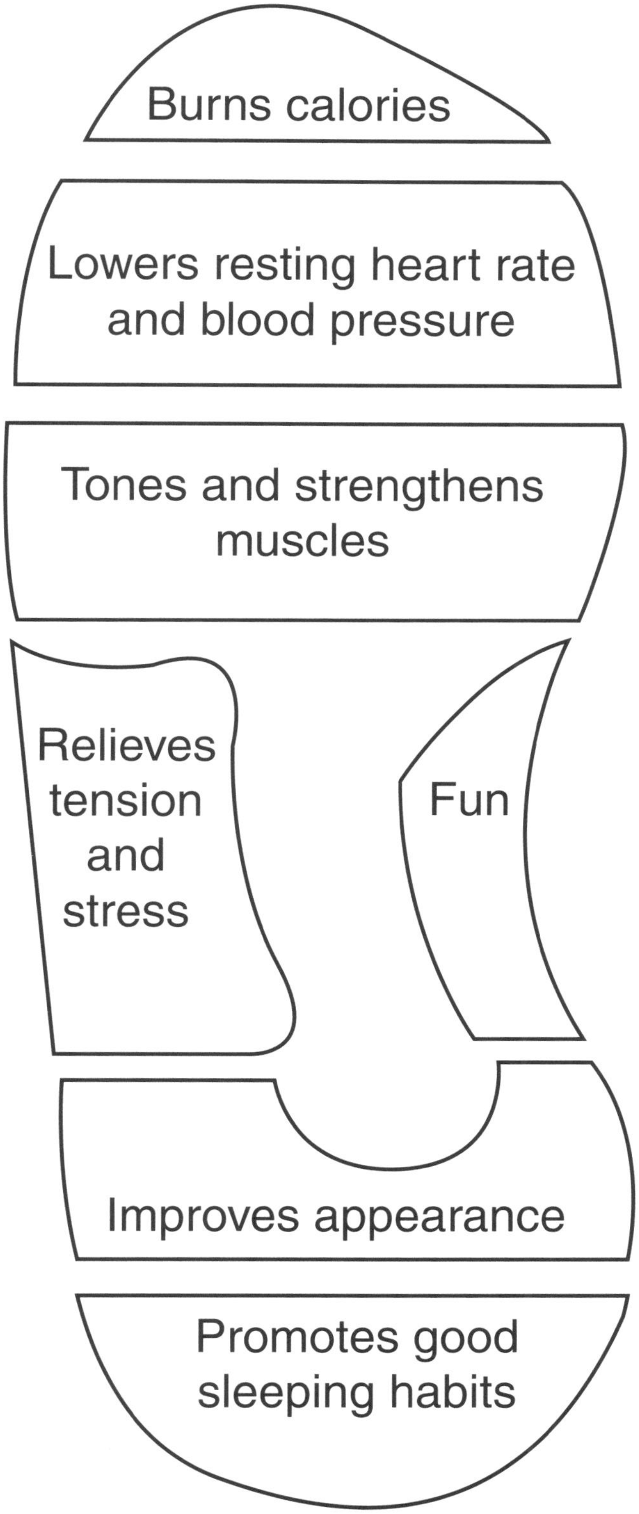

Burns calories

Lowers resting heart rate and blood pressure

Tones and strengthens muscles

Relieves tension and stress

Fun

Improves appearance

Promotes good sleeping habits

© Goodheart-Willcox

Name _____   Date _____   Period _____

Health- and Skill-Related Benefits of Exercise

Activity	Health-Related Benefits					Skill-Related Benefits					
	Cardio-respiratory Fitness	Muscular Endurance	Strength	Flexibility	Body Composition	Power	Agility	Balance	Coordination	Speed	Reaction Time
Bicycling	excellent	good	fair	poor	excellent	poor	fair	excellent	fair	fair	fair
Dancing (social)	fair/good	fair	poor	fair	fair/good	poor	good	fair	good	poor	fair
Rope Jumping	good	good	poor	poor	good	fair	good	fair	good	poor	fair
Skating (in-line)	good/excellent	good/excellent	poor	poor	good/excellent	fair	good	excellent	good	fair	fair
Swimming	excellent	good	fair	fair	excellent	fair	good	fair	good	poor	poor
Walking	good	fair	good	poor	good	poor	poor	poor	poor	poor	poor
Weight Training	poor	good	excellent	poor	fair	good	poor	fair	fair	poor	poor

© Goodheart-Willcox

What Makes an Exercise Right for You?

Name_____　**Date** _____　**Period** _____

Answer the following questions. Then, based on your responses, choose which types of exercise might be best for your lifestyle.

Which activities do you enjoy? (Check all that apply.)

_____ baseball	_____ gymnastics	_____ soccer
_____ basketball	_____ hiking	_____ swimming
_____ bicycling	_____ in-line skating	_____ tennis
_____ canoeing	_____ racquetball	_____ volleyball
_____ football	_____ running	_____ walking
_____ golf	_____ skiing	_____ weight training
_____ other:_____	_____ other: _____	

What is the most convenient time for you to exercise?

_____ before school　　_____ during lunch　　_____ after school
_____ in the evening　　_____ before bed

What is your current level of fitness?

_____ I am working to increase my activity level.
_____ I am active, but do not follow a consistent schedule.
_____ I have become increasingly active over the last few months.
_____ I am very active and will maintain this activity level.

How often do you like to exercise?

_____ once a day　　_____ every other day　　_____ other: _____
_____ twice a week　　_____ once a week

How long do your exercise sessions usually last?

_____ 20 minutes　　_____ 30 minutes　　_____ one hour
_____ several hours　　_____ other: _____

How much money do you budget for exercise activities and equipment? _____

With whom do you exercise?

_____ family member　　_____ friend　　_____ team
_____ other: _____

Based on my responses, the activities that best fit my lifestyle are _____
_____

© Goodheart-Willcox

Warm Up to Exercise

Name_____   Date _____   Period _____

Warming up is an important part of any exercise program. Stretching and toning your muscles before you start vigorous exercise prevents stiffness, aches, and pains. Warm-up exercises can also help prevent injuries. The following exercises will help you warm up before you start exercising.

Stretcher Stand facing wall arms' length away. Lean forward and place palms of hands flat against wall, slightly below shoulder height. Keep back straight, heels firmly on floor, and slowly bend elbows until forehead touches wall. Tuck hips toward wall and hold position for 20 seconds. Repeat exercise with knees slightly flexed.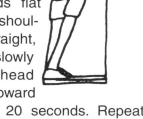

Reach and Bend Stand erect with feet shoulder-width apart and arms extended over head. Reach as high as possible while keeping heels on floor and hold for 10 counts. Flex knees slightly and bend slowly at waist, touching floor between feet with fingers. Hold for 10 counts. (If you can't touch the floor, try to touch the tops of your shoes.) Repeat entire sequence 2 to 5 times.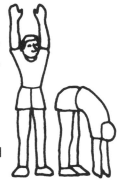

Knee Pull Lie flat on back with legs extended and arms at sides. Lock arms around legs just below knees and pull knees to chest, raising buttocks slightly off floor. Hold for 10 to 15 counts. (If you have knee problems, you may find it easier to lock arms behind knees.) Repeat exercise 3 to 5 times.

Sit-Up Several versions of the sit-up are listed in reverse order of difficulty (easiest one listed first, most difficult one last). Start with the sit-up you can do three times without undue strain. When you are able to do 10 repetitions of the exercise without great difficulty, move on to a more difficult version.

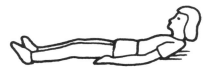

1. Lie flat on back with arms at sides, palms down, and knees slightly bent. Curl head forward until you can see past feet, hold for three counts, then lower to start position. *Repeat exercise 3 to 10 times.*

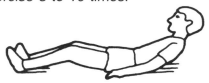

2. Lie flat on back with arms at sides, palms down, and knees slightly bent. Roll forward until upper body is at 45-degree angle to floor, then return to starting position. *Repeat exercise 3 to 10 times.*

3. Lie flat on back with arms at sides, palms down, and knees slightly bent. Roll forward to sitting position, then return to starting position. *Repeat exercise 3 to 10 times.*

4. Lie flat on back with arms crossed on chest and knees slightly bent. Roll forward to sitting position, then return to starting position. *Repeat exercise 3 to 10 times.*

5. Lie flat on back with hands laced in back of head and knees slightly bent. Roll forward to sitting position, then return to starting position. *Repeat exercise 3 to 15 times.*

© Goodheart-Willcox

Staying Physically Active: A Way of Life

Name_____

Date _____ **Period** _____ **Score** _____

Chapter 15 Test

Matching: Match the following terms and identifying phrases.

_____ 1. An activity that uses large muscles and is done at a moderate, steady pace for fairly long periods. The heart and lungs are able to meet the muscles' oxygen needs throughout the activity.

_____ 2. The range of heartbeats per minute at which the heart muscle receives the best workout.

_____ 3. The position of the body when standing or sitting.

_____ 4. The ability to do maximum work in a short time.

_____ 5. An activity in which the muscles are using oxygen faster than the heart and lungs can deliver it.

_____ 6. A state in which all body systems function together efficiently.

_____ 7. The highest speed at which the heart muscle is able to contract.

_____ 8. The ability of the muscles to move objects.

_____ 9. The number of times the heart beats per minute.

_____ 10. The body's ability to take in adequate amounts of oxygen and carry it efficiently through the blood to body cells.

A. aerobic activity
B. anaerobic activity
C. cardiorespiratory fitness
D. heart rate
E. maximum heart rate
F. physical fitness
G. posture
H. power
I. resting heart rate
J. strength
K. target heart rate zone

True/False: Circle *T* if the statement is true or *F* if the statement is false.

T F 11. Physical inactivity is a main reason many people lack physical fitness.

T F 12. The kinds of activities you do will not be affected by your goals for physical activity.

T F 13. The benefits of exercise can accumulate as a person moves from one physical activity to another throughout the day.

T F 14. Household tasks can count as part of your daily physical activity.

T F 15. The more active you are, the more active you will want to be.

T F 16. Reaching the goal of good health requires intense training designed to develop specific sports skills.

T F 17. A person who is flexible is equally strong.

T F 18. Agility is the ability to integrate the use of two or more parts of your body.

T F 19. The harder a person works out, the faster the heart will beat.

T F 20. Maximum heart rate is higher for a 50-year-old person than it is for a 16-year-old.

T F 21. The heart is a muscle that should be exercised like other muscles in the body.

T F 22. Fitness goals can usually be achieved within a week.

T F 23. Variety can help keep an exercise program enjoyable.

T F 24. The morning is really the best time to exercise.

T F 25. You should exercise until you feel pain because then you know you're working your muscles.

(Continued)

Name_____

Multiple Choice: Choose the best response. Write the letter in the space provided.

_____26. Tennis is an example of a(n) _____ activity.
  A. aerobic
  B. anaerobic
  C. strength-building
  D. warm-up

_____27. As cardiovascular fitness improves, the resting heart rate _____.
  A. slows down
  B. stays the same
  C. speeds up
  D. exceeds the target heart rate zone

_____28. Why is age a factor in computing the target heart rate zone?
  A. Older people are in poor health.
  B. Younger people's rates measure more accurately.
  C. Maximum heart rate decreases with age.
  D. Older people should not exercise at levels beyond resting heart rate.

_____29. Which of the following fitness goals is stated with specifically measurable outcomes?
  A. I want to be stronger.
  B. I will get motivated to exercise.
  C. I will lift weights after school on Monday, Wednesday, and Friday for 30 minutes.
  D. I will stay healthy until the day I die.

_____30. An exercise warm-up period _____.
  A. is unnecessary in hot, humid weather
  B. should last at least an hour
  C. should not involve muscles you will be using in your workout
  D. prepares your heart and other muscles for work

_____31. The workout period, the main part of your exercise program, should last at least _____.
  A. 5 minutes
  B. 20 minutes
  C. 1 hour
  D. 4 hours

_____32. Why should a person cool down after a strenuous workout?
  A. To let blood adequately reach the brain and avoid dizziness.
  B. To prevent muscles from shrinking.
  C. To avoid having to shower after exercise.
  D. To build motivation to continue with a strenuous exercise program.

Essay Questions: Provide complete responses to the following questions or statements.

33. What are three benefits of physical activity?

34. List the skill components of physical fitness and give an example of an exercise that would improve each area.

35. Tony is 21 years old. Calculate his maximum heart rate and his target heart rate zone.

Eating for Sports Performance

16

Objectives

After studying this chapter, students will be able to
*   explain an athlete's dietary and fluid needs.
*   plan a performance day or pregame meal for an athlete.
*   describe techniques athletes can use to safely lose or gain weight for competition.
*   state consumer cautions related to performance aids marketed to athletes.

Bulletin Boards

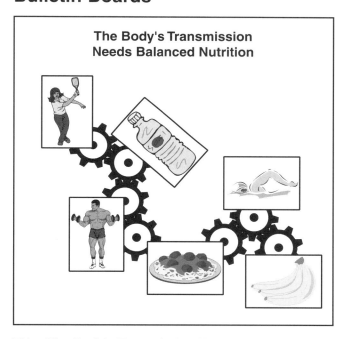

The Body's Transmission Needs Balanced Nutrition

Title: *The Body's Transmission Needs Balanced Nutrition*

Place several large photographs of teens involved in sports activities on the bulletin board. Between the sports photos, place photos of water and foods appropriate for pregame meals and snacks. (See Chart 16-6 on page 280 of the text.) Connect the photos with cutouts of mechanical gears.

Title: *Get the Edge on the Competition*

Place the title in the center of the bulletin board. Around the perimeter of the board, write words and place photos of items that optimize athletic performance, such as *fluids, training, nutritious snacks,* and *weight management.*

Teaching Materials

Text, pages 274-286
> *Learn the Language*
> *Check Your Knowledge*
> *Put Learning into Action*
> *Explore Further*

Student Activity Guide, pages 111-116
> A. *40-Fact Relay*
> B. *Analyze This*
> C. *Ask an Athlete*
> D. *Backtrack Through Chapter 16*

Teacher's Resources
> *Competition of Various Durations,* transparency master 16-1
> *Score Big Points in Sports Nutrition,* color transparency CT-16
> *The Mighty Dozen—Sports Myths and Facts,* reproducible master 16-2
> Chapter 16 Test

Introducing the Chapter

1. Survey students to find out how many participate in sports either recreationally or competitively. List the types of sports in which students are involved on the chalkboard.
2. Panel discussion. Invite a panel of student athletes to describe the benefits and drawbacks of sports participation. Also ask panel members to describe what is required to be a fit athlete in their sports. Have panel members explain the pressures they feel to perform better than the competition. Ask how these expectations influence diet and exercise behaviors.
3. In small groups, have students explore differences and similarities between diet and exercise patterns of athletes and nonathletes. List any myths students express. Have students research the accuracy of these myths throughout the study of this chapter.

Strategies to Reteach, Reinforce, Enrich, and Extend Text Concepts

The Nutrient Needs of an Athlete

4. **RT** Explain that because athletes use much energy in training, they have higher calorie needs than nonathletes. However, sources of energy in

the diets of athletes should be similar to those of nonathletes. Most people should be consuming 50 to 60 percent of their calories from carbohydrates, no more than 30 percent from fat, and the remaining 10 to 15 percent from protein. Ask students to name a good source of carbohydrates from each of the food groups.

5. Have students use *Personal Best* software to determine the energy they would expend by participating in each sport offered at your school. Discuss factors that affect individual energy expenditure.

6. **RT** *Competition of Various Durations,* transparency master 16-1. Use the transparency to explain the differences between anaerobic and aerobic activities. Discuss how glycogen stores are used differently.

7. **ER** Have students visit the Internet sites for the American Dietetic Association or the American College of Sports Medicine to find nutrition recommendations for better sports performance.

8. **ER** Have each student interview a high school athlete about his or her favorite foods. Then have students plan a day's menus for the athletes. Menus should be high in carbohydrates and supply a full range of vitamins and minerals. Menus should also include some of the athletes' favorite foods and provide approximately 3,000 calories to meet energy needs for training. Have students give completed menu plans to the athletes. Ask students to share the athletes' reactions in class.

9. Have students use *Personal Best* software to identify lowfat, high-carbohydrate snack foods that would make good choices for athletes following an exercise session. Have students distribute samples of these foods to members of a school team. Ask for feedback about which snacks team members preferred and why.

10. **ER** Guest speaker. Invite a sports nutritionist to discuss the unique nutritional needs of athletes participating in various sports activities. Ask the speaker to discuss the pros and cons of carbohydrate loading, use of sports drinks, and unusual dieting patterns.

11. Have students offer half the athletes at a team practice a sports drink while offering the other half water. Record the amounts of fluids consumed by each group at 15-minute intervals throughout the practice. After the practice, have students interview athletes about their fluid preferences and general sense of well-being. As a class, discuss the outcomes of this activity and the pros and cons of the use of sports drinks.

12. **ER** Have students gather refreshing drink recipes to serve athletes after a game.

13. **EX** Have students plan a menu for a pregame meal. Have the class offer to serve the meal 3 to 4 hours before a school sports event. Seek feedback from athletes about how the meal affected their performance levels.

14. **RF** Have students prepare posters titled *Food Power, Fluid Power,* or *Snack Power.* Have students place collages of magazine pictures on the posters to illustrate good choices of foods and beverages for athletes.

Weight Concerns of Athletes

15. **RT** Review the meaning of the terms *optimum weight* and *body composition.* Discuss why body composition is important to athletes.

16. **ER** Have students write a letter to the American College of Sports Medicine or check their Internet site to learn about their position on weight loss for athletes. Students should also find out what this organization has to say about the effects of weight training on growth patterns.

17. **ER** *Ask an Athlete,* Activity C, SAG. Students are to interview athletes about their choices of foods, beverages, and performance aids. Then students are to offer suggestions that would help the athletes improve their eating habits for sports performance.

18. **ER** Field trip. Plan a field trip to a sports medicine clinic so students can learn how the facility serves athletes. Have students collect educational materials for a display or bulletin board.

Harmful Performance Aids

19. **RT** *Score Big Points in Sports Nutrition,* color transparency CT-16. Use the transparency to emphasize how athletes can come out winners if they choose a balanced diet and training program over performance aids.

20. **RF** Gather news articles for students to read about athletes who have been found guilty of using banned substances to enhance their performance. Discuss health risks associated with use of steroids and other performance boosting drugs.

21. **ER** Have students check fitness magazines, Internet sites, and sporting goods stores to identify the types and costs of performance enhancing products on the market. Ask students to report their findings in class. Discuss why people are motivated to buy performance aids.

22. **ER** Obtain labels from a variety of performance aids. Have students read the labels to determine the contents of the products. Students should also evaluate label claims for believability. Ask students to write to the product manufacturers to gather evidence supporting label claims.

23. **EX** Have students evaluate ads for performance aids. Discuss what effect the ads have on consumers. Ask students what criteria consumers

can use to evaluate claims made in these ads. Also ask what can be done to make manufacturers more accountable for false claims.

24. **ER**   Guest speaker. Invite a member of a state or local athletic association to discuss the association's role in promoting the health and safety of athletes. Have the speaker describe any censures and/or penalties the association invokes on athletes found to be using performance enhancers.

25. **ER**   Guest speaker. Invite a sports psychologist to explain the role that attitude and confidence play in giving athletes a competitive edge. Ask the speaker to explain why some athletes believe they can get this edge from performance aids. Then have the speaker discuss techniques athletes can use to build a winning attitude without relying on bogus or harmful supplements.

26. **EX**   *Analyze This,* Activity B, SAG. Students are to complete an analysis of a news or feature article from a current general or fitness-related magazine that deals with eating for sports performance.

27. **RF**   *The Mighty Dozen—Sports Myths and Facts,* reproducible master 16-2. Have students write responses to help dispel the sports myths and support the facts listed on the handout.

Chapter Review

28. **RF**   In small groups, have students write two to three facts to add to a sports nutrition fact sheet. Each group can focus on a different area, such as fluid needs, energy sources, vitamin and mineral supplements, weight maintenance, and performance aids. Make the fact sheet available to other students in the school.

29. **RF**   *40-Fact Relay,* Activity A, SAG. Students are to identify true statements and correct false statements about eating for sports performance.

30. **RF**   *Backtrack Through Chapter 16,* Activity D, SAG. Students are to provide complete answers to questions and statements that will help them recall, interpret, apply, and practice chapter concepts.

Above and Beyond

31. **ER**   Find out how many males in the class are involved in school sports and how many females are involved in school sports. Then have students review the sports section of a local newspaper. Ask students to compare the number of articles that focus on male athletes with the number that focus on female athletes. Have each student conduct research to prepare an oral report about a particular female athlete and any obstacles she had to overcome to participate in her sport.

32. **ER**   Have students work together to write a position paper encouraging all students to participate in sports activities of their choice. The paper should explore solutions to the hurdles that make it difficult for some students to participate in sports events. Send the position paper to an appropriate school administrator for review and response.

33. **EX**   Have students prepare reports about special nutritional concerns for one of the following groups of athletes: pregnant women, senior citizens, children, or vegetarians.

34. **EX**   Remind students that few athletes become superstars and many do not aspire to fame and fortune. Then have the class make a *Bill of Rights for Winners* poster focusing on what it means to be individuals participating in sports that meet their unique needs for health, fitness, and recreation. Display the poster in a locker room or other appropriate area.

Answer Key

Text

Check Your Knowledge, page 285

1. body weight, type of activity, length of exercise period
2. glycogen
3. During anaerobic activity, the heart and lungs cannot keep up with the muscles' need for oxygen. Fat cannot be converted to energy without the presence of oxygen.
4. false
5. endurance activities requiring sustained muscle efforts for several hours at a time
6. two cups (500 mL) for every pound of body weight lost
7. (List two. Student response. See pages 279-281 in the text.)
8. males—10 to 15 percent, females—18 to 24 percent
9. An athlete's weight-gain goal is to add muscle, not fat. Muscle size cannot be increased by consuming more calories. Weight gain without training will be fat gain, not muscle gain.
10. Many coaches do not have adequate nutrition training to supervise an athlete's weight management program.

Student Activity Guide

40-Fact Relay, Activity A

1. true
2. fewer
3. true
4. fewer
5. true
6. a wide
7. is

8. true
9. carbon dioxide
10. true
11. true
12. true
13. carbohydrates
14. do not need
15. true
16. true
17. true
18. true
19. less
20. true
21. true
22. true
23. water
24. true
25. increase
26. poor
27. moderate
28. carbohydrates
29. underweight
30. true
31. weaken
32. does not
33. training
34. gradual
35. true
36. week
37. fat
38. true
39. cannot
40. true

Backtrack Through Chapter 16, Activity D

1. (List five:) relaxation, fun, health and wellness benefits, self-esteem, development of physical skills, social and emotional growth
2. the focus on competitiveness, the athlete's search for a winning edge
3. oxygen
4. because the body can stockpile fat
5. Lactic acid is a substance that results from an incomplete breakdown of glucose in the muscles.
6. These foods help them convert carbohydrates, fats, and protein to energy.
7. water retention, digestion distress, muscle stiffness, and sluggishness
8. throbbing headache, unsteadiness, nausea, dry skin, shivering, and confusion
9. 2 to 3 quarts
10. 2 hours before the event—3 cups water; 10 to 15 minutes before the event—1 to 2 cups water; 10 to 15 minute intervals during the event—½ cup to 1 cup water; after the event—2 cups water for every pound lost.

11. because they worsen dehydration, impair performance, irritate the stomach, and may cause vomiting
12. 2½ to 3
13. they are not true
14. the typical athlete burns more calories than the typical nonathlete
15. Lactic acid builds up in the muscles when you do not have enough oxygen to complete the breakdown of glucose. This produces a burning sensation and muscle fatigue that feels like "hitting a wall."
16. Too much body fat increases energy needs because it takes energy to move the excess weight. Too little body fat increases energy needs because it takes more energy to keep the body warm.
17. (Student response.)
18. (Student response. See pages 281-283 in the text.)
19. (Student response. See page 280 in the text.)
20. (Student response. See page 280 in the text.)

Teacher's Resources

The Mighty Dozen—Sports Myths and Facts,
reproducible master 16-2

1. Fact. Body composition will change for both men and women. However, men can bulk up more than women due to hormones.
2. Myth. Muscles and fat are two different types of tissue. Neither can turn into the other. However, muscles may decrease in size when training ends. Fat tissue may also accumulate if calorie intake is not reduced to meet the lower energy needs of a person no longer in training.
3. Myth. Carbohydrates should provide an athlete's primary source of energy.
4. Myth. Vitamins do not supply energy or improve performance. However, some vitamins help release energy from carbohydrates, proteins, and fats. Therefore, eating a balanced diet that meets daily vitamin needs is important.
5. Myth. Water is a critical nutrient and must be replenished to avoid dehydration, which will cause a decrease in performance.
6. Myth. Cramps are caused by severe fluid losses through sweating. Drinking plenty of water can help prevent cramps. Salt tablets can make the situation worse.
7. Myth. Sit-ups exercise the muscles of the stomach. Fat around the waist is reduced through energy expenditures being greater than energy intake.
8. Myth. Fat is an essential nutrient. Excess fat in the diet (over 30 percent of total calories) is associated with increased risk of some diseases, including obesity.

9. Myth. There is no such thing as a good or bad food. All foods are sources of energy. The key is balance, moderation, and variety in the foods chosen.
10. Myth. Steroids can be dangerous. Although they may help build muscle, they have risky side effects, such as liver disorders, kidney disease, and reproductive problems.
11. Fact. Athletes can replenish glycogen stores by eating a diet high in carbohydrates. All food groups include sources of carbohydrates.
12. Myth. Body composition does impact sports performance. Carrying excess fat decreases performance, but too little fat reduces energy levels and may stunt growth and cause amenorrhea.

Chapter 16 Test

1. D
2. E
3. C
4. A
5. B
6. T
7. T
8. F
9. T
10. T
11. F
12. T
13. F
14. T
15. F
16. T
17. T
18. F
19. F
20. T
21. A
22. C
23. C
24. D
25. A
26. D
27. D
28. C
29. B
30. A
31. (List two:) provide appropriate amounts of energy and fluid, avoid feelings of fullness, avoid digestive disturbances
32. (List four:) limit high-fiber foods, include moderate amounts of monounsaturated and polyunsaturated fats while avoiding saturated fats, reduce length and intensity of workout sessions, increase rest and sleep time, include weight training as part of exercise program, limit caffeine consumption, work with a registered dietitian
33. (List two. Student response. See text pages 283-284.)

Competition of Various Durations

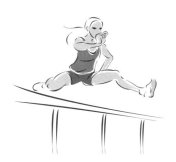
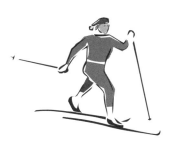
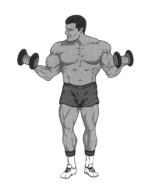
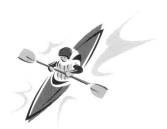
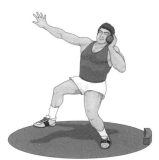
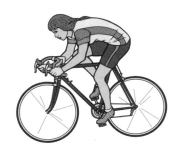

Anaerobic ← ———————————— → **Aerobic**

- bursts of activity
- lasts less than 90 seconds
- develops strength
- fueled mostly by muscle glycogen

- sustained activity
- lasts longer than 20 minutes
- develops cardiorespiratory fitness
- fueled by blood glucose and fat as well as muscle glycogen

© Goodheart-Willcox

The Mighty Dozen—Sports Myths and Facts

Name _____ **Date** _____ **Period** _____

For each sports myth or fact presented below, write a response to help dispel the myth or support the fact.

1. Strength training will improve muscle mass for women and men.
   _____

2. If a person stops weight training, muscle turns to fat.
   _____

3. Protein is the best source of energy for athletes.
   _____

4. Vitamin supplements enhance performance and give athletes more energy.
   _____

5. Water during exercise causes upset stomach and slows you down.
   _____

6. Muscle cramps are usually caused by a lack of salt.
   _____

7. Doing sit-ups will help get rid of fat around the waist.
   _____

8. Fat in the diet is unhealthy for athletes.
   _____

9. Some foods are good and some foods are bad when it comes to athletic performance.
   _____

10. Using steroids is one of the best ways to build muscle and add strength.
    _____

11. A good pregame meal is high in carbohydrates.
    _____

12. For an athlete to be competitive, he or she needs to reduce body fat to the lowest percentage possible.
    _____

In the space below, write three sports myths or facts you have heard.

A. _____

   _____

B. _____

   _____

C. _____

   _____

© Goodheart-Willcox

Eating for Sports Performance

Name_____

Date _____　　**Period** _____　　**Score** _____

Chapter 16 Test

Matching: Match the following terms and identifying phrases.

_____　1. A stored form of glucose found in the liver and muscle tissue.

_____　2. A product formed in the muscles as the result of the incomplete breakdown of glucose during anaerobic activity.

_____　3. An athlete involved in a sport that requires sustained muscle efforts for several hours at a time.

_____　4. A technique used by some athletes to trick the muscles into storing more glycogen for extra energy.

_____　5. A condition caused when body fluid levels drop too low.

A. carbohydrate loading
B. dehydration
C. endurance athlete
D. glycogen
E. lactic acid
F. stamina competitor

True/False: Circle *T* if the statement is true or *F* if the statement is false.

T　F　　6. Sam will use more calories running 4 miles in 30 minutes than his twin sister, Pam, who weighs 25 pounds less.

T　F　　7. Muscles use glucose as their main source of energy.

T　F　　8. For athletes involved in strength training, protein supplement drinks are essential.

T　F　　9. Carbohydrate loading is known to cause troublesome side effects for some athletes.

T　F　10. Symptoms of dehydration include dry skin, shivering, and dizziness.

T　F　11. Athletes can rely on their thirst as an indicator of when to consume fluids.

T　F　12. Cold water helps lower body temperature faster than warm water.

T　F　13. Research has shown that taking salt tablets is the most effective way to replace sodium lost during physical activity.

T　F　14. A pregame meal is recommended 3 to 4 hours before an event.

T　F　15. The recommended pregame meal is high in protein, high in fat, and low in carbohydrates.

T　F　16. Having a very low percentage of body fat can negatively affect an athlete's energy level for competition.

T　F　17. For teens who need to achieve a weight goal, gradual weight loss is always healthier than quick weight loss.

T　F　18. Athletes can rely on their coaches to provide sound advice about weight gain or loss for competition.

T　F　19. Athletes who are trying to gain weight should stop exercising to reduce the number of calories they burn.

T　F　20. Some products marketed as performance aids can actually have a negative effect on sports performance.

(Continued)

© Goodheart-Willcox

Name_____

Multiple Choice: Choose the best response. Write the letter in the space provided.

_____21. Which of the following does *not* affect the number of calories burned through exercise?
A. The age of the person exercising.
B. The body weight of the person exercising.
C. The intensity of the exercise.
D. The length of the exercise period.

_____22. Which of the following is *not* an end product of the breakdown of glucose in the body?
A. Carbon dioxide.
B. Energy.
C. Oxygen.
D. Water.

_____23. Which of the following is considered an endurance sport?
A. Basketball.
B. Hurdle jumping.
C. Marathon running.
D. Weight lifting.

_____24. What effect does training have on endurance athletes?
A. Delays muscle soreness and fatigue.
B. Develops the lungs' capacity to carry oxygen.
C. Improves the muscles' use of glucose.
D. All the above.

_____25. When should an athlete begin increasing fluid intake to avoid dehydration?
A. Two hours before a sports event.
B. Fifteen to thirty minutes before a sports event.
C. During a sports event.
D. After a sports event.

_____26. Which of the following beverages would be an athlete's best choice shortly before a competition?
A. Fruit juice.
B. Iced tea.
C. Milk.
D. Water.

_____27. Which of the following foods would be an athlete's best choice for a pregame meal?
A. Bacon cheeseburger and French fries.
B. Chocolate chip pancakes with syrup.
C. Fresh fruit salad and whole wheat rolls.
D. Spaghetti with marinara sauce.

_____28. The percentage ranges for body fat of physically fit male and female athletes are _____.
A. males 8-10%; females 15-17%
B. males 15-17%; females 8-10%
C. males 10-15%; females 18-24%
D. males 18-24%; females 10-15%

_____29. One of the recommended ways for an athlete to lose weight is to _____.
A. cut down on fluid intake
B. eat more complex carbohydrates while reducing fats in the diet
C. severely restrict calorie intake
D. skip meals occasionally

(Continued)

© Goodheart-Willcox

Name_____

_____30. What is an athlete's goal when trying to gain weight?
   A. To add muscle tissue.
   B. To build carbohydrate reserves.
   C. To expand fat stores.
   D. To increase water retention.

Essay Questions: Provide complete responses to the following questions or statements.

31. What are two goals of a pregame meal?

32. What are four tips for athletes who are trying to gain weight safely?

33. What are two cautions you would give an athlete who is considering buying performance aids?

Maintaining Positive Social and Mental Health

17

Objectives

After studying this chapter, the student will be able to
- determine the order in which a person will typically strive to meet specific human needs.
- list characteristics of a socially healthy person.
- explain techniques for promoting positive social health.
- summarize how self-concept and personality are related to mental health.
- identify strategies for promoting positive mental health.
- propose a self-management plan to make a positive life change.
- describe a situation that might require the help of a mental or social health care professional.

Bulletin Board

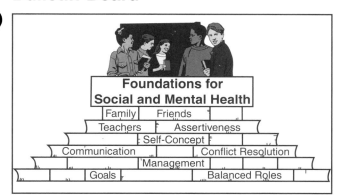

Title: *Foundations for Social and Mental Health*

Make bricks from various colors of poster board. Write words on the bricks describing the factors that support positive social and mental health. Ask students for word suggestions. Stack the bricks on top of one another to make a wall. Cut pictures of teens experiencing positive lifestyles from magazines and place them on top of the wall.

Teaching Materials

Text, pages 287-305
Learn the Language
Check Your Knowledge
Put Learning into Action
Explore Further

Student Activity Guide, pages 117-126
    A. *Applying Maslow's Hierarchy*
    B. *Communication Snapshot*
    C. *Dear Peacemaker*
    D. *Teams Work*
    E. *Countdown to Mental Health*
    F. *Managing Myself*
    G. *Backtrack Through Chapter 17*

Teacher's Resources
Characteristics of Successful Communicators, reproducible master 17-1
A Well of Resources, transparency master 17-2
Stepping Stones to Positive Social and Mental Health, color transparency master CT-17
Targeting Strength Areas, reproducible master 17-3
Chapter 17 Test

Introducing the Chapter

1. Have students list all the words that come to mind when they hear the words *social health* and *mental health*. Use this list of words to discuss how a person might become socially and mentally healthy.
2. Develop a class definition for the terms *positive social health* and *positive mental health*. Hang the definitions in the room where they can be seen frequently.
3. Have students form small groups. Ask them to discuss ways social and mental health are affected by daily choices. Have each group report their findings to the class.
4. Have students keep a journal while studying this chapter. Ask students to describe their feelings and activities that make them feel good or bad about themselves. Ask students to write about how they can handle bad situations in ways that will make them feel better.

Strategies to Reteach, Reinforce, Enrich, and Extend Text Concepts

Basic Human Needs

5. **ER** Review each of the levels of Maslow's hierarchy. Have students draw their own hierarchy. On the left side of the triangle, ask students to list

personal needs that are currently met. On the right side of the triangle, have students list needs they hope to have fulfilled. Explain that every person is always working for self-actualization.

6. **RF** Discuss the contributions Maslow's theory makes toward explaining human behavior. Include the idea that if needs are not met, social and mental health will be affected.

7. **RF** *Applying Maslow's Hierarchy,* Activity A, SAG. Students are to label each level of the hierarchy diagram and give two examples for each type of need. Students will then answer questions about human needs.

What Is Social Health?

8. **RF** Have students prepare a personal "circles of influence" diagram. Students should place their own names in the center circle. Have students draw circles in a ring around the center circle. These outer circles should be labeled with the names of people who have most influenced students' personal development. Ask students if they are surprised by the number of people who have influenced them.

9. **ER** Guest speaker. Invite a preschool educator to discuss the importance of meeting the social needs of children. Ask about words and actions that promote the positive social development of children. Discuss how to handle situations in which children require guidance. Have students prepare questions ahead of time.

10. **ER** Divide the class into groups. Instruct the groups to make a list of the ways social development can be affected by birth order. For example, oldest children may be more independent, while youngest children may be more social. Only children may express higher expectations in their associations with others. Have each group share their ideas in a classroom discussion.

11. **EX** Have students write a paper on how an important person has influenced who they are and who they want to be. Discourage students from writing about people they have not interacted with personally, such as movie stars or book characters.

Promoting Positive Social Health

12. **ER** Ask student volunteers to express various emotions through body language. Discuss the messages people send with body language. Ask what happens when nonverbal messages and verbal messages do not send the same message.

13. **ER** Divide students into groups. Have each group role-play a situation in which one student expresses disappointment, anger, or confusion. Have the other group members provide appropriate feedback. Discuss different ways communication can affect each situation.

14. **RF** *Characteristics of Successful Communicators,* reproducible master 17-1. Students are to rate themselves on given qualities of successful communicators.

15. **RF** *Communication Snapshot,* Activity B, SAG. Students are to read given conversations and determine if the communication is effective or ineffective. If the communication is ineffective, students should give suggestions for improvement.

16. **ER** Guest speaker. Invite a school peer mediator or guidance counselor to describe the processes used to resolve student conflicts. If possible, have students observe a peer mediation session in action. Highlight the importance of using "I" messages and compromising.

17. **RT** Review the definition of *assertiveness.* Have students practice using assertive responses to requests and difficult situations.

18. **ER** *Dear Peacemaker,* Activity C, SAG. Students are to write responses to people in conflict situations.

19. **RF** Have students write down qualities their friends have. Discuss how these qualities have influenced the social health of the students as well as their friends.

20. **RF** Have students give examples of compromise used in team projects. Ask why it is sometimes difficult for teams to function effectively.

21. **RF** *Teams Work,* Activity D, SAG. Students are to answer questions related to teamwork.

What Is Mental Health?

22. **ER** Have students research mental health on the Internet. They may visit the Web sites for the National Institutes of Health (NIH), National Library of Medicine, and National Mental Health Association. Have students request resources on mental health issues.

23. **RF** *A Well of Resources,* transparency master 17-2. Use the transparency to discuss ways people can help others build self-esteem. Ask students to share examples of times someone helped them build self-esteem.

Promoting Positive Mental Health

24. **RF** *Stepping Stones to Positive Social and Mental Health,* color transparency CT-17. Use the transparency to identify qualities possessed by socially and mentally healthy people.

25. **ER** Divide the class into pairs. Have the pairs of students talk with each other for five minutes about each other's interests. At the end of five minutes, go around the room and have each

person name one positive trait of his or her partner. Discuss how hearing positive statements about themselves affects the students' self-concepts.

26. **RF** *Countdown to Mental Health,* Activity E, SAG. Students are to answer questions that will help them assess their mental health. Students will determine areas they need to improve and list three goals they could set to help them improve.

27. **ER** Guest speaker. Invite a physician to class to discuss the relationship between physical and mental health. Have students prepare questions beforehand.

28. **EX** Have students determine the average time they usually spend each day on school, family, work, community, and self. Ask students to evaluate whether they think their roles are balanced. If not, ask them to evaluate what changes they might make in their schedules to distribute their roles more proportionately.

Making Positive Life Changes

29. **RF** Review the steps of the self-management plan. Ask students to apply the process to a life change example like getting more sleep.

30. **ER** *Targeting Strength Areas,* reproducible master 17-3. Students are to identify their strengths, areas to improve, and short-term and long-term goals for improvement.

31. **EX** *Managing Myself,* Activity F, SAG. Students are to prepare a self-management plan for making a positive behavior change.

Seeking Help for Social and Mental Health Problems

32. **ER** Guest speaker. Invite a psychologist to help dispel the myths about social and mental illnesses. Ask the speaker how people know when they need help, what resources are available to people with mental and social health problems, and what to expect from professional therapists.

Chapter Review

33. **RF** Draw three circles that overlap in the center. Label the three circles *social health, mental health,* and *physical health.* Discuss with students how the three areas impact each other. Have students suggest names for the area where the circles overlap.

34. **ER** Have each student choose a key term from the chapter, scramble the letters of the term, and write it on an index card. Collect, shuffle, and redistribute the cards. Have students unscramble the terms and discuss how they relate to positive social and mental health.

35. **RF** *Backtrack Through Chapter 17,* Activity G, SAG. Students are to provide complete answers to questions and statements that will help them recall, interpret, apply, and practice chapter concepts.

Above and Beyond

36. **ER** Start a "person of the week" program in the school. Each week, have students nominate a student or faculty member who has been instrumental in creating a positive learning environment. Stress that nominees should possess qualities discussed in the chapter.

37. **ER** Have students organize a "mental health week" for the school. Have students make posters promoting balance, support, and management to hang throughout the school.

38. **EX** Organize a school program that focuses on positive social and mental health. Create a resource center of materials for students and faculty to review.

Answer Key

Text

Check Your Knowledge, pages 304-305

1. (List four:) oxygen, water, food, shelter, clothing, sleep
2. After achieving one goal toward self actualization, you need to set new goals. Few people reach a point where they feel they have reached the highest level of achievement in every area.
3. (List three:) patience, empathy, courtesy, selflessness (Students may justify other responses.)
4. Most children in a physically safe and secure environment learn positive social skills by watching parents, family members, and caregivers.
5. (List five: Student response. See page 291 in the text.)
6. (List five: Student response. See page 292 in the text.)
7. B
8. false
9. Avoiding needless worrying can help a person reserve mental energy for times when he or she needs it most.
10. When someone feels physically well, he or she has the energy needed to face problems that can affect mental health. When someone is in a good state of mental health, his or her body can fight disease more effectively.
11. (List three each. Student response. See Figure 17-13 on page 299 in the text.)
12. This helps the person narrow his or her focus. He or she is less likely to be successful if his or her attention is scattered in too many directions.

13. time, money, physical energy
14. evaluate outcomes
15. Therapy often focuses on helping clients develop the social and mental tools they need to help themselves.

Student Activity Guide

Applying Maslow's Hierarchy, Activity A

(For level names and placements, see page 288. Examples are student response. For questions 1-5, sample answers include the following:)
1. Only by addressing these needs can a person reach his or her full potential.
2. The person will not be able to feel good about himself or herself (meet esteem needs) or reach his or her full potential (self-actualization needs). The person can work to form loving relationships in adulthood.
3. In a dangerous neighborhood, people fear for their lives. They worry about being hurt or killed. They worry their belongings will be stolen or destroyed. (Suggestions are student response.)
4. If a person cannot meet basic needs, most of his or her energy will be directed at trying to meet these needs. The person will not have time or energy to address higher needs. For instance, if a person is starving, he or she will not be concerned with setting and reaching lofty personal goals.
5. People can satisfy their esteem needs by developing positive relationships with people who value them. They can also meet these needs by learning to value themselves.

Communication Snapshot, Activity B

(Suggestions are student response.)
1. effective; rationale—he knew what he wanted to say, was honest, and avoided using slang and contradicting nonverbal messages
2. ineffective; rationale—he didn't think before he spoke, he did not use specific words to express his feelings, he used name-calling
3. ineffective; rationale—she didn't maintain eye contact, she did not use specific words to express her feelings
4. effective; rationale—she restated the message to make sure she understood
5. ineffective; rationale—he sent nonverbal messages (rolling eyes) that conflicted with what he said
6. ineffective; rationale—she did not speak loudly or clearly enough to be heard, she did not use specific words to express her feelings
7. effective; rationale—he listened carefully, he expressed understanding, he used specific words to express his own feelings, he was honest

8. ineffective; rationale—she was not honest; her nonverbal message (facial expression) did not match her words

Teams Work, Activity D

1. To cooperate means to work together.
2. To compromise means to find a solution that blends ideas from two differing parties.
3. (Student response.)
4. Without each member's help, the team's goal cannot be achieved.
5. (Student response.)
6. (Student response.)
7. (Student response.)
8. (Student response.)
9. Each person on the team has special talents and ideas to contribute. Also, having more people involved makes the work go faster.
10. (Student response.)

Backtrack Through Chapter 17, Activity G

1. a ranked series
2. in the family
3. friends
4. verbal
5. nonverbal
6. (Sample answer:) I feel angry when you say you will call but don't.
7. Assertiveness is the boldness to express what you think and feel in a way that does not offend others.
8. They focus on the team goals, show willingness to compromise, value the importance of each person's job to the team's success, cooperate and offer help when needed, and treat each person as a valued member by seeking his or her ideas and opinions.
9. all the characteristics that make you a unique person; your feelings and behaviors as you interact with your surroundings
10. self, family, school, job, and community
11. (List three of the following:)
    • Am I satisfied with the results of my choices and actions?
    • Do I feel better about myself than I did before?
    • Is my health status better now than it was before?
    • Do my friends and family show support of my newly developed behaviors and skills?
    • Does my overall quality of life seem to be improved?
12. Burnout means a lack of energy and motivation to work toward goals.
13. seek the help of mental and social health care professionals
14. Until lower needs are satisfied, people are unable to focus on higher-level needs. (Examples are student response.)
15. Learning about yourself helps you form stronger relationships, which increase your social health.

16. (Student response.)
17. Assertive means expressing yourself without offending others. Aggressive means expressing your feelings in a way that is pushy and offensive.
18. Self-concept is the image you have of yourself. Self-esteem is the worth or value you assign yourself.
19. (Student response.)
20. (Student response.)

Teacher's Resources

Chapter 17 Test

1.	E	12.	I	23.	T
2.	F	13.	T	24.	F
3.	G	14.	F	25.	F
4.	B	15.	T	26.	B
5.	A	16.	T	27.	C
6.	C	17.	F	28.	A
7.	J	18.	F	29.	B
8.	H	19.	F	30.	D
9.	K	20.	F	31.	C
10.	D	21.	T	32.	D
11.	L	22.	F	33.	A

34. (Describe five. See chart 17-10 on page 295 in the text.)

35. People with tense personalities tend to worry about unpleasant events before they happen. Needless worrying and unfounded anger can cloud a person's overall outlook. People with relaxed personalities aren't bothered by problems that *might* occur, only those that *do* occur. Avoiding needless worrying can help a person reserve mental energy for times he or she needs it most.

36. 1. List your strengths. 2. List your "needs improvement" behaviors. 3. Prioritize your "needs improvement" behaviors. 4. Clarify your goal. 5. List your alternatives for achieving your goal. 6. Evaluate the pros and cons of each alternative. 7. Make a choice and act on it. 8. Evaluate the outcomes of your choice. (Examples are student response.)

Characteristics of Successful Communicators

Name_____ **Date** _____ **Period** _____

For each statement about communication, circle the number that best describes your behavior. Then total your score below.

	Frequency		
	Rarely	**Sometimes**	**Usually**
1. I enjoy listening to people talk.	1	2	3
2. I write and speak clearly.	1	2	3
3. I avoid using slang.	1	2	3
4. My nonverbal communication agrees with what I communicate verbally.	1	2	3
5. I use words that convey my exact meaning.	1	2	3
6. I maintain eye contact when I am speaking with someone.	1	2	3
7. I am honest.	1	2	3
8. I show concern for the needs of others.	1	2	3
9. I listen for feelings and empathize with what others are saying.	1	2	3
10. I appreciate receiving ideas from others.	1	2	3
11. Patience is one of my strong points.	1	2	3
12. I am nonjudgmental when another person is talking.	1	2	3
13. I proofread my written and electronic messages carefully to be sure they do not contain spelling or grammar errors.	1	2	3
14. I evaluate the tone of my written and electronic messages to be sure they cannot be misinterpreted as offensive.	1	2	3
15. I keep my sentences short and limit my use of technical words in written and electronic messages.	1	2	3

Total score: _____

If your total score was over 34, you have characteristics of a successful communicator. If you scored lower, you may need to improve your communication skills. In the space that follows, describe three techniques people can use to improve their communication skills.

_____

_____

_____

_____

_____

_____

_____

© Goodheart-Willcox

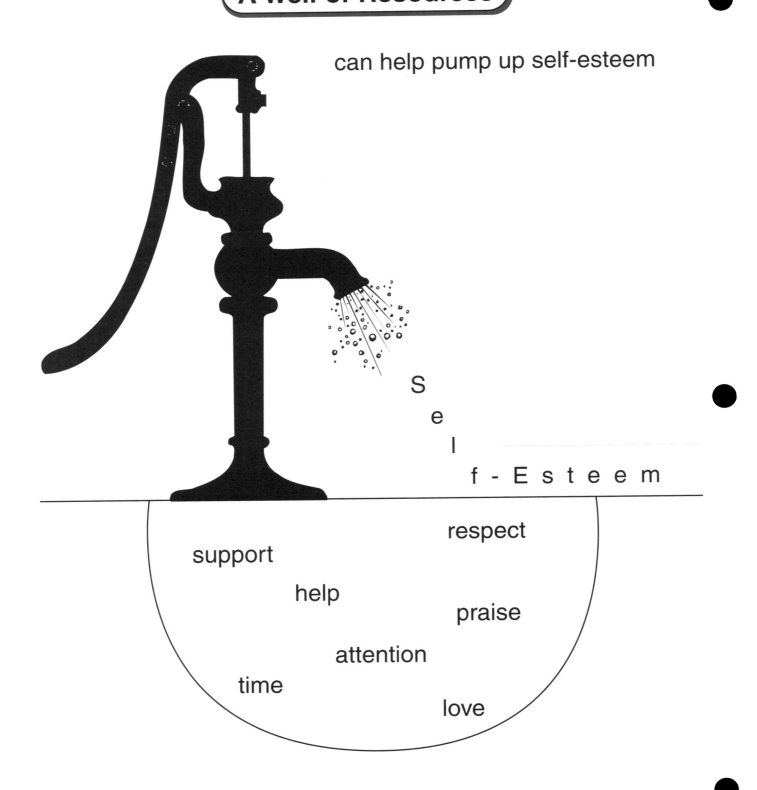

A Well of Resources

can help pump up self-esteem

Self-Esteem

respect

support

help

praise

attention

time

love

© Goodheart-Willcox

Targeting Strength Areas

Name_____   Date _____   Period _____

List your strengths in the center circle. In the next circle, list behaviors you need to improve. In the third circle, list short-term goals for improving these behaviors. List your long-term goals for improvement in the outer circle.

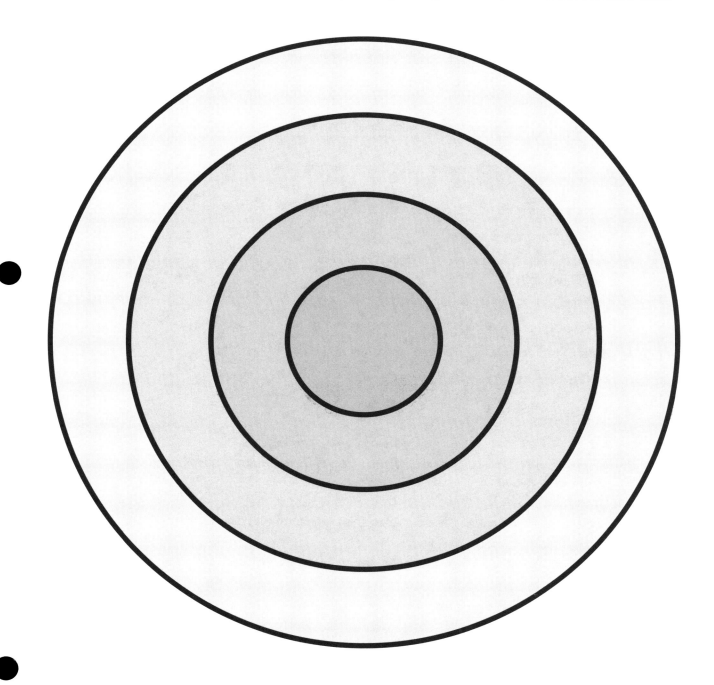

© Goodheart-Willcox

Maintaining Positive Social and Mental Health

Name

Date _____ Period _____ Score _____

Chapter 17 Test

Matching: Match the following terms and identifying phrases.

_____ 1. A solution to a problem that blends ideas from two differing parties.

_____ 2. The sending of a message from one source to another without the use of words.

_____ 3. All the characteristics that make each person unique.

_____ 4. A sense of proportional distribution given to life's roles and responsibilities.

_____ 5. A person's boldness to express what he or she thinks and feels in a way that does not offend others.

_____ 6. A lack of energy and motivation to work toward goals.

_____ 7. The worth or value a person assigns himself or herself.

_____ 8. A person's belief that he or she is doing his or her best to reach full human potential.

_____ 9. Learning how to get along with others.

_____ 10. The sending of a message from one source to another.

_____ 11. Effort of two or more people toward a common goal.

_____ 12. The idea a person has about himself or herself.

A. assertiveness
B. balance
C. burnout
D. communication
E. compromise
F. nonverbal communication
G. personality
H. self-actualization
I. self-concept
J. self-esteem
K. social development
L. teamwork
M. verbal communication

True/False: Circle *T* if the statement is true or *F* if the statement is false.

T F 13. A state of wellness is more likely to be achieved after basic needs are met.

T F 14. According to Maslow's theory, a person can experience self-actualization even if his or her physical needs are not met.

T F 15. Gangs can be a threat to teens' needs for safety and security.

T F 16. Socially healthy people enjoy the relationships they form with others.

T F 17. People first learn social skills in school.

T F 18. Communication occurs only through speaking.

T F 19. It is best to resolve a conflict in front of others so witnesses are present.

T F 20. People who are passive express their feelings in ways that are pushy and offensive.

T F 21. Developing the qualities of a friend will improve your social health by helping you form strong friendships.

T F 22. Team members can accomplish more individually than they can as a group.

T F 23. A high level of self-esteem enables you to set goals and take actions to achieve them.

(Continued)

© Goodheart-Willcox

Name_____

T F   24. Physical health does not affect mental health.

T F   25. The role of the professional mental health counselor is to provide people with solutions to their problems.

Multiple Choice: Choose the best response. Write the letter in the space provided.

_____26. Food, shelter, clothing, and sleep are all _____ needs.
   A. esteem
   B. physical
   C. love and acceptance
   D. safety and security

_____27. Social development _____.
   A. occurs at birth
   B. ends after marriage
   C. is a lifelong process
   D. All the above.

_____28. The closest and most continuous relationships most people have occur _____.
   A. within their families
   B. with friends
   C. over the Internet
   D. through group activities

_____29. Which is a guideline for effective communications?
   A. Use slang terms to make people feel included.
   B. Maintain eye contact to show interest.
   C. Use nonverbal signals that communicate boredom.
   D. Whisper.

_____30. If you do not understand a message someone is sending, _____.
   A. become angry with the person
   B. walk away
   C. try to interpret the message on your own
   D. restate the information that has been shared

_____31. Which is an example of assertiveness?
   A. "You're so unfair!"
   B. "I forgot to do my homework—let me see your answers."
   C. "I won't be able to serve on that committee. It will interfere with my basketball practice schedule."
   D. "I can't believe you want to see that stupid movie."

_____32. A team player _____.
   A. enjoys being the center of attention
   B. focuses on personal gains
   C. doesn't express personal opinions
   D. expresses appreciation of others' contributions

_____33. People with negative self-concepts _____.
   A. do not have accurate pictures of themselves
   B. have good mental health
   C. see both strengths and weaknesses
   D. have high self-esteem

(Continued)

© Goodheart-Willcox

Name_____

Essay Questions: Provide complete responses to the following questions or statements.

34. Describe five characteristics of a person with positive mental and social health.

35. Explain how personality can affect mental health.

36. List the steps of the self-management plan and give an example for each step.

© Goodheart-Willcox

Stress and Wellness

Objectives

After studying this chapter, students will be able to
- recognize potential sources of stress in their lives.
- describe the effects of stress on physical and mental health.
- explain how recognizing signs of stress, using support systems, relaxing, and using positive self-talk can help them manage stress.
- use strategies to prevent stress.

Bulletin Boards

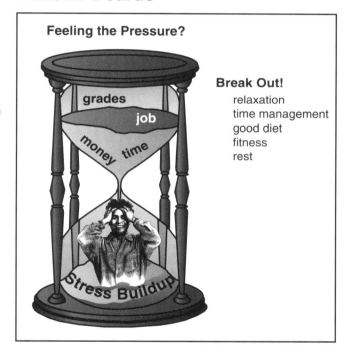

Feeling the Pressure?

grades

job

money time

Stress Buildup

Break Out!
relaxation
time management
good diet
fitness
rest

Title: *Feeling the Pressure? Break Out!*

Place a large cutout of an hourglass on the left side of the bulletin board. In the sand running from the top of the hourglass, list common stressors for teens, such as grades, time, money, and job. Sketch a person buried waist deep in the sand in the bottom of the hourglass with the words *Stress Buildup*. Place the title to the right of the hourglass with a list of stress relievers, such as relaxation, time management, good diet, fitness, and rest.

Title: *Read the Signs to Reduce Stress*

Place yellow caution signs on the bulletin board that warn of stress symptoms, such as frustration, irritability, depression, headache, upset stomach, and fatigue.

Teaching Materials

Text, pages 306-321
> *Learn the Language*
> *Check Your Knowledge*
> *Put Learning into Action*
> *Explore Further*

Student Activity Guide, pages 127-134
> A. *Do Not Stress Out!*
> B. *Stress Metaphors*
> C. *Good Stress/Bad Stress*
> D. *The Pileup Effect*
> E. *Straight Talk on Stress*
> F. *Friends in Need*
> G. *Backtrack Through Chapter 18*

Teacher's Resources
> *Optimal Stress,* transparency master 18-1
> *Are You Stressed Out?* reproducible master 18-2
> *Keys to Good Time Management,* color transparency CT-18
> Chapter 18 Test

Introducing the Chapter

1. Discuss how the following quote relates to stress:
Rule number 1 is: Don't sweat the small stuff.
Rule number 2 is: It's all small stuff, and if you can't fight and you can't flee, flow. (R.S. Eliot)
2. Ask each student to write his or her definition of stress. Have students read their definitions to the class as you tally how many definitions reflect positive stress and how many reflect negative stress. Explain that both types of stress affect social, emotional, and physical performance.
3. Have students think about life as it might have been 5,000, 1,000, and 10 years ago. Ask students how they think people's sources of stress have changed since these earlier eras.
4. Have students describe events they find stressful. Write responses on the chalkboard. Then ask students to rank items listed on the chalkboard

from least stressful to most stressful. Discuss why a given situation is more stressful to some people than to others.

Strategies to Reteach, Reinforce, Enrich, and Extend Text Concepts

Stress Is Part of Life

5. **RT** *Optimal Stress,* transparency master, 18-1. Use the transparency to illustrate how performance is related to degree of stress. Greatest performance is achieved when positive stress is high and negative stress is low. Too little positive stress or too much negative stress affect performance quality negatively. Invite students to share examples of times when positive stress improved their performance.

6. **EX** Divide the class into two groups to debate the statement *Change always produces stress.* Students should list points that support or refute the statement.

7. **EX** *Are You Stressed Out?* reproducible master 18-2. Have students complete the self-test to identify their levels of perceived stress. The lower the score, the greater the effects stress is likely to be having on personal wellness. Remind students that high levels of stress may indicate a need to think about strategies to reducing stress.

8. **RF** Have students bring in newspaper or magazine articles about crisis events in which people reacted with the fight or flight response. Place articles in a resource area within the room. Discuss the reactions hormones trigger in the body when a person is responding to a crisis or other stressful event.

9. **ER** Guest speaker. Invite an executive in a highly stressful working environment to discuss the kinds of stresses that exist in the work world. Ask the speaker to describe factors that make a job stressful. Encourage students to be aware of these factors when they look for jobs.

Effects of Stress on Health

10. **ER** Choose two students to be anonymous observers. Their task is to record signs of stress exhibited by the rest of the class when you announce that students have 5 minutes to study for a pop quiz worth 20 percent of their grades. After 5 minutes, ask the observers to report the signs of visible stress displayed by their classmates. Ask students to report how their bodies responded to the threat of a quiz. Summarize outcomes.

11. **RF** Provide students with crayons and markers. Ask students to draw a picture on one side of a sheet of paper showing what stress feels like physically, socially, and emotionally. On the other side of the paper, ask them to draw a picture showing what relaxed feels like. Encourage creativity. Play appropriate music to create moods of stress and relaxation while students draw. Invite students to describe their pictures to the rest of the class. Identify different ways people respond to stress and relaxation.

12. **ER** Have each student choose a topic related to stress he or she can research via the Internet. Ask students to summarize the results of their research in two-page papers.

13. **EX** *Stress Metaphors,* Activity B, SAG. After reading an example, students are to write an original metaphor for stress.

14. **RF** *Good Stress/Bad Stress,* Activity C, SAG. Students are to recognize positive or negative stress in given situations. For each situation of positive stress, students are to identify one good result that could occur. For each situation of negative stress, students are to identify one bad result that could occur.

15. **EX** *The Pileup Effect,* Activity D, SAG. After looking at an example, students are to create a diagram illustrating how one stressor can lead to a series of other stressors. Then students are to answer questions about cumulative stress.

Managing Stress

16. **ER** Guest speaker. Invite a school counselor to discuss strategies students can use to manage stress. Ask the speaker to emphasize school services available to students dealing with stress.

17. **RF** *Straight Talk on Stress,* Activity E, SAG. Students are to identify true statements and correct false statements about stress.

18. **RF** *Friends in Need,* Activity F, SAG. Students are to suggest positive ways people in given scenarios can manage stress.

Preventing Stress

19. **RT** *Keys to Good Time Management,* color transparency CT-18. Use the transparency to remind students of techniques they can use to control their use of time and avoid the stress created by rushing and failing to finish tasks.

20. **ER** Have each student prepare a four-column chart. The first column will be used to rank the priority of avoided tasks, which are listed in the second column. Tasks students list in the second column might include writing a paper, completing a scholarship application, or looking for a job. In the third column, students should write a solution for overcoming their procrastination of each task. Students should use the last column to identify a tentative time to begin tackling the task.

21. **ER** Have students keep "destress journals" for one week. Ask students to record their daily food choices, physical activities, and sleep patterns. At the end of the week, have students evaluate their stress level for the week. Ask students to share their journals in class to see if a relationship can be made between health habits and stress levels.

Chapter Review

22. **RF** *Do Not Stress Out!* Activity A, SAG. Students are to complete a word puzzle by filling in appropriate chapter vocabulary terms.

23. **RF** *Backtrack Through Chapter 18,* Activity G, SAG. Students are to provide complete answers to questions and statements that will help them recall, interpret, apply, and practice chapter concepts.

Above and Beyond

24. **ER** Have students work in groups to research an alternative technique for reducing stress, such as massage, hypnosis, or herbal therapies. Each group member should be responsible for a different part of the research. Research should include how the chosen technique is used, who supports its use, how effective it is, and any controversy involved in the use of the technique. Groups should share their findings in oral presentations.

25. **ER** Have students use the Internet to research stress reduction techniques used by people in other cultures. Ask students to share their findings by demonstrating the techniques to the class.

26. **EX** Have the class plan a "Time-Out Night" for all students during exam week. The class should plan a variety of activities to help students relieve stress.

27. **ER** Have students select favorite relaxation music to be played during the school's lunch hour.

28. **EX** Have students research how colors, textures, objects, and sounds in a physical environment can promote stress reduction. Then have students prepare an illustrated proposal incorporating their research into the redecoration of a student commons area. Submit the proposal to school administrators.

Answer Key

Text

Check Your Knowlegde, page 320

1. (Describe two:) when you see an event or situation as a threat to your well-being, when you experience a number of minor changes within a short period, when one change continues to affect you for a long time

2. (List three each. Student response. See Chart 18-3 on page 308 in the text.)

3. alarm, resistance, exhaustion

4. (List three:) breathe harder and faster, heart beats more rapidly, liver releases glucose into the bloodstream, fat cells release fat into the bloodstream, blood pressure increases

5. During periods of stress, immune system defenses can become lowered, making a person more vulnerable to infections.

6. Thoughts about a stressor and how to address it can interfere with peaceful sleep. This lack of rest can further add to stress.

7. (List three:) nibbling, bingeing, failing to eat due to focus on stressor, upset stomach, development of eating disorders

8. (List four. Student response. See page 313 in the text.)

9. (Give one example for each:) emotional—frustration, irritability, depression; behavioral—withdrawing from friends, grinding your teeth, forgetting details; physical—headaches, upset stomach, fatigue

10. (List three:) family members, friends, school counselors, social workers, psychologists

11. (Describe two. Student response. See pages 315-316 in the text.)

12. D

13. true

14. false

15. Alcohol and drugs only temporarily mask the symptoms of stress. At the same time, they create a huge new source of stress for people who abuse them.

Student Activity Guide

Do Not Stress Out! Activity A

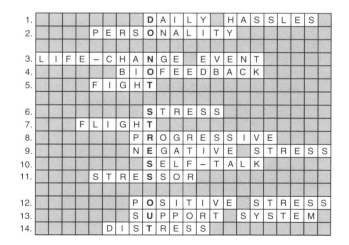

Good Stress/Bad Stress, Activity C

(Suggested answers follow. Accept other responses if supported.)
1. type—positive; result—peak performance
2. type—positive; result—best effort
3. type—negative; result—damage to relationship
4. type—negative; result—lessens work quality
5. type—negative; result—prevents rational action
6. type—negative; result—unhappiness

The Pileup Effect, Activity D

1. parents' divorce
2. (Student response.)
3. (List three. Student response.)
4. Having a support system can alleviate stress before it piles up. Having someone to talk to may reduce the stress a person feels. People in your support system can also provide insight into solving stressful situations.
5. Alleviating minor stress prevents it from becoming major stress. Letting a problem grow only leads to greater amounts of stress in the future.

Straight Talk on Stress, Activity E

1. resistance
2. physical
3. true
4. widening
5. resistance
6. true
7. true
8. true
9. bloodstream
10. release
11. true
12. true
13. lower
14. true
15. low
16. true
17. true
18. emotional
19. true
20. irritated by

Friends in Need, Activity F

(Suggested answers follow. Accept other responses if supported.)
1. Learn to read biofeedback; try to determine causes of stress.
2. Turn to people in your support system when you need help.
3. Use a relaxation technique, such as deep breathing or progressive muscle relaxation.
4. Use positive self-talk.
5. Keep a time-activity diary; then plan a time schedule.
6. Do not overlook physical needs, because this can bring on health problems and compound stress.

Backtrack Through Chapter 18, Activity G

1. tension or agitation
2. positive and negative
3. by making you fearful and making you perform poorly
4. by motivating you to accomplish challenging goals
5. daily hassle, because it is an everyday occurrence that produces stress
6. life-change event, because it is a major stressor that will change a person's lifestyle
7. The fight or flight response is a natural response to threatening situations. The body prepares to conquer danger or escape to safety.
8. (List an example for alarm stage, resistance stage, and exhaustion stage. Student response.)
9. coronary heart disease, hypertension, stroke
10. effects on the immune system, on sleep patterns, and on eating habits
11. (Student response. Answers may include the following.) recognize signs of stress, use support systems, learn how to relax, use positive self-talk, learn ways to prevent stress
12. learn to manage your time, stay physically fit, eat a nutritious diet, get adequate rest, avoid substance abuse
13. Biofeedback is a technique of focusing on involuntary bodily responses in order to control them.
14. (Student response.)
15. (Student response.)
16. (Student response. See page 314 in the text.)
17. (Student response. See page 314 in the text.)
18. no (Explanation is student response. See pages 314-315 in the text.)
19. (Student response.)
20. (Student response.)

Teacher's Resources

Chapter 18 Test

1. G	9. T	17. T	25. B
2. H	10. T	18. F	26. D
3. E	11. F	19. F	27. A
4. B	12. T	20. T	28. B
5. D	13. F	21. T	29. C
6. A	14. T	22. F	30. C
7. I	15. T	23. F	
8. F	16. T	24. B	

31. (Student response.)
32. (List two effects on physical health and one effect on emotional health. Student response. See pages 310-312 in the text.)
33. (List three:) manage time, eat a nutritious diet, stay physically fit, get adequate rest, avoid substance abuse

Optimal Stress

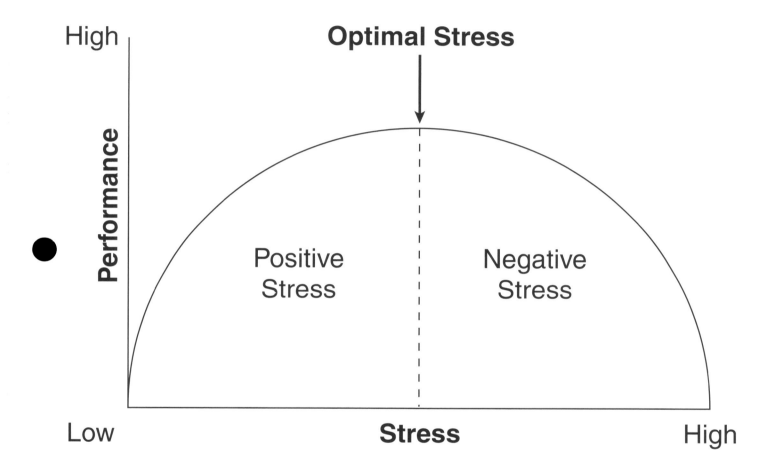

Optimal stress. The level of stress at which motivation is greatest to accomplish challenging goals.

Are You Stressed Out?

Circle the number that best describes your response to each question. Then answer the questions that follow.

	Never	Sometimes	Often
1. I can tell when I feel anxious, tense, or irritable.	1	2	3
2. I can relax my mind and body without the use of drugs.	1	2	3
3. I respect my accomplishments.	1	2	3
4. I enjoy my life.	1	2	3
5. I get enough sleep.	1	2	3
6. I can fall asleep within 20 minutes.	1	2	3
7. I eat a nutritious diet.	1	2	3
8. I take time to eat meals at a relaxed pace.	1	2	3
9. I feel in control of my mind. My body is relaxed.	1	2	3
10. I can make decisions without too much difficulty.	1	2	3

Everybody feels stressed sometimes. However, the lower your score, the more stressed you are likely to feel.

My score is _____

What causes people to become stressed? _____

_____

_____

In what ways do you think males and females react differently to stress? _____

_____

_____

What effect does stress within the family have on the children in the family?_____

_____

_____

How does the location of their homes affect people's stress?_____

_____

_____

© Goodheart-Willcox

Stress and Wellness

Name_____

Date _____   Period _____   Score _____

Chapter 18 Test

Matching: Match the following terms and identifying phrases.

_____ 1. The inner agitation a person feels when he or she is exposed to change.

_____ 2. A source of stress.

_____ 3. Major stressors, such as death, divorce, and legal problems, that can greatly alter a person's lifestyle.

_____ 4. Minor stressors that produce tension.

_____ 5. Physical reactions to stress that happen as the body gathers its resources to conquer danger or escape to safety.

_____ 6. A technique of focusing on involuntary bodily processes, such as breathing and pulse rate, in order to control them.

_____ 7. A group of people who can provide a person with physical help and emotional comfort.

_____ 8. A person's internal conversations about himself or herself and the situations he or she faces.

A. biofeedback
B. daily hassles
C. distress
D. fight or flight response
E. life-change events
F. self-talk
G. stress
H. stressor
I. support system

True/False: Circle *T* if the statement is true or *F* if the statement is false.

T   F   9. The effects of life's events can accumulate to cause a buildup of stress.

T   F   10. Positive stress increases performance effectiveness, whereas negative stress decreases it.

T   F   11. An example of a daily hassle is parents divorcing.

T   F   12. Stress increases the risk of heart disease.

T   F   13. During times of stress, the body's immune system becomes more effective in providing protection from diseases.

T   F   14. During stressful times, increased levels of mental activity have a tendency to decrease sleep quality.

T   F   15. For some people, stress suppresses appetite; for others it triggers excessive eating.

T   F   16. A circumstance that is stressful to one person may not be stressful to another.

T   F   17. The type B personality is more easy-going than the type A personality.

T   F   18. A person's attitude toward stressful situations has little to do with how stress will affect his or her health.

T   F   19. Stress is a silent condition that provides no physical clues it is occurring.

T   F   20. Personal stress levels can be reduced by simply sharing a problem with a listening friend.

T   F   21. Learning to relax the body helps reduce the health risks of stress.

T   F   22. The purpose of a time-activity diary is to learn how to accomplish more in less time.

T   F   23. Nutrition and diet patterns have little effect on levels of personal stress.

© Goodheart-Willcox

(Continued)

Name_____

Multiple Choice: Choose the best response. Write the letter in the space provided.

_____24. What kind of stress is created by fear of violence, threats, and danger?
   A. Annoying stress.
   B. Distress.
   C. Event-related stress.
   D. Positive stress.

_____25. The stage of stress when mental fatigue sets in and work performance is affected is called _____.
   A. alarm
   B. exhaustion
   C. flight
   D. resistance

_____26. Slowly tensing and then relaxing different groups of muscles is called _____.
   A. biofeedback
   B. deep breathing
   C. meditation
   D. progressive muscle relaxation

_____27. Which statement represents an example of positive self-talk?
   A. "If I take one step at a time, I'll get there."
   B. "I'll never be able to do this."
   C. "My nose is crooked."
   D. "Why am I so stupid?"

_____28. Which of the following is a recommended guideline for planning a time schedule?
   A. Reduce time scheduled for sleep to catch up on unfinished tasks.
   B. Schedule tasks with the highest priority first.
   C. Schedule tasks with the lowest priority first.
   D. When a special opportunity arises, cram it into the existing schedule.

_____29. What is the relationship between physical activity and stress?
   A. Physical activity makes stressors go away.
   B. Physical activity prevents stress.
   C. Physical activity refreshes the mind to allow clearer thinking about solutions to problems.
   D. A and B above.

_____30. Which of the following statements about alcohol and stress is a myth?
   A. Alcohol can be a source of tension in relationships.
   B. Alcohol can increase the possibilities of stress due to fights, accidents, and arrests.
   C. Alcohol eases stress.
   D. Alcohol only temporarily masks the symptoms of stress.

Essay Questions: Provide complete responses to the following questions or statements.

31. What are five possible sources of stress for teens?

32. Describe two effects stress can have on physical health and one effect stress can have on emotional health.

33. What are three strategies for preventing stress?

© Goodheart-Willcox

The Use and Abuse of Drugs

19

Objectives

After studying this chapter, students will be able to
* describe appropriate uses of drugs as medicine.
* distinguish between drug misuse and drug abuse.
* identify health risks associated with the abuse of stimulants, depressants, hallucinogens, and anabolic steroids.
* suggest ways to offer help for someone with a substance abuse problem.

Bulletin Board

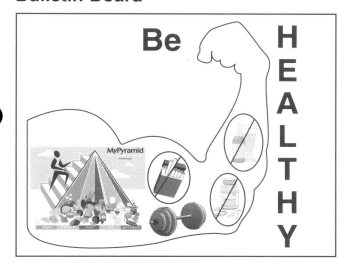

Title: *Be Healthy*

Prepare large letters for the words *Be Healthy*. Create a poster board drawing of a large arm muscle. Within the muscle, place a small copy of MyPyramid and pictures of exercise equipment. Place the "do not use" circle/slash around cigarettes, alcohol, and drugs.

Teaching Materials

Text, pages 322-342
    Learn the Language
    Check Your Knowledge
    Put Learning into Action
    Explore Further
Student Activity Guide, pages 135-142
    A. *What's the Question?*
    B. *Drugs Crossword*
    C. *Psychoactive Drugs*

    D. *Common-Sense Comebacks*
    E. *What Do You Think?*
    F. *Backtrack Through Chapter 19*
Teacher's Resources
    My Thoughts About the Use and Abuse of Drugs, reproducible master 19-1
    Take as Directed, transparency master 19-2
    Any Combination Spells Danger, color transparency CT-19
    Make a Table Tent, reproducible master 19-3
    Chapter 19 Test

Introducing the Chapter

1. Bring in items such as vitamin C supplement, diet drink mix, aspirin, oranges, and coffee. Ask students to pick out the drugs included in the group. Discuss the definition of *drug.*
2. *My Thoughts About the Use and Abuse of Drugs,* reproducible master 19-1. Have students answer the questions on the handout. Then have students form small groups to discuss each of the questions.
3. Ask students to bring in newspaper articles that describe drug and alcohol abuse situations, treatment programs, or the effects of drugs and alcohol. Keep the news display area updated weekly. Use the articles to discuss why people should choose a healthy lifestyle.
4. Discuss with students the Dietary Guidelines for Americans. Ask students why they think there is a guideline about alcohol.

Strategies to Reteach, Reinforce, Enrich, and Extend Text Concepts

Drugs as Medicine

5. **RF** Discuss with students the differences between over-the-counter and prescription drugs.
6. **ER** Guest speaker. Invite a licensed pharmacist to discuss consumer rights to prescription information. Also discuss the differences between generic and trade name drugs, and over-the-counter and prescription drugs. Have students prepare questions about the research and marketing efforts of the pharmaceutical industry.

7. **ER** Demonstrate how to use resources for looking up information about drugs, usage, and side effects. You may wish to use *The Physicians Desk Manual, The Pill Book, Consumer's Drug Digest,* or the Internet.

8. **RT** Discuss absorption and elimination of drugs. (You may want to refer students to Figure 3-7 on page 49 of the text, a diagram of the digestive system.) Stress the relationship of food to medications. Discuss negative and positive interactions with specific drug effectiveness.

9. **EX** Have students debate whether the beneficial effects of medications outweigh side effects. Discuss what happens when people have reactions to medications.

Drug Misuse and Abuse

10. **RF** Tell students prescription drugs kill more people each year than automobile and airplane accidents combined. Have students work in small groups to list potential risks associated with prescription drugs.

11. **RT** *Take as Directed,* transparency master 19-2. Review with students the guidelines for proper use of medications.

12. **ER** Have students generate a list of consumer rights and responsibilities regarding the correct use of medications. Post the rights and responsibilities for other classes to read.

13. **ER** Arrange for students to conduct an experiment with preschool children. Have students give several different types of empty medication bottles to a group of preschoolers. See which lids the children can remove and which they cannot. Ask the preschool teacher to discuss ways to keep children safe from harmful medications in the household.

14. **RF** *Any Combination Spells Danger,* color transparency CT-19. Use the transparency to reinforce the dangers of combining alcohol, drugs, and medications.

Stimulants

15. **ER** Conduct a taste test in class. Have students sample regular and caffeine-free soft drinks and indicate which tastes better. Cover containers so students have a blind test. Tally the results. Then discuss why some people choose caffeinated soft drinks while others choose caffeine-free.

16. **ER** Have students keep a one-day diary of beverages consumed. Have the students analyze their caffeine consumption. Discuss what moderate use of caffeine means. Review when and how a person can cut back on caffeine intake.

17. **ER** Have students research where coffee or tea comes from, how it is made, and why it is popular in many cultures. Discuss why cappuccino and specialty teas continue to grow in popularity among consumers.

18. **ER** Guest speakers. Invite a panel of students and trainers involved in peer counseling to discuss the responsibilities of peer counselors. Have students prepare questions for the panel ahead of time.

19. **ER** Have students research diet pills and write a report on their effectiveness in helping people maintain healthy weight.

20. **ER** Have students research the effects of cocaine on the body and make posters to hang around the school.

21. **ER** Have students check the school's policy on smoking and drugs. Review the stated consequences for offenders of the policy. Find out the school's system for reporting illegal sales or use of drugs.

22. **ER** Have students compute how much a person spends on cigarettes in one year if he or she smokes one pack a day. Multiply that number by 45 as an estimate of what people might spend on cigarettes in their lifetimes. Ask students to discuss better ways they could put that amount of money to use.

23. **ER** Guest speaker. Invite a speaker from the American Lung Association, American Cancer Society, or the American Heart Association to discuss the harmful effects of smoking.

24. **RF** *Psychoactive Drugs,* Activity C, SAG. Have students complete the chart as each drug is discussed in class.

Depressants

25. **RF** Show students two nutrient fact panels: one from beer and one from orange juice. Have students examine the nutrient contents from both products. Discuss which nutrients are higher and which are lower in each. Relate the risk of missing vital nutrients in the diet if calories from alcohol replace nutrient-dense foods.

26. **RF** Have students find several examples of alcohol advertisements. In discussion groups, have students answer the following questions: What message is being communicated in the ad? To whom is the ad appealing? What methods were used to attract consumer interest? What effect will the ad have? Have students prepare an alternate "ad" or poster on alcohol use.

27. **EX** Have students organize and participate in a Students Against Drunk Driving event. If your school or community does not have a SADD chapter, have students find out how they can start one.

28. **ER** Have students research diseases and other health hazards associated with the use of alcohol,

inhalants, and narcotics. Students may wish to use library or Internet resources. Have students prepare an oral report of their findings. Require one visual to be used with their presentations to help explain the effect of the depressant on health.

29. **ER** Guest speaker. Invite a representative from the March of Dimes organization to discuss the effects of alcohol and other drugs on the fetus during pregnancy.

Hallucinogens

30. **RF** Discuss the tendency of drugs to lead to a dependency. Emphasize that recovery is possible through a process of working through the dependency habit.
31. **EX** Have students debate the idea of doctors using illegal drugs such as marijuana as medications.
32. **RF** Have students discuss designer drugs that have been prominent in the news. Ask students what the effects of the drugs are, and how they differ from other better-known hallucinogens.
33. **ER** Guest speaker. Invite a drug counselor to discuss how to determine if there is a dependency problem.
34. **EX** Have students form small groups to discuss how the sale and use of illegal drugs affects the entire community. Discuss the impact of drugs on quality of life. Have each group report to the class and summarize points on the board.

Drugs and Athletes

35. **ER** Discuss the problems associated with steroid use for males and females.
36. **ER** Arrange a field trip to an athletic club. Have a certified fitness educator discuss the best ways to build muscle and gain strength. The educator should also stress the harmful effects of using steroids and other body enhancing drugs.

Getting Help for a Substance Abuse Problem

37. **ER** Have students give examples of ways the following groups can help people overcome substance abuse problems: parents, schools, students, law enforcement authorities, religious groups, social service agencies, community organizations, media.
38. **ER** Guest speakers. Invite a panel of counselors who work in drug and alcohol rehabilitation programs. Have the panel discuss how drugs affect the person, family members, and society. Ask the panel to explain the process of drug/alcohol rehabilitation and the programs and services available in the community. Students should write a summary of the content of the presentation for the school newspaper.

39. **RF** *Common-Sense Comebacks,* Activity D, SAG. Students are to write responses to given statements urging alcohol or drug use.

Chapter Review

40. **RF** *What's the Question?* Activity A, SAG. Students are to write questions for provided answers about drug use and abuse.
41. **RF** *Drugs Crossword,* Activity B, SAG. Students are to complete the crossword puzzle using terms from the chapter.
42. **ER** *What Do You Think?* Activity E, SAG. Students are to respond to opinion questions on drug use.
43. **RF** *Backtrack Through Chapter 19,* Activity F, SAG. Students are to provide complete answers to questions and statements that will help them recall, interpret, apply, and practice chapter concepts.

Above and Beyond

44. **EX** Have students form groups. Ask each group to research a different drug and report findings to the class. The report should include origins of the drug, its harmful effect on the body, and the complications of addiction.
45. **EX** Have students prepare skits on responding to peer pressure to use alcohol, drug, and tobacco. Have the students present the skits to elementary students. Include a discussion session to review appropriate ways to say no.
46. **EX** *Make a Table Tent,* reproducible master 19-3. Have students form groups to prepare table tent cards on drug use. Students might use the cards to highlight positive aspects of making safe lifestyle choices. Place the table tents in the cafeteria.
47. **EX** Ask local grocery stores to provide the class with paper grocery bags. Have students illustrate the bags with drug awareness messages. Return the illustrated bags to the grocery stores for use.

Answer Key

Text

Check Your Knowledge, page 341

1. Any substance other than food or water that changes the way the mind or body operate is a drug. A medicine is a drug used to treat an ailment or improve a disabling condition.
2. false
3. liver
4. appetite, absorption, metabolism
5. (List three:) taking more/less medicine per dose; taking medicine more/less often per day than directions state; taking medicine for longer/shorter periods than directions state; taking someone

else's medicine; sharing your medicine with others; leaving medicine within children's reach
6. true
7. alcohol
8. heroin
9. (List three:) desire to experiment, pressure from friends, stress, personal/social problems (Students may justify other answers.)
10. physician, school counselor, self-help groups, Yellow Pages

Student Activity Guide

What's the Question? Activity A

(The following questions are appropriate for the answers given. Consider other student responses on an individual basis.)
1. What are the two kinds of legal drugs?
2. What is a side effect?
3. What three types of names do drugs have?
4. What are the five forms of drug products?
5. Where in the body are drugs absorbed?
6. How does the liver react to drug chemicals?
7. What does caffeine do?
8. What is the recommended limit on caffeine consumption?
9. Where are amphetamines found?
10. What is a tolerance?
11. What is the major cause of lung cancer?
12. What are some health risks of long-term alcohol abuse?
13. What are four types of opiates?
14. What are hallucinations?
15. What are anabolic steroids?

Drugs Crossword, Activity B

Psychoactive Drugs, Activity C

(See pages 329-337 in the text.)

Backtrack Through Chapter 19, Activity F

1. because doctors have the training to decide which prescription drugs best fit the medical needs of their patients
2. No, the composition and quality are the same for each type.
3. Brand name drugs usually cost 20 to 70 percent more.
4. the person's age, health status, and diet; the timing and content of meals; genetics
5. Drug misuse means using a drug in a way that was not intended. Drug abuse means using a drug for other than medical reasons.
6. stimulants, depressants, and hallucinogens
7. irritability, nervousness, sleeplessness, nausea, vomiting, trembling, and cramps
8. nicotine
9. seven
10. Smokers need 35 milligrams more vitamin C than nonsmokers. Smoking increases the rate at whcih the body breaks down vitamin C.
11. Smokeless tobacco products also contain nicotine. They are just as addictive and harmful to a person's health.
12. Designer drugs are made in illegal laboratories without regard to purity. They often contain contaminants or stronger, highly unsafe amounts of the drug chemicals.
13. Alcoholics Anonymous, Al-Anon, and Alateen (Other student responses may also be valid.)
14. headache, drowsiness, and irritability; by gradual withdrawal
15. Amphetamines only reduce appetite while they are being taken. The dieter does not learn new eating behaviors and quickly regains lost weight after he or she stops taking the drugs.
16. Tar can cause chronic swelling in the lungs and lead to coughs and bronchial infections.
17. Alcoholics have no control of their alcohol intake. They do not realize they have a disease and find it hard to seek help.
18. Anabolic steroids can lead to coronary artery disease, liver tumors, and death. They've been known to cause acne, stunted growth, and sterility. In women, they have caused baldness, increased body hair, voice deepening, and decreased breast size.
19. (Student response.)
20. (Student response.)

Teacher's Resources

Chapter 19 Test

1. B	12. C	23. T	34. T
2. D	13. B	24. F	35. F
3. I	14. A	25. T	36. T
4. E	15. C	26. F	37. C
5. G	16. B	27. T	38. A
6. C	17. C	28. F	39. D
7. H	18. A	29. T	40. B
8. A	19. T	30. F	41. A
9. A	20. F	31. T	42. C
10. C	21. F	32. F	43. A
11. A	22. T	33. T	

44. Alcohol alters the effects of drugs. Depending on the quantity consumed and the frequency of use, alcohol can dull or magnify a drug's effects. Also, too much alcohol can damage the liver, making it less able to process certain drugs.

45. Stimulants speed up the nervous system. They increase heart rate, blood pressure, and breathing rate. Depressants decrease the activity of the nervous system. They slow down body functions and reactions. Hallucinogens cause the mind to create images that do not really exist.

46. medical treatment, inpatient therapy, self-help groups

My Thoughts About the Use and Abuse of Drugs

Name_____ **Date** _____ **Score** _____

Answer the following questions. Then discuss your answers in small groups.

1. What have your parents/guardians discussed with you regarding the use of drugs and alcohol? _____
   _____
   _____
   _____

2. Do your friends' parents allow you to drink or use drugs at their homes?_____
   _____

3. What boundaries are set for you pertaining to alcohol and drugs? _____
   _____
   _____

4. What are your personal boundaries for drinking or using drugs? _____
   _____
   _____

5. What are the consequences if you are caught drinking and driving? _____
   _____
   _____

6. At what age do you think most people start to consume alcohol? _____

7. What influences teens' decisions to drink or use drugs?_____
   _____
   _____
   _____

8. What would impact teens' decisions not to drink and drive or use drugs? _____
   _____
   _____
   _____

9. Do you feel your peers have a problem with drinking or drug use?_____

10. How do your peers get alcohol and/or drugs? _____
    _____

11. What problems do you think school-age children face regarding drugs or drinking? _____
    _____
    _____

12. When should programs begin for educating children about drugs and alcohol?_____
    _____

© Goodheart-Willcox   *(Continued)*

Name_____

Summarize your conclusions from the group's discussion.

_____

_____

_____

_____

_____

_____

_____

_____

_____

_____

_____

_____

_____

_____

_____

_____

_____

_____

_____

_____

_____

_____

_____

_____

Take as Directed

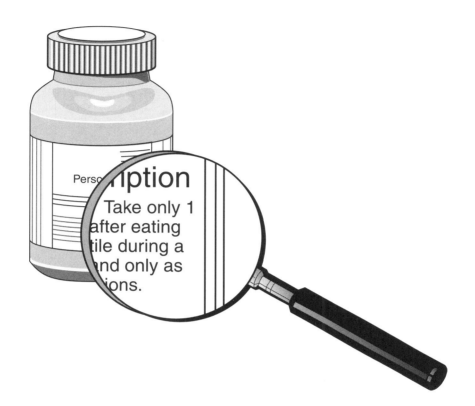

- Read instructions
- Take only medicines prescribed for you
- Report adverse effects to your doctor immediately
- Do not consume alcohol while taking medications
- Dispose of out-of-date prescriptions

© Goodheart-Willcox

Reproducible Master 19-3

Make a Table Tent

Using the directions below, make a table tent to place in the school cafeteria. Illustrate the table tent with pictures and information on drug abuse. Highlight the positive aspects of making safe lifestyle choices.

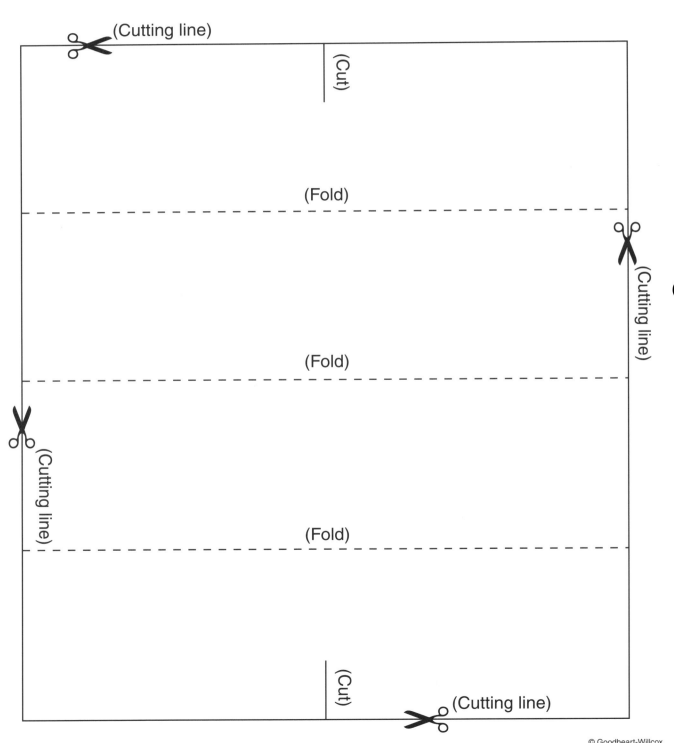

© Goodheart-Willcox

The Use and Abuse of Drugs

Name_____

Date _____   **Period** _____   **Score** _____

Chapter 19 Test

Matching: Match the following terms and identifying phrases.

_____ 1. The use of a drug for other than medical reasons.

_____ 2. The officially accepted name of a drug.

_____ 3. The name manufacturers use to promote a drug.

_____ 4. A drug that is unlawful to buy or use.

_____ 5. A legal drug sold without a prescription.

_____ 6. Using medicine in a way that was not intended.

_____ 7. A medicine that can only be obtained from a pharmacy with a written or phoned order from a doctor.

_____ 8. Any substance other than food or water that changes the way the body or mind operates.

A. drug
B. drug abuse
C. drug misuse
D. generic drug name
E. illegal drug
F. medicine
G. over-the-counter drug
H. prescription drug
I. trade name

Matching: Match the following drugs and categories. Each category can be used more than once.

_____ 9. Inhalants.

_____ 10. Caffeine.

_____ 11. Narcotics.

_____ 12. Nicotine.

_____ 13. Marijuana.

_____ 14. Alcohol.

_____ 15. Amphetamines.

_____ 16. LSD.

_____ 17. Cocaine.

_____ 18. Barbiturates.

A. depressant
B. hallucinogen
C. stimulant

True/False: Circle *T* if the statement is true or *F* if the statement is false.

T   F   19. Most drugs produce some side effects in some people.

T   F   20. OTC drugs are not regulated by any government agency.

T   F   21. Generic drugs contain less of the active ingredients than brand name drugs.

T   F   22. As drugs are absorbed, they are carried throughout the body in the bloodstream.

© Goodheart-Willcox   *(Continued)*

Name_____

T F   23. Long-term use of some drugs can alter a person's nutritional status.

T F   24. Sharing prescription drugs with a friend is an example of drug abuse.

T F   25. When people stop taking an addictive drug, they are likely to go through withdrawal.

T F   26. Caffeine is an addictive drug.

T F   27. As tolerance builds, larger doses are required to obtain the drug's effect.

T F   28. Smokeless tobacco is much safer to use than cigarettes.

T F   29. Alcohol can be absorbed in the mouth and stomach.

T F   30. The effects of a hangover can be reduced by drinking coffee.

T F   31. Alcoholics do not always realize they have a disease.

T F   32. A person cannot die from first-time inhalant use.

T F   33. Some opiates are available with a doctor's prescription.

T F   34. Short-term effects of marijuana include mood swings and loss of concentration.

T F   35. Designer drugs are safer than other street drugs because they are created in a lab.

T F   36. Even brief use of steroids can have harmful effects on a growing body.

Multiple Choice: Choose the best response. Write the letter in the space provided.

_____37. The _____ regulates the manufacture and sale of drugs.
    A. American Medical Association
    B. America Drug Manufacturer's Association
    C. Food and Drug Administration
    D. Bureau of Alcohol, Tobacco, and Firearms

_____38. It is best to take medicines with _____.
    A. water
    B. juice
    C. milk
    D. cola

_____39. Long-term use of antibiotics can destroy _____.
    A. vitamin A
    B. vitamin B
    C. vitamin D
    D. vitamin K

_____40. Which drug kills the most people?
    A. Marijuana.
    B. Nicotine.
    C. Alcohol.
    D. Cocaine.

_____41. Secondhand smoke is most harmful to _____.
    A. infants and young children
    B. teens
    C. middle-age people
    D. older adults

(Continued)

© Goodheart-Willcox

Name_____

_____42. What part of the body is first affected by alcohol consumption?
   A. Heart.
   B. Liver.
   C. Brain.
   D. Digestive system.

_____43. Which of the following descriptions best defines cirrhosis?
   A. Scarring of the liver; an irreversible condition.
   B. Loss of kidney function; a reversible condition.
   C. Scarring of heart tissue; a reversible condition.
   D. Loss of brain cells; an irreversible condition.

Essay Questions: Provide complete responses to the following questions or statements.

44. Why should alcohol and drugs never be consumed together?

45. What are the main differences among stimulants, depressants, and hallucinogens?

46. What sources of help are available for a person with a drug problem?

Keeping Food Safe

20

Objectives

After studying this chapter, students will be able to
- list common food contaminants.
- practice preventive measures when shopping for, storing, and preparing food to avoid foodborne illness.
- identify population groups that are most at risk for foodborne illness.
- recognize symptoms of foodborne illnesses.
- discuss the roles of food producers, food processors, government agencies, and consumers in protecting the safety of the food supply.

Bulletin Board

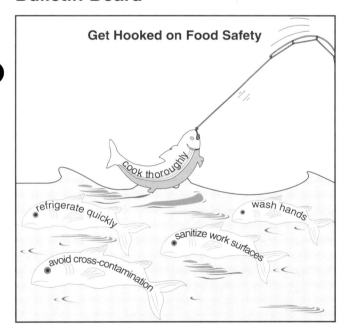

Get Hooked on Food Safety

cook thoroughly
refrigerate quickly
wash hands
sanitize work surfaces
avoid cross-contamination

Title: *Get Hooked on Food Safety*

Place cutouts of a large fishing hook and a number of fish on a blue background. Label each of the fish with a basic food safety guideline, such as *wash hands, sanitize work surfaces, avoid cross-contamination, refrigerate quickly,* and *cook thoroughly.*

Teaching Materials

Text, pages 344-359
Learn the Language
Check Your Knowledge

Put Learning into Action
Explore Further
Student Activity Guide, pages 143-148
A. *Safe Shopping List*
B. *Food at Home and on the Go*
C. *The Contaminators*
D. *Backtrack Through Chapter 20*
Teacher's Resources
Growing Microorganisms, reproducible master 20-1
Zap Bacteria, color transparency CT-20
Store Food Safely, transparency master 20-2
Everyone Has a Responsibility to Keep Foods Safe, transparency master 20-3
Chapter 20 Test

Introducing the Chapter

1. Tell students to imagine they run into friends at a park and receive an impromptu invitation to join them for a picnic. What questions might students ask, at least in their minds, to evaluate the safety of the food before deciding whether to accept the invitation? List student responses on the chalkboard. As you study the chapter, encourage students to add other appropriate questions to the list.
2. Refer to a recent news report of foodborne illness or a food recall. Ask how many students have ever been affected by foodborne illness. Inform students that study of chapter material will help them avoid such illnesses.

Strategies to Reteach, Reinforce, Enrich, and Extend Text Concepts

Common Food Contaminants

3. **RT** Have students list the different types of food contaminants discussed in the chapter and give an example of each.
4. **ER** *Growing Microorganisms,* reproducible master 20-1. Have lab groups complete the experiment as directed on the master. Students will be observing the growth of bacteria from various surfaces. Prepare the gelatin mixture as follows: for each petri dish, bring ¼ cup of water to a boil. Add 2 teaspoons of sugar and 1 packet of unflavored gelatin. Stir until the gelatin dissolves. Remove the pan from heat and cool for 2 minutes.

Pour the mixture into the petri dish and chill until firm. Following the experiment, discuss results and answers to the questions.

5. **ER** Have students develop an illustrated trifold brochure on how to limit intake of pesticide residues. Make the brochure available to the student body.

6. **RF** *The Contaminators,* Activity C, SAG. Students are to choose the best responses to multiple choice items about food contaminators.

Outwitting the Food Contaminators

7. **RT** *Zap Bacteria,* color transparency CT-20. Use the transparency to introduce the behaviors food handlers need to follow to zap bacteria before they have a chance to cause foodborne illness.

8. **RF** *Safe Shopping List,* Activity A, SAG. Students are to use ideas from food shopping scenarios to develop a list of tips for safe food shopping.

9. **EX** Have students role-play a couple of bacteria describing their perfect home for growing and multiplying. The bacteria should also describe environments they would hate.

10. **ER** Guest speaker. Invite a representative from a power company or a county extension agent with food and nutrition background to speak to the class about food safety issues that arise during a power outage in the home. Discuss how to evaluate whether foods are safe and how to maintain food quality as long as possible.

11. **EX** Have students write 20-second songs or raps about proper hand washing. Encourage students to teach their songs or raps to children or friends who work in foodservice.

12. **RF** *Store Food Safely,* transparency master 20-2. Use the transparency to discuss proper storage of cold foods.

13. **RF** Have the class develop a checklist for use in evaluating food safety concerns in a kitchen. Then have students use the checklist to assess the foods lab or their home kitchens. Discuss how students would go about addressing each concern they identify.

14. **RF** *Food at Home and on the Go,* Activity B, SAG. Students are to identify true statements and correct false statements about food handling at home and away from home.

When Foodborne Illness Happens

15. **ER** Guest speaker. Invite the school nurse to review the symptoms and treatment of foodborne illness.

16. **RF** Ask students why it is important to report an incident of foodborne illness when the source of contamination is suspected to be a public foodservice agency. Also ask what information students should be prepared to relate when filing a report.

People and Public Food Safety

17. **RT** *Everyone Has a Responsibility to Keep Foods Safe,* transparency master 20-3. Use the transparency to introduce the responsibilities people at each point along the food chain have for keeping foods safe.

18. **ER** Guest speaker. Invite someone from a local or state health department or regional FDA office to speak to the class. Ask the speaker to discuss methods used and precautions taken to maintain food safety and quality during production, processing, and distribution.

19. **ER** Field trip. Organize a field trip to a restaurant. Ask the owner or manager to provide a tour to show students the sanitation procedures that are followed throughout the establishment. Also ask the owner or manager to discuss state regulations and health inspections that affect the foodservice industry.

Chapter Review

20. **RF** Assign pairs of students different food items. Have each pair create a safe food handling label for its assigned item.

21. **RF** *Backtrack Through Chapter 20,* Activity D, SAG. Students are to provide complete answers to questions and statements that will help them recall, interpret, apply, and practice chapter concepts.

Above and Beyond

22. **RF** Have each student survey the primary meal manager in the student's household to find out the main question the meal manager has about food safety. Then have students use the text and Internet resources to prepare reports that provide well-researched answers to the meal managers' questions.

23. **ER** Have students set up a food safety information table for a community center. The table should provide fact sheets about how to store and prepare foods safely. It might also offer free literature gathered from county extension offices, county health departments, the USDA, and the FDA.

24. **ER** Have each student research the food safety standards in another country. Have students compile their findings into an informational bulletin about food safety precautions to follow when traveling internationally.

25. **EX** Have students develop a questionnaire to assess food handling habits and awareness of safe food handling practices. Have students use the questionnaire to survey 10 percent of the student body. Then have students write an article for the school newspaper summarizing the data they collected. The article should also include basic food safety guidelines.

26. **EX** Guest speaker. Invite a county extension agent to demonstrate how to safely can homegrown food products, such as fresh green beans and other low-acid foods. As part of the demonstration, ask the speaker to discuss how to look for signs of spoilage in home-canned foods.

Answer Key

Text

Check Your Knowledge, page 358

1. Trichinella in pork can be prevented from causing disease by cooking pork to an internal temperature of 160°F (71°C).
2. D
3. Some types of fish, such as tuna and blue marlin, produce scombroid toxin when they begin to spoil.
4. (List three: Student response. See Chart 20-3 on page 347 in the text.)
5. leaky packages, misshapen packages, heavy layer of frost on packages, watermarks on packages
6. 20 seconds
7. Keep hot foods above 140°F (60°C). Keep cold foods at or below 40°F (4°C).
8. infants, children, pregnant women, older adults, substance abusers, people with immune disorders
9. vomiting, stomach cramps, diarrhea
10. To help prevent dehydration, replace the fluids lost through diarrhea and vomiting by drinking plenty of water. Get a lot of rest. If symptoms continue for more than two or three days, call a physician.
11. Food distributors must be sure food is kept at safe temperatures during shipping.
12. U.S. Department of Agriculture (USDA) and Food Safety and Inspection Service (FSIS)

Student Activity Guide

Safe Shopping List, Activity A

(Answers may vary—sample answers follow)

Shop at stores that are known for food safety and cleanliness.

Check food freshness dates.

Be sure raw meats are wrapped tightly and bagged separately.

Check store fixtures for cleanliness.

Be sure foods are properly stored in refrigerator and freezer cases.

Beware of odors indicating spoiled foods.

Avoid frozen foods that are covered with frost.

Check canned foods for dents, rust, and swelling. Note that disorder and uncleanness in stores may indicate improper food handling.

Food at Home and on the Go, Activity B

1. in the interior
2. true
3. 40
4. freezer
5. a cool, dry place
6. true
7. true
8. three to four days
9. aluminum foil
10. is not
11. true
12. true
13. cut
14. true
15. true
16. true
17. most
18. true
19. as soon as possible
20. in the refrigerator
21. use a meat thermometer to check the internal temperature of
22. salmonella
23. true
24. true

The Contaminators, Activity C

1. D	11. B
2. D	12. D
3. C	13. B
4. B	14. A
5. D	15. C
6. C	16. D
7. B	17. C
8. D	18. B
9. A	19. B
10. D	20. D

Backtrack Through Chapter 20, Activity D

1. because people mistake their symptoms for "stomach flu"
2. harmful bacteria
3. *E. coli* 0157:H7, *Salmonella, Listeria monocytogenes, Campylobacter jejuni,* and *Staphylococcus aureus*
4. hepatitis A and Norwalk virus
5. shop with safety in mind, store foods safely, keep clean in the kitchen, prepare foods safely, and pack foods safely
6. by not accepting foods they suspect are tainted, keeping facilities clean, keeping foods at proper temperatures during shipping, and setting and monitoring guidelines for handling food

7. poultry, eggs, and meat products
8. all foods other than poultry, eggs, and meats
9. local health departments
10. choosing wholesome foods, handling foods properly, reporting foodborne illnesses
11. no, many contaminated foods look, smell, and taste wholesome
12. no, trichinella is only destroyed when pork is cooked well done
13. because some molds produce toxins that are poisonous to the human body
14. so foods can be taken home and stored quickly, to keep cold foods cold and hot foods hot
15. (List two:) do not put cooked meat on the same plate as uncooked meat; brush sauces only on cooked surfaces of meat; do not use marinade as meat sauce unless it has been kept separate from the raw meat
16. because their immune systems are not mature enough to fight bacteria easily
17. so health officials can examine it if a product recall becomes necessary
18. by washing produce thoroughly and by removing outer leaves of leafy vegetables
19. select leaner fish and eat freshwater fish no more than once a week
20. (Student response.)

Teacher's Resources

Growing Microorganisms, reproducible master 20-1
1. Data will vary, but even washed surfaces may produce some bacterial growth. (Section 8, which had no bacteria transferred to it, should be free of bacteria.)

2. Answers will vary depending on which surfaces were the most unclean.
3. Risk of foodborne illness due to bacteria can be reduced by keeping hands, utensils, and work surfaces as clean as possible when handling foods.

Chapter 20 Test

1. C	10. D	19. T	28. B
2. B	11. T	20. T	29. C
3. E	12. F	21. F	30. A
4. A	13. F	22. T	31. C
5. J	14. T	23. T	32. D
6. F	15. F	24. F	33. B
7. K	16. F	25. T	34. A
8. G	17. F	26. C	35. A
9. I	18. F	27. C	

36. (List four. Student response. See pages 351-352 in the text.)
37. The symptoms of most foodborne illnesses appear within a day or two after eating tainted food. However, some illnesses take up to 30 days to develop. Symptoms of most illnesses last only a few days.
38. Consumers have a responsibility to choose wholesome food, handle it properly, and report foodborne illnesses to the appropriate agencies.

Growing Microorganisms

Name_____   Date _____   Period _____

Objective: To show the presence of bacteria on surfaces.

Supplies:

     felt-tip pen
 2 petri dishes filled with gelatin mixture
     tape
     plastic wrap

Procedure:

1. Use a felt-tip pen to draw two intersecting lines on the bottom of the petri dishes, dividing each dish into quarters. Number the quarters 1 through 8.
2. You will be transferring bacteria from each item listed in the table below. Use the following process to transfer bacteria. Tear off a 2-inch strip of tape. Place the sticky side of the tape on the first item listed in the table. Pull off the tape and lay it, sticky side down, on the gelatin in the section marked number 1. Gently lift off the tape. Repeat the process with clean tape for each item. As a control, do not touch the gelatin in or transfer any bacteria to the section marked number 8. (A *control* is a standard of comparison in judging experimental effects.)
3. Cover the petri dishes with plastic wrap and place in a warm environment for three days. Then describe what you see in each section.

Section	Item	Observations
1	**dishcloth**	
2	**quarter**	
3	**floor**	
4	**cutting board**	
5	**washed hand**	
6	**unwashed hand**	
7	**doorknob**	
8	**control**	

Questions:

1. Were any surfaces free of bacterial colonies? _____

2. Which surfaces produced the most bacterial growth? Why do you think this occurred?_____

    _____

    _____

3. How do your observations relate to food safety?_____

    _____

© Goodheart-Willcox

Store Food Safely

- Check refrigerator and freezer temperatures with a refrigerator thermometer. Refrigerator should be 40°F or below. Freezer should be 0°F or below.
- Keep refrigerator and freezer clean.
- Store foods in covered containers.
- Use foods within recommended storage times.
- Refrigerate leftovers promptly. Discard food left at room temperature for more than two hours.
- Use shallow storage containers to help foods cool quickly.

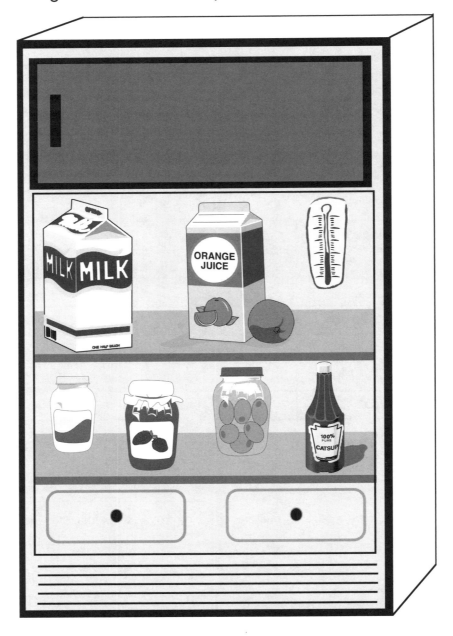

© Goodheart-Willcox

Everyone Has a Responsibility to Keep Foods Safe

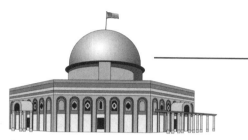

Government agencies
- regulate
- inspect
- educate

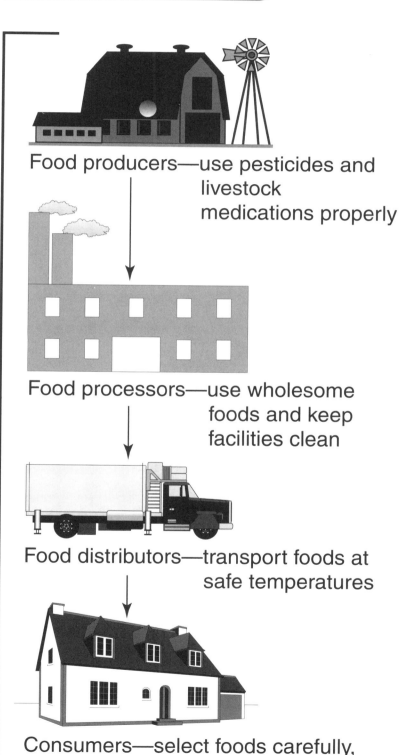

Food producers—use pesticides and livestock medications properly

Food processors—use wholesome foods and keep facilities clean

Food distributors—transport foods at safe temperatures

Consumers—select foods carefully, store foods properly, and prepare foods safely

© Goodheart-Willcox

Keeping Food Safe

Name_____

Date _____   **Period** _____   **Score** _____

Chapter 20 Test

Matching: Match the following terms and identifying phrases.

_____ 1. A disease transmitted by food.

_____ 2. An undesirable substance that unintentionally gets into food.

_____ 3. A living being so small it can be seen only under a microscope.

_____ 4. Single-celled microorganisms that live in soil, water, and the bodies of plants and animals.

_____ 5. Poison.

_____ 6. An organism that lives off another organism, which is called a host.

_____ 7. A disease-causing agent that is the smallest type of life-form.

_____ 8. Particles of chemical insect repellents left in food after it is prepared for consumption.

_____ 9. Maintaining clean conditions to help prevent disease.

_____ 10. Practices that promote good health.

A. bacteria
B. contaminant
C. foodborne illness
D. hygiene
E. microorganism
F. parasite
G. pesticide residue
H. protozoa
I. sanitation
J. toxin
K. virus

True/False: Circle *T* if the statement is true or *F* if the statement is false.

T F   11. Food poisoning is often mistaken for stomach flu.

T F   12. Foods that contain illness-causing bacteria can usually be detected by changes in appearance, odor, and flavor.

T F   13. If mold is removed from liquids or soft foods, the foods will still be safe to eat.

T F   14. Large fish are likely to have stored more environmental contaminants than small fish.

T F   15. Outwitting food contaminators is nearly impossible for consumers.

T F   16. Buying food in dented cans that have been reduced in price is a good way to save money at the grocery store.

T F   17. It is a good idea to cool a leftover meat loaf at room temperature for 2 to 3 hours before refrigerating it.

T F   18. Most leftover stored foods can stay in the refrigerator at least a week.

T F   19. Using the same unwashed knife to cut uncooked chicken and a head of lettuce could result in cross-contamination.

T F   20. A thermometer can be used to check the internal temperature of meat.

T F   21. Eating raw or undercooked eggs poses no risks for healthy people.

T F   22. Using insulated bags and ice packs will help keep cold foods safe when carrying them away from home.

T F   23. Symptoms of foodborne illness that include double vision, inability to swallow, or difficulty speaking require immediate hospital care.

(Continued)

© Goodheart-Willcox

Name_____

T F   24. Because foods can be contaminated during processing and handling, food producers have little responsibility for assuring food safety.

T F   25. Fish processors are not required to have their products inspected by a government agency.

Multiple Choice: Choose the best response. Write the letter in the space provided.

_____26. How can trichinosis be prevented when preparing pork?
    A. Add spices to the meat to kill microorganisms.
    B. Broil the meat instead of baking it.
    C. Cook meat to an internal temperature of 160°F (71°C).
    D. Marinate the meat for several hours.

_____27. How do leavening agents affect food products?
    A. They are used to age some cheeses.
    B. They give yogurt its tangy taste and creamy texture.
    C. They produce a gas that causes batters and doughs to rise.
    D. They contaminate food products and cause foodborne illness.

_____28. To get foods from store to home safely, which principle should be followed?
    A. Complete grocery shopping, then start other shopping errands.
    B. Freeze frozen foods as quickly as possible.
    C. Keep frozen foods and warm baked breads in the same grocery bag.
    D. Keep warm deli foods on the kitchen counter until ready for use.

_____29. What is the recommended time required to thoroughly wash hands before preparing food?
    A. 5 seconds.
    B. 10 seconds.
    C. 20 seconds.
    D. 2 minutes.

_____30. Which of the following food practices may be considered the safest?
    A. Wear gloves to prepare foods if you have an infection on your hand.
    B. Dry hands using the same towel used for drying utensils.
    C. Sneeze into a dishcloth rather than sneezing on foods.
    D. Let long hair drape over food being prepared.

_____31. In which temperature range does bacteria grow most rapidly?
    A. 0° to 40°F (-18 to 4°C)
    B. 40° to 140°F (4° to 60°C)
    C. 60° to 125°F (16° to 52°C)
    D. 140° to 165°F (60° to 74°C)

_____32. The safest way to thaw frozen meat is to _____.
    A. defrost it on the kitchen counter
    B. place it in warm water
    C. put it in direct sunlight
    D. set it in the refrigerator

_____33. Who is most at risk for danger from food poisoning?
    A. Athletes.
    B. Pregnant women.
    C. Sedentary adults.
    D. Teenagers.

(Continued)

© Goodheart-Willcox

Name_____

_____34. Removing a product from store shelves and warning the public not to use the product describes
_____.
   A. a product recall
   B. consumer carelessness
   C. distributor irresponsibility
   D. legislative actions

_____35. Which government agency is responsible for the truthful advertising of food claims?
   A. Federal Trade Commission (FTC).
   B. U.S. Department of Agriculture (USDA).
   C. U.S. Environmental Protection Agency (EPA).
   D. U.S. Food and Drug Administration (FDA).

Essay Questions: Provide complete responses to the following questions or statements.

36. Your neighbor has a frozen steak he wants to marinate and cook on the grill. What are four food safety guidelines he should follow?

37. When do the symptoms of most foodborne illnesses appear and how long do they usually last?

38. As the last link in the food chain, what responsibilities do consumers have for keeping food safe?

Meal Management

21

Objectives

After studying this chapter, students will be able to
- plan menus that include a variety of food flavors, colors, textures, shapes, sizes, and temperatures.
- use the MyPyramid system, the Dietary Guidelines for Americans, and meal patterns to plan nutritious menus for their families.
- describe techniques for controlling food spending to stay within the family food budget.
- identify methods for saving time when preparing foods.
- explain how to meet meal management goals when eating meals away from home.

Bulletin Board

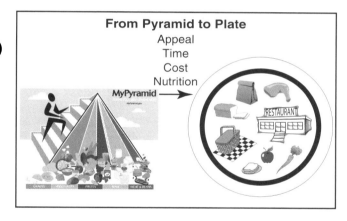

From Pyramid to Plate
Appeal
Time
Cost
Nutrition
MyPyramid →

Title: *From Pyramid to Plate*

Place a picture of MyPyramid on one side of the bulletin board. On the other side, place a large plate cut from construction paper. Connect the Pyramid to the plate with a black arrow. Cut pictures of food from magazines and place them on the plate. Include pictures of packed lunches, picnic baskets, restaurants, and fast-food restaurants. Above the arrow, place the words *appeal, time, cost,* and *nutrition.*

Teaching Materials

Text, pages 360-373
Learn the Language
Check Your Knowledge
Put Learning into Action
Explore Further

Student Activity Guide, pages 149-156
A. *A Meal Manager in the Making*
B. *Meal Makeovers*
C. *Three Squares Plus*
D. *Budgeting Dilemmas*
E. *Eating Out and About*
F. *Backtrack Through Chapter 21*

Teacher's Resources
Cultural Aspects of Food Appeal, reproducible master 21-1
Pyramid Menu-Planning Game, reproducible master 21-2
Stretching the Food Dollar, CT-21
Time Management Skills in Meal Preparation, transparency master 21-3
Chapter 21 Test

Introducing the Chapter

1. Ask students to write down their all-time favorite meals. Have students volunteer to share their meal descriptions. Ask what makes the meals their favorites. Then ask how their preferences have changed over the years.
2. Have students write short stories describing a "disaster meal." Have students read the stories out loud and explain what went wrong in each instance. Use the stories to stimulate discussion of what it means to plan satisfying meals.
3. Show students pictures of a modern kitchen and a kitchen from the early twentieth century. Ask students what technological advances are evident in the picture of the modern kitchen. Ask students how they think these advances have affected life for family members today.

Strategies to Reteach, Reinforce, Enrich, and Extend Text Concepts

Planning for Appeal

4. **RT** Show colorful magazine pictures of several meals. List on the board the five factors that affect the appeal of a meal. Discuss how the factors apply to each picture.
5. **RF** List several different foods on the board. Have students suggest foods they would serve with each food listed. Encourage students to name

foods that would add interest to meal flavor, color, shape and size, texture, and temperature. Then ask students to name foods that would detract from the appeal if they were served with the listed foods.

6. **RF** *A Meal Manager in the Making,* Activity A, SAG. Students are to read diary entries and identify the advantage of meal planning not being met. Students will then offer tips for preventing each problem.

7. **ER** Guest speaker. Invite a dietitian or retirement home food manager to describe the process used to plan menus for large groups. Have the speaker discuss the problems of planning variety into meals every day.

8. **ER** *Cultural Aspects of Food Appeal,* reproducible master 21-1. Students are to use illustrated cookbooks for two ethnic cuisines to complete the chart. They will describe typical flavors, colors, textures, shapes, sizes, and temperatures of the food in each cuisine. Students will then answer additional questions.

9. **RF** *Meal Makeovers,* Activity B, SAG. Students are to read each given menu and determine how it is lacking in variety. Students will then rewrite the menu to improve variety.

10. **ER** Discuss why garnishes are used and how they relate to food appeal. Place students in pairs and have each pair learn how to make a garnish. Have students demonstrate how to make the garnish and explain how it might be used.

Planning for Nutrition

11. **RF** Ask students to explain how food likes and dislikes relate to nutrition. Stress that all nutrients can be found in many different foods.

12. **RF** Have students list their 10 most favorite and least favorite foods. List responses on the board in two columns. Have students identify the food group to which each belongs. Which food groups are most and least represented? What might this indicate about the nutrition of teens?

13. **RF** *Three Squares Plus,* Activity C, SAG. Students are to plan three meals and a snack for one day's menu.

14. **EX** Have students exchange their meals planned in Activity C with another student. Have students evaluate their partners' meal plans for nutrition and variety.

15. **RF** *Pyramid Menu-Planning Game,* reproducible master 21-2. Divide the class into groups of three or four. Give each group a set of cards and game rules. Have students play the game and then use the foods listed on the winner's cards to plan a nutritious, appealing meal.

16. **EX** Ask how many times a week students eat meals together with their families. Discuss how individual snacking throughout the day may lead to a less-nutritious diet. Then have the class debate the following topic: the decrease in family meals is a major reason for decreased nutrition in teen diets.

17. **ER** Survey the number of students who ate breakfast that morning. Discuss nutrients found in typical breakfast foods. Have students describe how they feel after missing breakfast. Complete a list of pros and cons for eating breakfast. Suggest ways to build breakfast into a busy lifestyle.

18. **EX** Using a pyramid representing another culture, prepare a day's menu using foods from that culture.

Controlling Food Costs

19. **RT** Discuss factors that affect a family's food budget.

20. **ER** Ask students to form teams. Have each team prepare two menus that are comparable in nutrition. For one menu, students should use low-cost food items. The other menu should include higher-priced foods. Have students price the foods at a local store to compare dollar differences in the two meals. Discuss how a to feed a family healthful foods at a lower cost.

21. **RF** *Stretching the Food Dollar,* CT-21. Use the transparencies to review tips for saving food dollars. Ask students to identify other tips for saving costs when food shopping.

22. **ER** Have students compare price and appeal of fresh, frozen, canned, boxed, and prepared products. Discuss when food items are worth extra money and when cost-cutting is wise.

23. **EX** *Budgeting Dilemmas,* Activity D, SAG. Students are to read each given situation and decide if it will fit into a $50 food budget. Students will then answer questions to evaluate their budgets and food choices.

24. **EX** Have students work in pairs to plan one week's menus for themselves. Have the teams estimate how much it will cost to buy the food on the week's menu. (They may need to check prices at a local store.) Have each team present its menu plan for the class to evaluate. Ask students to identify cost differences and decide how menus could be modified to cut food dollars.

Saving Time

25. **RF** Have students list factors that affect time involved in shopping, planning, and preparing meals for a family. Ask students why it is important to be time-efficient.

26. **RT**   Ask students to identify resources used by meal managers to save time in meal preparation.

27. **RF**   *Time Management Skills in Meal Preparation,* transparency master 21-3. Use the transparency to identify time management tips. Have students add other time-saving ideas as they observed their parents/friends cook.

28. **ER**   Have students search the Internet for new food products designed to save time in meal preparation. Add gathered information reports and pictures to a bulletin board labeled *Look for New Meal Conveniences.*

29. **EX**   Divide students into teams to work in the foods lab. Have the teams prepare a cake from scratch and a boxed cake mix. Compare the preparation and cleanup time. Also have students evaluate cost, nutrition, and appeal of each product. Have each group prepare a report.

30. **ER**   Guest speaker. Invite a restaurant chef to talk to the class about the importance of time management in restaurant operations. Have the person describe time-wasters that need to be corrected and rewarding time-savers.

Meals Away from Home

31. **RF**   Have students develop menus for packed lunches for a young child and an adult. Have students evaluate the lunches for nutrition and appeal.

32. **RT**   Review safety tips for packing lunches covered in Chapter 20.

33. **ER**   Have students use cookbooks and Internet recipe sources to locate a creative choice for a packed lunch. Discuss the problems associated with finding nutritious foods for packing.

34. **RF**   Ask students to suggest ways to organize for early morning lunch preparations.

35. **RT**   Discuss ways a person can enjoy eating out and still eat a healthful diet.

36. **RF**   *Eating Out and About,* Activity E, SAG. Students are to prepare tips for nutritional eating when packing lunches and eating out.

Chapter Review

37. **RF**   *Backtrack Through Chapter 21,* Activity F, SAG. Students are to provide complete answers to questions and statements that will help them recall, interpret, apply, and practice chapter concepts.

38. **RF**   Have students recall all they ate yesterday. Write the foods on a paper and have them evaluate the "menu" according to the recommendations learned in this chapter.

Above and Beyond

39. **EX**   Have students complete a one week's menus for the school cafeteria. Make sure students recommend appealing foods moderate in fat, sugar, and sodium.

40. **EX**   Conduct a school-wide survey to determine the top 10 favorite foods of the student body. If the cafeteria does not already serve these items, have students find out if it would be possible to include these foods on the menu.

41. **EX**   Have students schedule, plan, and prepare the evening meal for their families. Students should choose a nutritious meal, shop for foods, prepare the meal, and clean up. Have students discuss the results of the project. Review how teens can take an active role in preparing family meals.

42. **EX**   Have students volunteer to food shop for the elderly, prepare a meal in a soup kitchen, or buy foods for a food bank. Have students write a short report for the school newspaper on their volunteer efforts.

Answer Key

Text

Check Your Knowledge, page 372

1. (List two:) introduce new foods from time to time, include a variety of flavors in every meal, balance strongly flavored foods with those that are more subtle

2. B

3. Foods are safer when they are served at the correct temperatures.

4. false

5. A meal pattern based on MyPyramid plan for 2,000 calories includes the following portions at each meal: two to three portions from the grains group; one to two portions from the vegetable group; one to two portions from the fruit group; one portion from the milk group; one to three ounces from the meat and beans group (five to six portions per day).

6. Fixed expenses are the same each month. Flexible expenses vary from month to month.

7. (Give one example for each of three food groups. Student response. See page 366 in the text.)

8. (List two. Student response. See page 366 in the text.)

9. (List three:) require only a few common ingredients, have a small number of preparation steps, require only a few utensils, rely on fast cooking techniques

10. (Give one advantage and one disadvantage. Student response. See page 368 in the text.)

11. (List two:) Pack lunches the night before and keep them in the refrigerator. Store leftovers in serving-sized containers and put them directly into lunch

bags. Set up an assembly line to make sandwiches for the whole family.
12. (List five. Student response. See pages 370-371 in the text.)

Student Activity Guide

A Meal Manager in the Making, Activity A

(Following are suggested answers; other answers may be given.)
1. saving time and effort
2. organize tools and equipment; plan ahead to have needed ingredients on hand; select quick and easy recipes when time is short
3. appeal
4. add variety of color, flavor, and texture; freeze leftovers for later use; plan creative, enjoyable uses for leftovers
5. nutrition
6. serve a variety of foods; plan one menu for everyone; plan vegetarian menus to include all the needed nutrients
7. economy
8. plan menus ahead; shop for a week or more at each time; don't go to the store hungry; select low-cost foods; buy vegetables in season; plan a budget and follow it

Meal Makeovers, Activity B

1. color
2. shape and size
3. flavor
4. texture
5. temperature

(Other answers may be accepted if students support their answers. Menus are student response.)

Backtrack Through Chapter 21, Activity F

1. appeal, good nutrition, economy, saving time and effort
2. flavor, color, texture, shape and size, and temperature
3. MyPyramid, Dietary Guidelines for Americans, and meal patterns
4. fat, saturated fat, cholesterol, sugar, sodium, and alcohol
5. an outline of what to serve at each meal
6. Microwave cooking is quick and requires little water. This minimizes destruction of nutrients by heat and loss of water-soluble nutrients.

7. a spending plan
8. (Student response. Sample answers include the following:) slow cooker, microwave, food processor, pressure cooker, bread machine
9. food items that are purchased partially or completely prepared
10. (Student response.)
11. to supply a variety of nutrients and make meals more enjoyable
12. Expenses that are the same each month are fixed, while those that vary are flexible. (Examples are student response.)
13. (List three. Student response. See page 366 in the text.)
14. (Student response.)
15. simple to prepare, taste good, and offer creative variations
16. often cost more, may be high in sodium and fat
17. (List one:) include your favorites, meet Dietary Guidelines, save money
18. (Student response.)
19. (Student response.)
20. (Student response.)

Teacher's Resources

Chapter 21 Test

1. A	10. T	19. F
2. C	11. F	20. F
3. B	12. T	21. B
4. F	13. T	22. B
5. E	14. F	23. A
6. T	15. F	24. C
7. F	16. T	25. D
8. T	17. T	26. D
9. F	18. F	27. A

28. The MyPyramid system, the Dietary Guidelines for Americans, basic meal patterns
29. organize work space and equipment, use time-saving appliances, select quick and easy menu items, use convenience foods
30. (Name two. Student response. See page 367 in the text.)
31. (List five. Student response. See pages 370-371 in the text.)

Cultural Aspects of Food Appeal

Name_____   Date _____   Period_____

Use illustrated cookbooks for two ethnic cuisines to help you complete the chart below. Describe typical flavors, colors, textures, shapes, sizes, and temperatures of the food in each cuisine. You may include the names of specific dishes to support your descriptions. Then answer the questions at the bottom of the page.

Food Characteristics	
Cuisine: _____	Cuisine: _____
Flavors	
Colors	
Textures	
Shapes and Sizes	
Temperatures	

1. What is different about food appeal between the two ethnic cuisines? _____

_____

_____

_____

2. Why does appeal of foods vary from culture to culture? _____

_____

_____

_____

3. What aspects of food appeal seem to stay the same in most cultures? _____

_____

_____

_____

_____

© Goodheart-Willcox

Reproducible Master 21-2

Pyramid Menu-Planning Game

Name_____   Date _____   Period_____

Game rules:

In a group of three or four players, one player will begin the game by shuffling the cards and dealing six cards to each player. The dealer will place the remaining cards facedown to form a draw pile. He or she will turn up one card to form a discard pile.

Play begins with the player to the left of the dealer and moves clockwise around the table. Each player takes a turn by drawing the top card from either the draw pile or the discard pile. Each player ends his or her turn by placing a card faceup on the discard pile. Play continues until one player collects a set of cards representing a meal pattern based on the MyPyramid system:

- 2 Grains cards
- 1 Vegetable card
- 1 Fruit card
- 1 Milk card
- 1 Meat and Beans card

After a player is declared the winner, the group should use the foods listed on the winner's cards to plan a nutritious, appealing menu.

(Cut cards apart on dotted lines.)

Grains	**Grains**	**Grains**
Tortillas	Rye bread	Whole wheat rolls
Grains	**Grains**	**Grains**
Barley	Biscuits	Couscous
Grains	**Grains**	**Grains**
Matzos	Polenta	Muffins

(Continued)

© Goodheart-Willcox

Grains	**Grains**	**Grains**
Cornbread	Noodles	Rice

Grains	**Vegetables**	**Vegetables**
Bagels	Potatoes	Lettuce

Vegetables	**Vegetables**	**Vegetables**
Tomatoes	Onions	Carrots

Vegetables	**Vegetables**	**Vegetables**
Celery	Corn	Broccoli

Fruits	**Fruits**	**Fruits**
Bananas	Apples	Watermelon

Fruits	**Fruits**	**Fruits**
Oranges	Cantaloupe	Grapes

(Continued)

© Goodheart-Willcox

Fruits

Grapefruit

Fruits

Strawberries

Milk

Calcium-fortified soy milk

Milk

Cheddar cheese

Milk

Cottage cheese

Milk

Fat free milk

Milk

Lowfat Ice cream

Milk

Pudding

Milk

Yogurt

Milk

Swiss cheese

Meat and Beans

Ground turkey

Meat and Beans

Roast beef

Meat and Beans

Ground beef

Meat and Beans

Pork chops

Meat and Beans

Pork sausage

Meat and Beans

Lamb chops

Meat and Beans

Veal cutlets

Meat and Beans

Chicken breasts

© Goodheart-Willcox

Time Management Skills in Meal Preparation

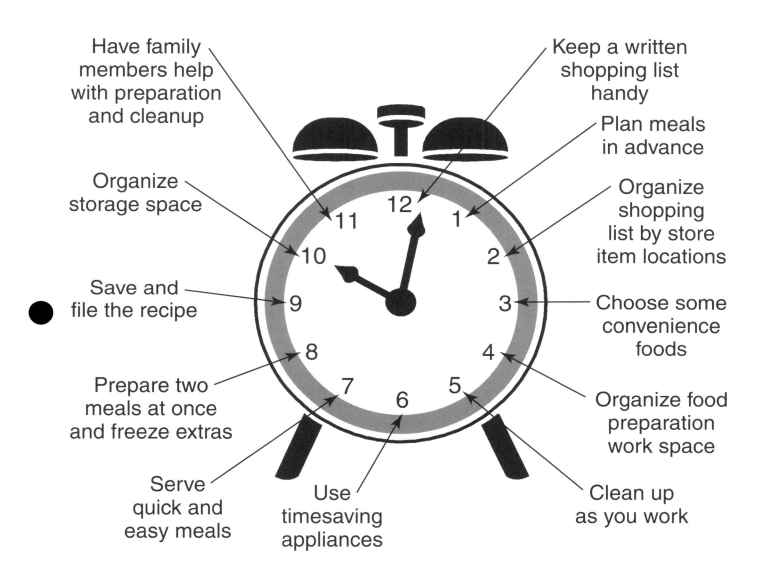

Have family members help with preparation and cleanup

Organize storage space

Save and file the recipe

Prepare two meals at once and freeze extras

Serve quick and easy meals

Use timesaving appliances

Keep a written shopping list handy

Plan meals in advance

Organize shopping list by store item locations

Choose some convenience foods

Organize food preparation work space

Clean up as you work

Meal Management

Name_____

Date _____   Period _____   Score _____

Chapter 21 Test

Matching: Match each meal with the appeal factor it is lacking.

_____ 1. Poached fish, scalloped potatoes, and steamed cabbage.

_____ 2. Fish sticks, French fries, and green beans.

_____ 3. Tomato juice, salad with tomatoes, and spaghetti with tomato sauce

_____ 4. Pancakes, warm syrup, and hot chocolate.

_____ 5. Creamed turkey, mashed sweet potatoes, and applesauce.

A. color
B. flavor
C. shape and size
D. smell
E. texture
F. temperature

True/False: Circle *T* if the statement is true or *F* if the statement is false.

T F   6. Variety adds interest and appeal to meals.

T F   7. As long as you serve different meals every day, it doesn't matter if the meals themselves lack variety.

T F   8. Strongly flavored foods can be balanced with those that are more subtle.

T F   9. For variety in temperature, it's a good idea to serve foods lukewarm instead of cold or hot.

T F   10. Meal planning helps meal managers provide for their families' nutritional needs.

T F   11. Meal managers do not need to consider the different nutrient needs of family members when planning menus.

T F   12. All family members can usually enjoy the same meal in different size portions.

T F   13. Following a meal pattern based on the MyPyramid system can help people meet their recommended daily amounts from each food group.

T F   14. Breakfast, lunch, and dinner should each furnish one-third of the day's nutrient and calorie needs.

T F   15. The high heat used in a microwave oven can increase losses of heat-sensitive vitamins.

T F   16. Keeping fruits and vegetables in large pieces can reduce the amounts of nutrients these foods lose during cooking.

T F   17. Eating out increases food spending.

T F   18. Stopping to jot down items you need on a shopping list is a time-wasting activity.

T F   19. Use of convenience foods saves time and money.

T F   20. Registered dietitians suggest avoiding fast-food restaurants.

Multiple Choice: Choose the best response. Write the letter in the space provided.

_____21. Family members are more likely to accept new food tastes that are introduced _____.
   A. at every meal
   B. now and then
   C. when guests are present
   D. without considering family preferences

(Continued)

© Goodheart-Willcox

Name_____

_____22. The major purpose of preparing a food budget is to _____.
  A. force people to eat nutritious foods
  B. control food costs
  C. discourage use of food coupons
  D. avoid buying what people really need

_____23. Which of the following is the best example of a fixed expense?
  A. Car payment.
  B. Movies.
  C. Clothing.
  D. Dining out.

_____24. Which would be the best way to cut food costs?
  A. Buy foods that are not in season.
  B. Use fresh foods instead of frozen or canned.
  C. Use nonfat dry milk in recipes.
  D. Avoid buying food advertised as store specials.

_____25. Which of the following is *not* a convenience food?
  A. Cake mix.
  B. Canned soup.
  C. Frozen dinner.
  D. Fresh corn on the cob.

_____26. When packing lunches, _____.
  A. include foods from only two food groups
  B. avoid packing fruit
  C. include only foods low in dietary fiber
  D. use a thermos to keep drinks cool

_____27. Jenny is at a restaurant and wants to order an item that is relatively low in fat. Which is her best choice?
  A. Baked potato with salsa sauce.
  B. Large fries.
  C. Double burger.
  D. Creamy potato salad.

Essay Questions: Provide complete responses to the following questions or statements.

28. What nutrition information resources are available for the meal manager?

29. List four ways to save time in meal preparation.

30. Name two timesaving appliances and explain how they help save preparation and cooking time.

31. List five tips for meeting goals for good nutrition when eating out.

Making Wise Consumer Choices

Objectives

After studying this chapter, students will be able to
- describe at least six types of stores that sell food.
- explain how advertising, food processing, organic foods, and prices can affect consumer choices.
- use information on food labels to make healthful food choices.
- evaluate the quality of fitness products and services.
- identify your consumer rights and responsibilities.

Bulletin Board

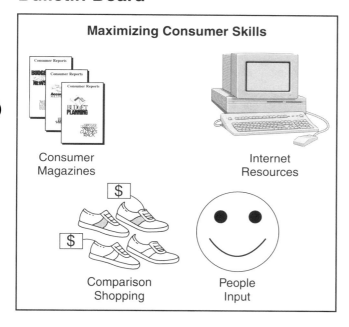

Maximizing Consumer Skills

Consumer Magazines

Internet Resources

Comparison Shopping

People Input

Title: *Maximizing Consumer Skills*

Display the resources available to help consumers make informed decisions. Use the cover of magazines such as *Consumer Reports,* pictures of running shoes with price tags attached, a picture of a computer terminal, and a smiling face to indicate people as an information source. Label the pictures appropriately.

Teaching Materials

Text, pages 374-395
Learn the Language
Check Your Knowledge
Put Learning into Action
Explore Further

Student Activity Guide, pages 157-164
    A. *Where to Shop?*
    B. *What Influences Shopping Decisions?*
    C. *Design a Label*
    D. *Savvy Shopper or Careless Consumer?*
    E. *Backtrack Through Chapter 22*

Teacher's Resources
Computer Shopping: Technology Trade-Offs, transparency master 22-1
Organic Farming: The Natural Way to Control Pests and Fertilizer, CT-22
Lean on the Label, reproducible master 22-2
The Right Shoe, transparency master 22-3
Chapter 22 Test

Introducing the Chapter

1. Ask students to raise their hands if they are consumers. Ask them to define the word *consumer.*
2. Discuss why it is important to be a skilled consumer. Ask for examples of times students were wise consumers and times they made poor consumer choices.
3. Have students form groups. Ask each group to think of 10 questions they have about the consumer skills needed to make food and fitness product choices. Place questions in an envelope and save these questions to be used for review.
4. Brainstorm reasons it is difficult to be a smart consumer in today's world. List the reasons on the board. Ask students if they think of these reasons as challenges or obstacles. Remind students there are tools and skills that help people make satisfying consumer decisions.

Strategies to Reteach, Reinforce, Enrich, and Extend Text Concepts

Where to Shop for Food

5. **RF** Have students name the kinds of food stores that exist in the community. Discuss the advantages and disadvantages of shopping at the various types of stores.
6. **RF** *Where to Shop?* Activity A, SAG. Students are to match terms and identifying phrases. Students will then identify the type of store that

would satisfy each person's needs in given scenarios.

7. **ER** Gather back issues of grocery and marketing magazines often sent to local supermarkets. (Store managers may be willing to give back issues to the school for educational use.) Have students examine the magazines to determine at least one new marketing trend in the food distribution industry. Discuss how the trends will affect life for families in the future.

8. **EX** Have students describe a "supermarket of the future" based on current trends.

9. **RF** *Computer Shopping: Technology Trade-Offs,* transparency master 22-1. Use the transparency to identify pros and cons of Internet shopping. Discuss the meaning of *trade-offs*.

10. **RF** Ask students if they know anyone who has purchased merchandise over the Internet. If so, ask if the people were satisfied with their purchases and explain why.

11. **ER** Have students research different grocery services available on the Internet. Have students report on the services' prices and policies.

Factors That Affect Consumer Food Choices

12. **ER** *What Influences Shopping Decisions?* Activity B, SAG. Students are to interview the food shoppers in their homes and answer the questions on the worksheet.

13. **ER** Have students look through popular magazines. Ask students to count the number of food product advertisements shown. Tally the number of ads for each group in the MyPyramid system. Determine if there is one food group that is advertised more frequently. Discuss why manufacturers might choose to promote certain foods and not others.

14. **RF** Display an example of a persuasive food advertisement. Ask students to write down 10 words the ad brings to mind. Have students share their lists and identify commonly identified words. Discuss the effects ads can have on buying behaviors.

15. **ER** Make a display of food ads that show information advertising and persuasive advertising. Discuss the value of each. Ask what consumers can do to encourage the use of more informational advertising in the marketplace.

16. **RF** Have students list the foods they ate at their last meal. Ask them to determine if each food was processed or nonprocessed. Discuss how most foods that people eat today are processed to some degree.

17. **RT** Have students list the pros and cons of buying processed foods. Discuss the reasons foods are processed.

18. **ER** Ask students to bring in food labels. Have students generate a list of food additives from the ingredients lists. Then have the students research the additives to develop a glossary of food additive terms. (Students may wish to use an FDA list of food additives.)

19. **RF** Have students discuss the major purposes for use of additives in food products.

20. **RF** *Organic Farming: The Natural Way to Control Pests and Fertilizer,* color transparency CT-22. Use the transparency to discuss the means used by organic food growers to raise crops. Discuss the pros and cons in buying organically grown or commercially grown produce.

21. **ER** Arrange a field trip to an organic farm to learn about the processes used in growing crops organically.

22. **RT** Ask students what it means to comparison shop. Discuss the challenges of comparison shopping.

23. **ER** Have students practice determining unit prices. Display food items of similar content but with varying sizes, qualities, forms, and brands. (For example, you might bring in cans of name-brand peas in different sizes, a can of generic peas, and a box of frozen peas.) Have students decide which is the best buy and justify their selection.

24. **RF** Compare the prices and nutrient values of four snacks. Ask which one the students would choose and why.

25. **RF** Ask students how many use a shopping list when going to the store. Discuss why a shopping list is helpful. Ask students how they organize their lists.

Using Food Labels

26. **RF** Have students read health claims that appear on food labels. Ask students to explain what each claim actually means.

27. **RF** Have students compare a label from a canned product with a label from a smaller food item such as gum. Ask students what the differences are and why they believe the smaller item warranted a different label.

28. **ER** *Lean on the Label,* reproducible master 22-2. Have students compare the two Nutrition Facts panels and answer the questions on the handout.

29. **EX** *Design a Label,* Activity C, SAG. Students are to design canned food labels according to criteria discussed in this section.

30. **EX** Have students debate whether the government should require manufacturers to include sell by and use by dates on all food products.

Being a Consumer of Fitness Products and Services

31. **RF** *The Right Shoe,* transparency master 22-3. Use the transparency to highlight the features of athletic shoes that support and cushion the feet. Remind students to wear supportive shoes during all forms of exercise.

32. **ER** Have each student choose a piece of exercise or sports equipment they would be interested in buying. Ask students to research and evaluate different styles and brands of their chosen product. (Students should use the questions on page 390 of the text to evaluate the equipment.) Have students report their evaluations to the class.

33. **RF** Have students think of 10 questions to ask about an exercise video tape before buying it. Then have students critique two videos according to their questions. Have students determine if there are other points they need to consider when purchasing an exercise video.

34. **ER** Guest speakers. Invite a panel of fitness trainers to discuss points to consider when selecting a health club. You may also wish to discuss the cost and practicality of hiring a personal trainer. Have students prepare questions beforehand.

Your Consumer Rights

35. **RF** Ask if any students ever bought a defective product. Have students tell the class what they did about the product. Discuss whether the students should have done something differently to receive a more satisfactory response.

36. **EX** Have students develop and perform role-plays about returning defective food and fitness items. Have students be sure to include any consumer rights and responsibilities that apply to each situation.

37. **RT** Review with students the steps for filing a consumer complaint.

Chapter Review

38. **ER** Have students design their own crossword puzzle using terms from the chapter.

39. **RF** *Savvy Shopper or Careless Consumer?* Activity D, SAG. Students are to read given situations and determine if each person was a savvy shopper or a careless consumer. Students are then to justify their answers.

40. **RF** *Backtrack Through Chapter 22,* Activity E, SAG. Students are to provide complete answers to questions and statements that will help them recall, interpret, apply, and practice chapter concepts.

Above and Beyond

41. **ER** Organize a field trip to the supermarket. Have students gather information about services offered, marketing techniques, changes expected in the grocery industry, and career opportunities in the grocery business. Ask students to present their findings to the class.

42. **EX** Have students make posters of the labels they designed in SAG Activity C, *Design a Label.* Display the posters throughout the school.

43. **ER** Have students prepare complimentary letters for a local store that does an excellent job on informational advertising.

Answer Key

Text

Check Your Knowledge, pages 394-395

1. (List five:) supermarkets, warehouse stores, convenience stores, cooperatives, outlet stores, specialty stores, roadside stands, farmers' markets (Advantages and disadvantages are student response. See pages 375-376 in the text.)
2. (Describe three. Student response. See pages 376-377 in the text.)
3. Informational advertising tends to focus on facts, such as ingredients, prices, and nutrients. Persuasive advertising appeals to your human needs and desires for love, approval, fulfillment, and happiness.
4. preserve food; enhance colors, flavors, or textures; maintain or improve nutritional quality; aid processing
5. Small organic farms cannot produce and ship foods as economically as large farming operations.
6. D
7. (List five. Student response. See page 382 in the text.)
8. in descending order by weight
9. false
10. The percent Daily Values listed on food labels are based on a 2,000-calorie diet.
11. true
12. (List three:) provide support for your feet, be flexible, be lightweight, not create any sore spots on your feet, provide adequate traction, be cushioned
13. (List five. Student response. See pages 389-390 in the text.)
14. (List four:) atmosphere, clients, instructors, equipment, services, cleanliness, costs, location, hours
15. the right to safety, the right to be informed, the right to choose, the right to be heard

Student Activity Guide

Where to Shop? Activity A

1. C
2. H
3. G
4. D
5. A
6. B
7. E
8. roadside stand
9. convenience store
10. cooperative
11. supermarket
12. farmers' market
13. wholesale store
14. specialty store
15. outlet store

Savvy Shopper or Careless Consumer? Activity D

1. CC. Practice: buying shoes without trying them on
2. SS. Practice: considering function in selecting shorts
3. SS. Practice: selecting clothing for comfort
4. CC. Practice: ignoring fit and comfort, being influenced by sales price
5. CC. Practice: purchasing something other than your preferred style
6. SS. Practice: setting up a home gym at a minimal cost for convenience
7. SS. Practice: boosting the motivation to work out by joining a health club
8. SS. Practice: comparing pieces of equipment before purchasing
9. CC. Practice: failing to read instructions for safe use of equipment
10. SS. Practice: planning ahead to be sure equipment will fit available space
11. CC. Practice: purchasing with little or no product information
12. SS. Practice: previewing video before purchasing
13. CC. Practice: hiring a trainer without checking credentials or references
14. CC. Practice: choosing a health club that was inconveniently located
15. SS. Practice: doing a cost comparison before making a choice
16. CC. Practice: accepting defective merchandise, not protecting his right to be heard
17. SS. Practice: following the appropriate procedure for making a complaint, keeping his receipt
18. SS. Practice: keeping her receipt so she could return the item, contacting the appropriate person about the problem
19. CC. Practice: not keeping his receipt
20. CC. Practice: not protecting her rights to safety and information, not making a complaint about the problem

Backtrack Through Chapter 22, Activity E

1. someone who buys and uses products and services
2. (List three:) preserves food for long-term storage, kills bacteria, saves consumers time, makes foods more nutritious, and improves appearance of foods

3. (List two. Student response. See page 378 in the text.)
4. Food and Drug Administration (FDA)
5. no
6. on tags attached to shelves beneath food products
7. The U.S. Department of Agriculture is responsible for meat and poultry products, while the U.S. Food and Drug Administration is responsible for all other food products.
8. foods prepared by small businesses, such as bakeries; restaurant and deli foods; custom processed fish and meats; donated foods; and individual foods from multiunit packages
9. in descending order by weight
10. to avoid substances to which they are allergic, to avoid foods for religious or cultural reasons, to know what they are eating, to make wise food choices
11. sturdy, comfortable shoes and nonbinding clothes
12. right to safety, right to be informed, right to choose, and right to be heard
13. (Student response.)
14. (Student response.)
15. (Student response.)
16. If quality is very important in the intended use, you can buy national or store brands. If quality is not important in your intended use, you can buy generic products and save money.
17. The *sell by* date shows how long the manufacturer recommends grocers keep the item on the shelf. The *use by* date is the last day the manufacturer recommends consumers use the product for peak quality.
18. the local store, the manufacturer, and a government agency
19. (Student response.)
20. (Student response.)

Teacher's Resources

Chapter 22 Test

1. D	11. B	21. T	31. F
2. E	12. A	22. T	32. T
3. C	13. D	23. F	33. B
4. B	14. G	24. T	34. C
5. H	15. T	25. F	35. C
6. G	16. F	26. F	36. B
7. F	17. F	27. F	37. A
8. C	18. F	28. T	38. D
9. H	19. F	29. T	39. C
10. E	20. T	30. F	

40. (List three:) advertising, food processing, whether the food is organic, price
41. preserve food; enhance colors, flavors, or textures; maintain or improve nutritional quality; aid processing
42. (List five. Student response. See pages 389-390 in the text.)

Computer Shopping: Technology Trade-Offs

Online shopping isn't for everyone!

Advantages

- Fast and easy
- Convenient
- Timesaving
- Helpful to homebound people

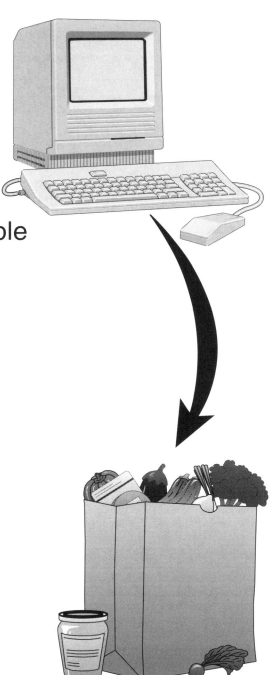

Disadvantages

- Higher food costs
- Membership fees
- Limited availability
- Limited information
- Tips for delivery persons

© Goodheart-Willcox

(Lean on the Label)

Name_____ **Date** _____ **Period** _____

Compare the two Nutrition Facts panels below to answer the questions at the bottom of the page.

Instant Lunch-in-a-Cup

Nutrition Facts

Serving Size 1 Package (64g)
Servings Per Container 1

Amount Per Serving	
Calories 230	Calories from Fat 25

	% Daily Value*
Total Fat 3g	**4%**
Saturated Fat 0g	**0%**
Trans Fat 0g	**0%**
Cholesterol 0mg	**0%**
Sodium 480mg	**20%**
Total Carbohydrate 46g	**15%**
Dietary Fiber 8g	**31%**
Sugars 5g	
Protein 10g	

Vitamin A	30%	•	Vitamin C 60%
Calcium	6 %	•	Iron 15%

*Percent Daily Values are based on a 2,000 calorie diet.

Nutrition Bar

Nutrition Facts

Serving Size 1 Bar (74g)
Servings Per Container 1

Amount Per Serving	
Calories 280	Calories from Fat 50

	% Daily Value*
Total Fat 6g	**10%**
Saturated Fat 1g	**6%**
Trans Fat 0g	**0%**
Cholesterol 0mg	**0%**
Sodium 250mg	**10%**
Total Carbohydrate 52g	**18%**
Dietary Fiber 2g	**6%**
Sugars 12g	
Protein 4g	

Vitamin A	30%	•	Vitamin C 0%
Calcium	40%	•	Iron 20%

*Percent Daily Values are based on a 2,000 calorie diet.

1. Which product would you choose if you were trying to limit you calorie intake? _____

2. Which product would you choose if you were trying to limit your fat intake? _____

3. Which product would you choose if you were trying to limit your sodium intake? _____

4. Which product would you choose if you were trying to increase your fiber intake? _____

5. Which product is lower in sugar? _____

6. Which product is higher in protein? _____

7. Which product is a better source of vitamin C? _____

8. Which product is a better source of calcium? _____

9. Which product is a better source of iron? _____

10. Suppose you are buying this product to have on hand for a busy day when you will not have time to make and eat a full meal for lunch. The products have the same price, and you find both of them appealing. Which product would you choose? Explain your choice.

_____

_____

_____

© Goodheart-Willcox

The Right Shoe

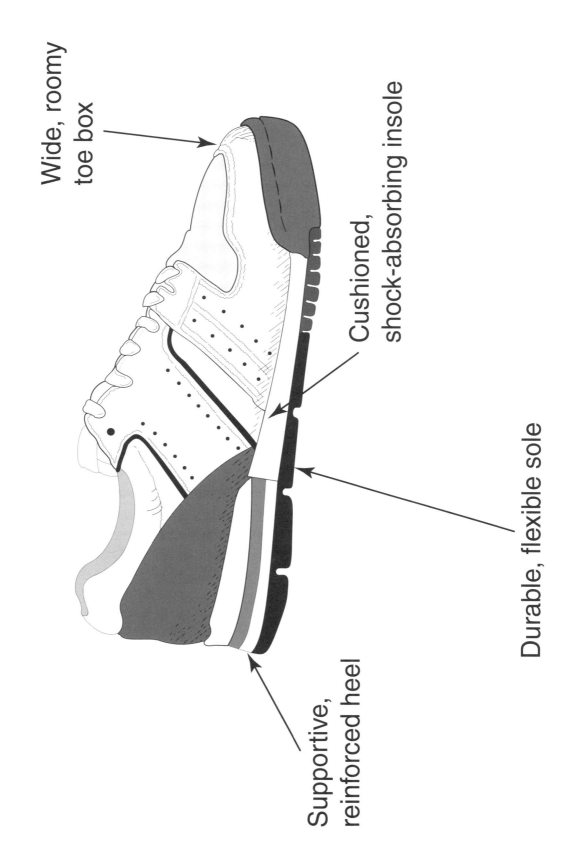

Wide, roomy toe box

Cushioned, shock-absorbing insole

Durable, flexible sole

Supportive, reinforced heel

© Goodheart-Willcox

Making Wise Consumer Choices

Name_____

Date _____ **Period** _____ **Score** _____

Chapter 22 Test

Matching: Match the following terms and identifying phrases.

_____ 1. Stores that sell products made by one food manufacturer.

_____ 2. Produce stand offered by an individual farmer.

_____ 3. Group of produce stands offered by a group of farmers, often in a city location.

_____ 4. Food store that is open only to members who pay an annual fee and volunteer their services.

_____ 5. Store that often sells food items in large containers and multiunit packages.

_____ 6. Grocery store that may offer many other products and services.

_____ 7. Store that specializes in selling one type of product.

A. convenience store
B. cooperative
C. farmers' market
D. outlet store
E. roadside stand
F. specialty store
G. supermarket
H. warehouse store

Matching: Match the following terms and identifying phrases.

_____ 8. A substance added to food products to cause desired changes in the products.

_____ 9. A brand that is sold in only specific chains of food stores.

_____ 10. An unbranded product, which can be identified by plain, simple packaging.

_____ 11. Someone who buys and uses products and services.

_____ 12. Assessing prices and quality of similar products to choose those that best meet a consumer's needs and price range.

_____ 13. Any procedure performed on food to prepare it for consumers.

_____ 14. A brand that is distributed and advertised throughout the country by a major company.

A. comparison shopping
B. consumer
C. food additive
D. food processing
E. generic product
F. impulse buying
G. national brand
H. store brand

True/False: Circle *T* if the statement is true or *F* is the statement is false.

T F   15. Electronic shopping is done using home computers.

T F   16. Persuasive advertising focuses on facts, such as ingredients, prices, and nutrients.

T F   17. A can of corn has not been exposed to food processing.

T F   18. If a food additive is proven harmful to health, it can still be placed on the GRAS list.

T F   19. It has been proven that organic foods are more nutritious than nonorganic foods.

T F   20. If a carton of a dozen eggs costs $1.20, the unit price of each egg is $.10.

T F   21. Generic food items are generally equal in nutritional value to name brand food items.

T F   22. Picking up a candy bar from the checkout counter is an example of impulse buying.

(Continued)

© Goodheart-Willcox

Name_____

T F   23. When grocery shopping, pick up milk and frozen items first.

T F   24. By law, all processed and packaged foods are required to have food labels.

T F   25. The Food and Drug Administration (FDA) governs labels on meat and poultry products.

T F   26. The percent Daily Values listed on food labels are based on a 1,500-calorie diet.

T F   27. The use by date on a can of peas is February 8. This means it is not safe to use the peas on February 9.

T F   28. The only items required for taking part in physical activity are sturdy, comfortable shoes and nonbinding clothes.

T F   29. Athletic shoes should have cushioning to absorb shock and reduce jarring to the body.

T F   30. Safety gear is only necessary for inexperienced athletes.

T F   31. You should not ask a personal trainer for credentials or references because you will insult the trainer.

T F   32. As a consumer, you have the right to make complaints about products.

Multiple Choice: Choose the best response. Write the letter in the space provided.

_____33. _____ is information about people in the communities in which stores are located.
   A. research
   B. demographic data
   C. interviews
   D. study analysis

_____34. Which food processing technique involves adding microbes to a food product to cause specific enzymatic changes?
   A. Aseptic canning.
   B. Dehydration.
   C. Fermentation.
   D. Pasteurization.

_____35. Which can of green beans would be the best buy?
   A. A 10-oz. can for $1.99.
   B. A 9-oz. can for $1.50.
   C. A 20-oz. can for $2.50.
   D. A 3-oz. can for $.75.

_____36. The ingredients in a food product are listed on the label _____.
   A. in ascending order by size
   B. in descending order by weight
   C. in descending order by volume
   D. in ascending order by density

_____37. Which of the following health claims would be permitted on a food label?
   A. A diet low in total fat is linked to a reduced risk of cancer.
   B. Calcium prevents osteoporosis.
   C. Folic acid causes birth defects.
   D. All the above.

_____38. Before purchasing a piece of exercise equipment, it is best to _____.
   A. hire a personal trainer
   B. sign a contract
   C. join a health club
   D. try it out personally

(Continued)

© Goodheart-Willcox

Name_____

_____39. If you buy a piece of fitness equipment that does not operate as advertised, you should _____.
   A. do nothing
   B. call the FDA
   C. take the product and receipt back to the store
   D. threaten to sue the manufacturer

Essay Questions: Provide complete responses to the following questions or statements.

40. List three factors that influence food choices made by consumers.

41. What are four functions of food additives?

42. List five questions that will help you evaluate a fitness equipment purchase.

© Goodheart-Willcox

Food and Fitness Trends

Objectives

After studying this chapter, students will be able to
- identify four food preferences that indicate trends.
- outline the pros and cons of nonnutrient supplements.
- list three ways that bioengineering may affect food and nutrition.
- explain the potential of functional foods.
- describe four technologies that will help keep food safe.
- identify five aspects of the growing fitness industry.

Bulletin Boards

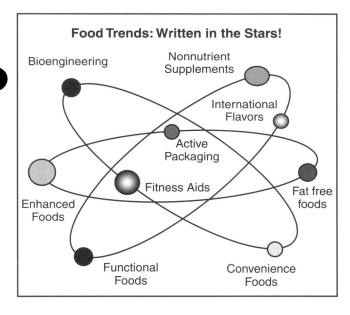

Food Trends: Written in the Stars!

Bioengineering
Nonnutrient Supplements
International Flavors
Active Packaging
Fitness Aids
Fat free foods
Enhanced Foods
Functional Foods
Convenience Foods

Title: *Food Trends: Written in the Stars!*

Using planets cut from construction paper, prepare a solar system. Use string to connect the planets. On or near each planet, write words describing future trends.

Title: *What's Cooking for the Future?*

Sketch a large dome cover lifted from a serving dish. On the lid, write future dates such as 2010, 2030, 2050. On the dish, write phrases such as *vitamin enhanced foods, international flavors, convenience, active packaging, fat free,* and *nonnutrient supplements.* Use other food trends currently identified in the news.

Teaching Materials

Text, pages 396-414
  Learn the Language
  Check Your Knowledge
  Put Learning into Action
  Explore Further
Student Activity Guide, pages 165-170
  A. *This Word or That*
  B. *Assemble the Evidence*
  C. *Comparing Nonnutrient Supplements*
  D. *Backtrack Through Chapter 23*
Teacher's Resources
  Preferences and Science Point the Way to Food Trends, CT-23
  Be Safe—Know Your Product, transparency master 23-1
  New Product Development, reproducible master 23-2
  Chapter 23 Test

Introducing the Chapter

1. Define the term *trend.* Ask students to list several modern food or fitness trends. Discuss which trends are positive and which seem to create problems. Discuss how people learn about trends and who is most likely to adopt a trend.
2. Have students locate all the terms in the chapter that sound "futuristic." Ask students to find the definitions for those terms. Place terms and definitions on large index cards, which can be used for review at the completion of the chapter.
3. Show the class pictures of high-tech fitness equipment advertised in fitness magazines. Ask students to describe how they think the equipment was developed. Relate the equipment to current trends in exercise aid preferences.

Strategies to Reteach, Reinforce, Enrich, and Extend Text Concepts
Food Preferences

4. **EX** Have students brainstorm ideas about future food or fitness products they would like to see on the market. Have them name their products and sketch the product design. Then have students identify reasons this product may be desired by the public. Post the creative sketches for others to see.

5. **RF** Have students identify some of the food innovations from the last 50 years. Discuss why each innovation was or was not accepted well. Also discuss how food technology has changed to meet current consumer needs and interests.

6. **ER** Have students survey their family members to determine five food characteristics that influence buying decisions. Combine preferences from all the surveys into one list. Discuss the relationship between preferences and trends in the marketplace. Discuss the causes of changes in trends.

7. **RF** *Preferences and Science Point the Way to Food Trends,* color transparency CT-23. Use the transparency to identify major factors that influence food development trends.

8. **RF** Have students name local restaurants that specialize in international cuisines. List all the countries represented. Discuss reasons people enjoy ethnic foods.

9. **ER** Have students participate in a taste test by sampling fat free, reduced fat, and regular versions of the same food product. Have students compare taste and mouth feel for each food sample. See if students can identify the differences. Discuss reasons fat free foods are a popular trend.

10. **RF** Highlight the benefits and myths associated with selecting fat free products. Common myths include the following: fat free means calorie free; fat free and reduced fat foods are the solution to obesity; Americans have successfully cut the amount of fat in their diet by using fat free products. Discuss how and for whom fat free products are useful.

11. **ER** Have students visit food company Web sites to identify new products the companies are offering. Have students use contact links to inquire about steps the companies take to develop and market new products. Have students use the information they gather to prepare a display entitled *From Idea to Market: How New Foods Are Created for the Marketplace.* Discuss the techniques used by the food industry to promote new foods. Ask students how they feel about trying new products.

12. **ER** Plan a visit to the food store to identify new food items. Have students complete a list of the names of the new food products. Ask the store manager how companies acquire shelf space in stores for their products. Have the manager identify the factors involved in deciding what products to sell.

13. **RF** *Be Safe—Know Your Product,* transparency master 23-1. Use the transparency to discuss the claims and cautions associated with the use of herbs and other botanicals. Use the list on page 401 in the textbook to discuss cautions for use of nonnutrient supplements.

14. **ER** Guest speaker. Invite a registered dietitian to discuss why $\frac{1}{3}$ of Americans are using herbal pills, powders, teas, and tonics as a supplement to the diet or a replacement for medicine. Include a discussion of the pros and cons of consuming various herbs and botanicals.

15. **RF** *Comparing Nonnutrient Supplements,* Activity C, SAG. Students are to compare the product labels on two brands of the same nonnutrient supplements. Students will then answer questions that follow.

16. **ER** Have students write a report on the laws regarding product selling and labeling for herbal products. Check the Web sites from the Food and Drug Administration concerning adverse effects from herbal products as reported to the FDA. (The FDA hot line number is 1-800-332-1088.)

17. **ER** Have students search the Internet to learn about safe use of botanicals. Evaluate the source of the Web site for its credibility as a resource since this topic is particularly vulnerable to sales pitches and exaggerated claims.

18. **EX** Conduct a class debate on whether botanicals are a nonnutrient supplement or a medicine. List the reasons they are frequently used for both.

19. **ER** Provide sample pills and powders of herbal products that are advertised as "natural." Have students read the ingredients label and the product label claims. Discuss what is believable and what is not. Discuss the meaning of *natural.* Discuss FDA regulations for herbs and botanicals, which state these products must not be harmful and cannot make medical claims unless approved as a medicine by the FDA.

20. **ER** *Assemble the Evidence,* Activity B, SAG. Students are to use various resources to gather evidence supporting each of the listed trends.

Food Science Trends

21. **EX** Have students list three words that come to mind when they think of the word *bioengineering.* Categorize the word associations as positive, neutral, or negative. Discuss if the perceptions have greater tendency to be positive or negative.

22. **RF** Review the definition of *bioengineering* and discuss synonyms such as *genetic engineering* and *biotechnology.*

23. **ER** Display the food products of cheese, yogurt, and bread. Ask how these products relate to the bioengineering definition. Tell students that enzymes are used to make cheese and yogurt, and yeast modifies the taste, texture, and flavor of bread.

24. **ER** Plan for a joint class meeting with the chemistry students to explore issues related to bioengineering. Have the classes debate cautions versus potentials. Summarize the major issues.

25. **RF** Identify the characteristics of a functional food. List the names of typically identified functional foods. They contain phytochemicals including carotenoids (carrots, fruits, vegetables, tomatoes), flavonoids (tea, onions, soy), and sulfur compounds (garlic, onions, and leek). Foods containing fatty acids (tuna and other fish oils) are also considered functional.

26. **EX** Have small teams of students prepare an advertisement for a functional food of their own invention. Make sure they incorporate the benefits listed on page 407 of the textbook. Display the ads.

27. **EX** Assign students to groups of four. Have each group research one of the following topics: use of competitive bacteria, DNA fingerprinting, active packaging, and irradiation. Have the groups give an oral presentation to the class on their topics.

Fitness Trends

28. **ER** Have students research statistics on the percentages of Americans who are physically active and inactive. Discuss the recent trends that relate physical fitness to quality of life and health.

29. **ER** Have students think of excuses people give for not exercising. For each excuse, have other students give a statement that refutes the excuse.

30. **ER** Conduct a field trip to a local health care center that works with clients to improve health through physical fitness. Discuss how the growth of fitness information has influenced the type of services provided to consumers over the last ten years.

31. **ER** Have students draw a floor plan design for an ideal workplace that provides a variety of wellness resources for employees. Discuss perceived costs and added benefits of such a program to the company or organization. Have the students think about their own work environment and what effect an employee wellness program would have on them and other employees. Brainstorm ideas about how to be an employee advocate for fitness in the worksite.

32. **ER** Have each student identify and describe one new fitness trend researched through use of the library or Internet. Prepare a class fact sheet that lists the major trends along with the source of information. Share the fact sheet with other health and physical education professionals in the school.

33. **RF** *This Word or That,* Activity A, SAG. Students are to determine if given statements are true or false. If the statement is true, the student will write the letter *T* on the line before each number. If the statement is false, the student will write the letter of the word choice that will make it true.

Chapter Review

34. **EX** Have students suggest names for future foods, such as broccoflower. Students should relate their names to apparent food trends.

35. **RF** *Backtrack Through Chapter 23,* Activity A, SAG. Students are to provide complete answers to questions and statements that will help them recall, interpret, apply, and practice chapter concepts.

Above and Beyond

36. **EX** *New Product Development,* reproducible master 23-2. Have student teams complete the activity by developing new food products. Have teams present their products to the class.

36. **ER** Guest speakers. Invite representatives from consumer and environmental groups and the biotechnology industry to present an all-school presentation on bioengineering. Stress the question of how to attain a safe, nutritious, and sustainable food supply for all people.

38. **EX** Have students write research reports on trends and issues in food, nutrition, and technology. Encourage students to use current news articles and food, nutrition, and technology journals and textbooks for topic ideas.

39. **ER** Have students use the Yellow Pages to identify fitness trainers, programs, centers, and other fitness facilities in your community. Prepare and distribute a class directory of local fitness resources.

Answer Key
Text

Check Your Knowledge, page 413

1. false
2. cleaning, trimming, cutting, and packaging
3. true
4. olestra (or the Olean brand product)
5. advocates: They are nature's answer to staying healthy. They are completely safe.
   opponents: They can be harmful. They have not been tested to find if health benefits really exist.
6. when the following is on the ad or label: "This statement has not been evaluated by the Food and Drug Administration. This product is not intended to diagnose, treat, cure, or prevent any disease."
7. DNA (or genes)
8. D
9. false
10. milk from special goats
11. when the food causes an allergic reaction in some people, has a change in its nutrient content, or is new to the diet

12. through the traditional crossbreeding of cauliflower and broccoli
13. (List two:) phytochemicals, dietary fiber, some fatty acids
14. Neutraceuticals is a term that combines the words *nutrition* and *pharmaceuticals*, which are drugs. This implies that a nutrition source has druglike health effects.
15. false
16. fights food spoilage and provides information about the safety of the product for eating
17. B
18. The U.S. population was very active 100 years ago but is very sedentary today.
19. (List four:) fitness aids are increasing; sports and fitness apparel options are increasing; corporations are encouraging employees to stay fit; health care institutions are sponsoring fitness programs; career opportunities in the fitness field are expanding
20. by providing on-site exercise programs and facilities available, by giving discounts for using nearby health clubs

Student Activity Guide

This Word or That, Activity A

1. B	11. C		
2. A	12. T		
3. T	13. C		
4. D	14. A		
5. T	15. T		
6. T	16. C		
7. A	17. D		
8. C	18. T		
9. T	19. T		
10. B	20. B		

Backtrack Through Chapter 23, Activity D
1. The industry responds by trying to address as many trends as possible.
2. strong interest in international foods and new flavors, preference for freshness with convenience, effort to reduce dietary fat intake, and reliance on supplements
3. herbs, spices, and other flavorings
4. eat-in restaurants, nutrition consulting services, and diet planning services
5. over one in three
6. soybean or cottonseed oil and sugar
7. nonnutrient
8. headaches, dizziness, vomiting, strokes, seizures, and death

9. new technology at the cellular level and advances in food preservation and safety
10. genetic engineering and biotechnology
11. about five years
12. increase quantity and quality of food, enhance the nutrient content of food, and prevent possible diseases
13. tomatoes that do not rot quickly
14. because fat affects every aspect of food quality—texture, color, flavor, and mouth feel
15. "This statement has not been evaluated by the Food and Drug Administration. This product is not intended to diagnose, treat, cure, or prevent any disease." Nonnutrient supplements are forbidden to claim they can treat a disease because there is no scientific proof of these claims.
16. A vaccine creates an immunity by introducing a small amount of a weakened strain of a disease-causing agent into the body. The body can easily fight this agent and builds its defenses against this particular disease. This is called an immunity.
17. Bioengineering is producing and identifying functional foods.
18. because of the general fear of consumers that irradiation may be unsafe
19. (Student response.)
20. (Student response.)

Teacher's Resources

Chapter 23 Test

1. E	9. I	17. F	25. B
2. L	10. A	18. T	26. D
3. C	11. J	19. F	27. C
4. B	12. D	20. T	28. D
5. F	13. T	21. F	29. D
6. H	14. F	22. T	30. A
7. K	15. T	23. T	31. B
8. M	16. F	24. T	32. A

33. international foods and flavors—people desire something new and different; freshness with convenience—busy people require food that takes little time and effort to prepare, but that looks and tastes fresh; foods with less—people are focusing on lowfat and fat free foods in order to lose weight; nonnutrient supplements—people wish to stay healthy in natural ways
34. (List two. Student response. See pages 407-409 in the text.)
35. (List three. Student response. See pages 410-412 in the text.)

Be Safe—Know Your Product

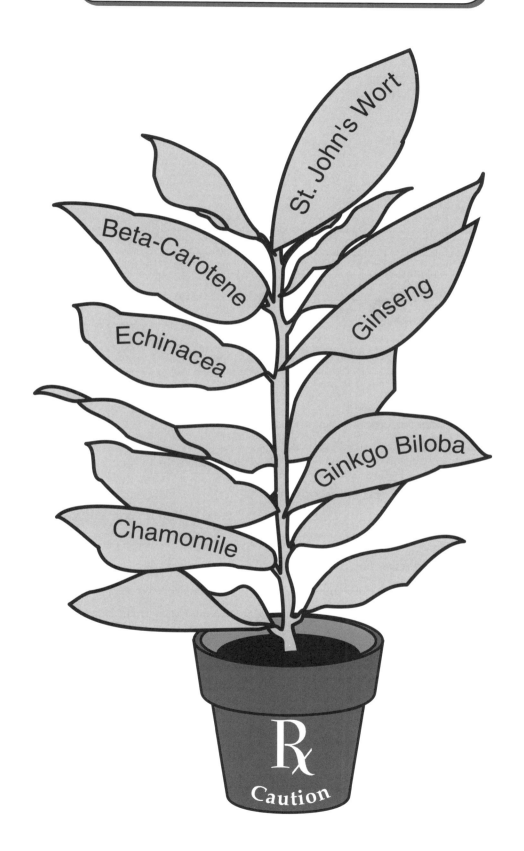

© Goodheart-Willcox

New Product Development

Name_____   Date _____   Period _____

Develop a new food product based on one of the following factors driving food science:

- increased food quality
- enhanced nutrient content
- possible disease prevention
- advance in food safety

Then answer the following questions.

1. Product name: _____

2. Ingredient list: _____

_____

_____

3. Nutrients provided from ingredients: _____

_____

_____

Plan how you will sell your product.

4. Why will the consumer want to purchase this product?_____

_____

_____

5. Are there any health benefits associated with this product? _____

_____

_____

6. How would you promote and advertise this product? _____

_____

_____

A. What slogan might you use for your product? _____

_____

B. What guarantees or health claims might you put on the product label? _____

_____

C. Sketch a sample product label or logo for the product below.

© Goodheart-Willcox

Food and Fitness Trends

Name_____

Date _____   Period _____   Score _____

Chapter 23 Test

Matching: Match the following terms and identifying phrases.

_____ 1. A process that traces the cause of a food poisoning or impurity.

_____ 2. A general pattern or direction.

_____ 3. A plant material or part of a plant.

_____ 4. The science of changing the genetic makeup of an organism.

_____ 5. A food or food ingredient that provides health benefits beyond basic nutrition.

_____ 6. The exposure of food to ionizing energy.

_____ 7. A pill, powder, or liquid that claims to promote health but has not been proven to do so.

_____ 8. A weakened strain of a disease-causing organism.

_____ 9. A concentrated level of a substance many times higher than its natural occurrence in the diet.

_____ 10. A type of food package that interacts with the food or the atmosphere inside.

_____ 11. The sensation perceived by the tongue to different foods.

_____ 12. Bacteria that prevent the growth of pathogens.

A. active packaging
B. bioengineering
C. botanical
D. competitive bacteria
E. DNA fingerprinting
F. functional food
G. immunity
H. irradiation
I. megadose
J. mouth feel
K. nonnutrient supplement
L. trend
M. vaccine

True/False: Circle *T* if the statement is true and *F* if the statement is false.

T F 13. The food industry addresses as many trends as possible by bringing hundreds of new products to market each year.

T F 14. One eating trend in the U.S. is an increased lack of interest in ethnic foods.

T F 15. Busy families look for convenience foods as one way to solve time management problems.

T F 16. Nonnutrient supplements can be substituted for food.

T F 17. The FDA safety checks that are required of new foods and drugs also apply to nonnutrient supplements.

T F 18. Scientists are working to replace laboratory-prepared vaccines with edible vaccines.

T F 19. Special labeling will be required on all bioengineered foods.

T F 20. Broccoli is an example of a functional food.

T F 21. New technologies such as competitive bacteria replace routine sanitation practices.

T F 22. The FDA requires a special symbol on the labels of irradiated food.

T F 23. People's lifestyles today are more inactive than they were 100 years ago.

T F 24. Career opportunities in the fitness field are rapidly expanding.

© Goodheart-Willcox   *(Continued)*

Name_____

Multiple Choice: Choose the best response. Write the letter in the space provided.

_____25. Which of the following is used by manufacturers as a fat replacement ingredient?
  A. Aspartame.
  B. Olestra.
  C. Water.
  D. Herbs.

_____26. What is the predicted population age trend in the U.S. for the next three decades?
  A. Birth rate will double.
  B. The number of teenagers will triple.
  C. The middle-aged population will decline by one-half.
  D. The number of people age 65 and older will triple.

_____27. Which of the following claims is most reliable?
  A. "This product is guaranteed to raise IQ."
  B. "Eyesight will improve with use of this product."
  C. "This food is an excellent source of vitamin A."
  D. "One pill a day will halt the aging process."

_____28. Why is bioengineering more effective than traditional cross-breeding methods for changing food characteristics?
  A. Bioengineering is a less-costly process.
  B. Bioengineered food never spoils.
  C. Bioengineered products are not regulated by any government agencies.
  D. Bioengineering requires less time to get desired results.

_____29. Why are people interested in consuming functional foods?
  A. Rising health care costs.
  B. Desire to use food rather than drugs to maintain health.
  C. Science has revealed new facts about ways to promote good health using food.
  D. All the above.

_____30. When a food source that causes contamination is identified through DNA fingerprinting, the manufacturer will likely _____.
  A. announce a product recall
  B. close down
  C. ship the product out of the country
  D. All the above.

_____31. Which one of the following occupational lifestyles involves using the least amount of physical activity?
  A. Farm management.
  B. Data processing.
  C. Landscape maintenance.
  D. Building construction.

_____32. What is the U.S. population trend regarding weight management?
  A. The number of overweight people is rising.
  B. The number of overweight people is declining.
  C. The number of overweight children is declining.
  D. Interest in weight management is declining.

Essay Questions: Provide complete responses to the following questions or statements.

33. Name four current food trends and explain why the trends are gaining followers.
34. List two advances in foods safety and explain how they increase food safety.
35. List three trends current in the fitness industry.

© Goodheart-Willcox

Nutrition and Health: A Global Concern

Objectives

After studying this chapter, students will be able to
- define terms related to global hunger.
- explain the major causes of hunger.
- refute common misconceptions about global hunger.
- describe how a nation's hunger problem can be solved through the following factors: economic progress, science and technology advances, effective infrastructure, slower population growth, and education.
- identify the primary organizations working to combat hunger in the United States and throughout the world.
- propose several ways individuals can help fight hunger.

Bulletin Board

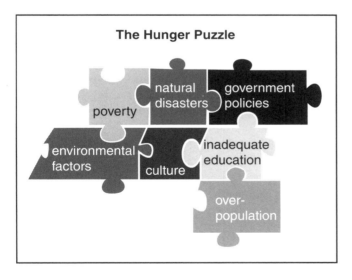

The Hunger Puzzle

Title: *The Hunger Puzzle*

Use construction paper to make cutouts of seven large puzzle pieces that fit together. Label each piece with one of the primary causes of global hunger: poverty, overpopulation, natural disasters, government policies, environmental factors, culture, and inadequate education. Place the pieces on the bulletin board one by one as you study these topics in class.

Teaching Materials

Text, pages 415-438
> *Learn the Language*
> *Check Your Knowledge*
> *Put Learning into Action*
> *Explore Further*

Student Activity Guide, pages 171-180
> A. *Meanings in Action*
> B. *It All Adds up to Hunger*
> C. *Hunger—Why Do I Care?*
> D. *A Case in Point*
> E. *Portrait of the Hungry*
> F. *Stepwise Solutions to Hunger*
> G. *Backtrack Through Chapter 24*

Teacher's Resources
> *Populations at Risk of Inadequate Nutrition,* transparency master 24-1
> *Trends in Undernutrition,* transparency master 24-2
> *The Poverty Web,* transparency master 24-3
> *Emergency Food Assistance Survey,* reproducible master 24-4
> *The Food Chain,* color transparency CT-24
> *Chapter 24 Test*

Introducing the Chapter

1. Ask students to list five world problems they regularly hear reported in the news. Have students rank the items in their lists, with number one being the most serious. Invite students to share their lists in class. Discuss which problems people have influence over. Also discuss how one problem often relates to others. Focus on responses that relate to the global hunger problem.
2. Ask students to imagine how their lives would be affected if they had no food available to them. Ask them to list words describing what it feels like to be hungry. Write responses on the chalkboard.
3. Discuss how students feel about living in a world where some people go hungry and others are overfed. How do dual standards of health and wellness affect society?

Strategies to Reteach, Reinforce, Enrich, and Extend Text Concepts

The Hunger Problem

4. **RT** Review the definitions of the following terms: *developing nation, hunger, undernutrition, malnutrition,* and *starvation.*

5. **ER** Guest speaker. Invite a historian to discuss the roles wars and political upheavals have played in creating famines for civilians. Discuss how people battle malnutrition in these instances and the role of food aid in times of crisis.

6. **RT** Review the health consequences of undernutrition.

7. **RT** *Populations at Risk of Inadequate Nutrition,* transparency master 24-1. Use the transparency to pinpoint areas of the world where malnutrition is a concern. Have students refer to a current world map to identify individual countries that lie within shaded areas.

8. **RT** *Trends in Undernutrition,* transparency master 24-2. Use the transparency to compare trends in undernutrition in developing countries from 1969 through 1992. Discuss where undernutrition is expected to increase and where it is expected to decrease by 2010.

9. **EX** Ask students what a typical teen in the United States might have for lunch. Write a menu on the chalkboard and have students use diet analysis software or Appendix B, *Nutritive Values of Foods,* to determine the nutrient content of the meal. Ask students to compare this nutritional analysis with the analysis of a lunch composed of 1 cup cooked rice, ½ cup milk, and 1 banana, which might be typical of a teen living in a developing country. Have students identify which nutrients are lacking in each meal. Then discuss how the diet patterns relate to culture, land resources, and economy.

10. **EX** Ask students what effects a nutritionally deficient diet might have on pregnancy, the healing of a broken leg, or recovery from pneumonia.

11. **EX** Have students review Figure 24-3 on page 418 in the text. Then ask students to brainstorm ideas about how to break the hunger cycle.

12. **RF** *Hunger—Why Do I Care?* Activity C, SAG. Students are to list the reasons they care about the hunger problem and identify whether each reason is primarily humanitarian, political, or economic. Then students are to compare and contrast their lists with classmates and summarize their findings.

13. **ER** Panel discussion. Invite a panel of volunteers who work with hunger relief agencies in your community to speak to the class. Ask panel members to discuss why they want to help people in need. Have students summarize comments of panel members in an article for the school newsletter encouraging students to become involved in hunger relief.

14. **EX** *The Poverty Web,* transparency master 24-3. Use the transparency to show the interrelationship of factors related to poverty that results in the complex issue of hunger. Divide the class into six groups. Have each group complete a web diagram for one of the other factors that leads to hunger (overpopulation, natural disasters, government policies, environmental factors, culture, and inadequate education). Ask each group to share its diagram with the rest of the class.

15. **EX** Have students compare environmental conditions in developing nations with those in industrialized nations.

16. **EX** Ask each student to find a magazine, newspaper, or Internet article about hunger. Have students summarize their articles in brief oral reports.

Working Toward National Solutions

17. **ER** Guest speaker. Invite a resource person from a national food assistance program to speak to the class. Ask the speaker to describe the population groups served by the program and the effects the program has had on people's lives.

18. **RF** Have students gather brochures related to food and nutrition services within the community. Also sign up to receive agency newsletters. Arrange collected materials in a reading center or a bulletin board display.

19. **ER** *Emergency Food Assistance Survey,* reproducible master 24-4. Have students use the handout to interview people from a variety of emergency food assistance agencies. Ask students to share their findings in groups to determine how well the needs of the community are being met.

Working Toward Global Solutions

20. **RF** *Portrait of the Hungry,* Activity E, SAG. Students are to list traits on the left side of the sketch that describe hungry people in the United States. Students are to list traits on the right side of the sketch that describe hungry people elsewhere around the globe. Then students are to compare and contrast the two groups of descriptors they used.

21. **ER** Guest speaker. Invite a county agricultural agent to discuss the effects of technology on increasing crop yields. Ask the speaker to bring samples of regular rice or grain and technologically improved rice or grain. Discuss technology's role in helping to meet the food needs of all people. Also discuss why agricultural assistance programs are often more helpful than food assistance programs.

22. **EX** Have students debate the statement "Technology is the key to solving world hunger." Debate teams should conduct research to support their arguments about how technology can improve or deteriorate conditions for people. Debate might also focus on the inequitable distribution of technological resources throughout the world.

23. **ER** Field trip. Arrange a visit to an aquaculture center where fish farming occurs. Discuss the contributions of aquaculture to the world food supply.

24. **RF** *It All Adds up to Hunger,* Activity B, SAG. Students are to write responses to or interpretations of statistics about world hunger.

25. **ER** Define the term *myth.* Have students list each of the seven hunger myths presented in the text on pages 427-429. Have students ask three friends outside your class if they think each statement is a myth or fact. Have the class total results to learn which myths are most commonly held by schoolmates. Discuss other myths about hunger and poverty that may exist among students.

26. **RF** Turn each myth statement on pages 427-429 in the text into a question. Ask students to respond to each question with an answer based on facts.

27. **RF** *Stepwise Solutions to Hunger,* Activity F, SAG. Students are to write given steps and strategies in the appropriate diagrams to describe the five major fronts on which hunger needs to be attacked.

28. **RF** Use the Internet to locate reports of the World Food Summit from the Food and Agricultural Organization of the United Nations (FAO). Identify the food goals for the world listed in the reports. Read the goal statements to students and discuss whether goals are being met.

What Can One Person Do?

29. **ER** Have students write to one of the hunger-relief agencies identified in Figure 24-22 on page 435 in the text. Students should request material describing the work of the organization and the contributions they make to relieving world hunger. Display materials gathered.

30. **EX** In small groups, have students brainstorm ways in which they can participate in helping to solve hunger problems. Ask each group to share its ideas with the rest of the class.

31. **RF** *A Case in Point,* Activity D, SAG. Students are to research the hunger problem in another country and list possible causes under various categories. Then students are to write letters to government officials in their chosen countries suggesting ways to address the problem.

32. **EX** *The Food Chain,* color transparency CT-24. Use the transparency to generate a discussion on the impact eating lower on the food chain would

have on economics, the environment, and the food supply. You may wish to have students refer to the copy on vegetarianism on pages 115-116 in the text.

33. **RT** Highlight the need for people and relief organizations to work collaboratively to help solve global hunger problems.

34. **EX** Have students write at least three action statements focusing on what students can do to help solve the world hunger problem. Each statement should begin with the words *We can.* Then have students design a colorful poster listing their action statements. Display the poster in a location that will be seen by the entire student body.

Chapter Review

35. **RF** *Meanings in Action,* Activity A, SAG. Students are to match terms related to hunger with examples of their meanings.

36. **RF** Have each student write one new piece of information he or she learned through the study of this chapter. Go around the room, asking each student to share what he or she wrote. Discuss the value of studying world hunger.

37. **RF** *Backtrack Through Chapter 24,* Activity G, SAG. Students are to provide complete answers to questions and statements that will help them recall, interpret, apply, and practice chapter concepts.

Above and Beyond

38. **ER** Have students plan a collaborative project involving Internet or library research to find information on the underlying reasons for malnutrition in a specific country or region. Have pairs of students research one of the following factors used to indicate quality of life: land size, population, projected population growth within the next 5 to 10 years, birth rate, infant mortality rate, family income, typical diet, educational levels, life expectancy, health care services, sanitation standards, land suitability, quality of water, religious influence on life and economics, and political attitudes. Have students share findings by making poster presentations connecting researched factors with food-related issues in the country or region.

39. **EX** Have students plan an activity in observance of World Food Day or some other national or international day that focuses on world hunger. Activity plans should help increase awareness of the entire study body about the problem of world hunger. Resources may be available through sponsoring organizations.

40. **ER** Have each student draft a letter to a government official who has a record of supporting

hunger-relief programs. Students may choose to thank the officials for support of current programs. Students may also wish to encourage the officials to sponsor new legislation targeted at specific hunger-relief efforts. After reviewing the drafts and asking students to make any necessary revisions, mail letters to the officials. When replies are received, discuss the responses in class and/or post them on a bulletin board.

41. **EX** Make arrangements for students to volunteer in a community food and nutrition program or event.

Answer Key

Text

Check Your Knowledge, pages 437–438

1. low calorie intake
2. low protein intake
3. underweight, stunted, wasted
4. (List five:) carbohydrates, protein, vitamin A, iodine, iron, zinc
5. (List five:) infant and child mortality rate, life expectancy, percent of population with safe water, percent of population with adequate sanitation, primary school enrollment rate, per capita GDP
6. lack of access to food due to poverty
7. (List five:) overpopulation, natural disasters, government policies, environmental factors, culture, inadequate education
8. (List five:) Food Stamp Program, School Breakfast Program, National School Lunch Program, Special Milk Program, WIC Program, Congregate Meals Program, Commodity Distribution Program
9. true
10. Poor farmers do not have the economic resources to take advantage of new technologies and often are replaced by them.
11. Many people do not want to end hunger because they benefit financially from it.
12. Giving food to needy people does not ensure their future ability to buy or grow food. This solution does not solve the problems that cause hunger.
13. Seeds, fertilizer, and other supplies are easily moved to where they are needed. Food can be stored under safe and sanitary conditions.
14. false
15. (List four:) With education, people can learn to read, develop job skills, earn a living, improve the land, raise food, apply nutrition and sanitation principles, protect their health, and support change.
16. United Nations International Children's Emergency Fund (UNICEF)
17. (List five:) investigate hunger in the local

community, support groups that attack the underlying causes of hunger, volunteer time, help fundraising efforts, donate money or material items, communicate your views in writing to policy makers, educate others, be a spokesperson for change, find creative ways to help hungry families

Student Activity Guide

Meanings in Action, Activity A

1. B	10. C	19. B
2. A	11. A	20. A
3. C	12. D	21. D
4. B	13. D	22. B
5. D	14. C	23. C
6. A	15. A	24. A
7. A	16. B	25. B
8. C	17. C	26. A
9. D	18. A	27. C

Stepwise Solutions to Hunger, Activity F

Economic—make food policies, convert to market economies, view hunger as an obstacle to growth

Infrastructure—improve schools, improve waterways, improve highways

Population growth—improve health, improve health education, improve nutrition

Education—teach people to read, teach job skills, teach gardening

Research and technology—produce new food varieties, increase food yields, have a green revolution

Backtrack Through Chapter 24, Activity G

1. 83
2. South and East Asia and parts of Africa
3. In the past, crop diseases and natural disasters were the main causes. Today, famines are caused by war conditions where food is withheld from the enemy.
4. lack of access to food due to poverty
5. They get sick quicker, lack energy, and have decreased motivation, intellectual ability, and drive to succeed.
6. (Name one:) vitamin A, iodine, iron, and zinc (Explanation is student response. See page 419.)
7. infant and child mortality rate, life expectancy, primary school enrollment rate, percent of population with safe water, percent of population with adequate sanitation, and per capita GDP
8. earthquakes, hurricanes, and floods
9. over 10 percent
10. the green revolution
11. October 16, the United States National Committee for World Food Day

12. Even though enough food is available, people lack the money to buy it.
13. because protein foods are scarce
14. Women of poor health have low-birthweight babies with health problems. The cycle is repeated from generation to generation.
15. because it strains food resources, deteriorates the environment, and the quality of life
16. without education, people cannot learn ways to improve their lives
17. Even though the United States has only six percent of the world's population, it uses 30 to 40 percent of the world's resources. A person in a developed nation consumes 30 times as much food as one born in a developing nation.
18. The goal is to reduce the number of undernourished people in the world at least 50 percent by 2015. (Reaction is student response.)
19. (Student response.)
20. (Student response.)

Teacher's Resources

Chapter 24 Test

1. G	11. H	21. F	31. D
2. M	12. C	22. T	32. A
3. I	13. T	23. F	33. D
4. D	14. T	24. F	34. C
5. F	15. T	25. T	35. C
6. L	16. T	26. F	36. D
7. J	17. F	27. T	37. D
8. K	18. F	28. D	
9. A	19. F	29. B	
10. E	20. T	30. B	

38. (Student response. See page 429 in the text.)
39. (Describe two U.S. programs and one international organization. Student response. See pages 425-426 and 433-434 in the text.)
40. (List three. Student response. See pages 435-436 in the text.)

Populations at Risk of Inadequate Nutrition

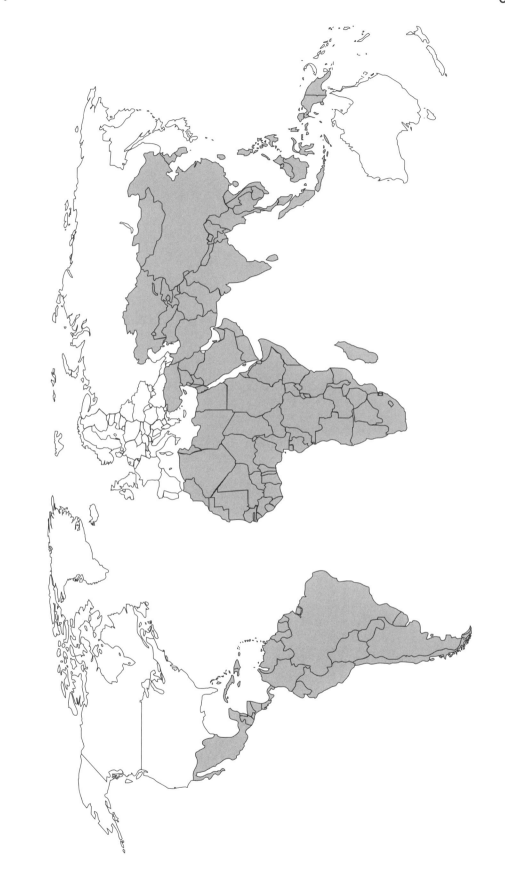

Countries with populations at risk of inadequate nutrition

© Goodheart-Willcox

Trends in Undernutrition

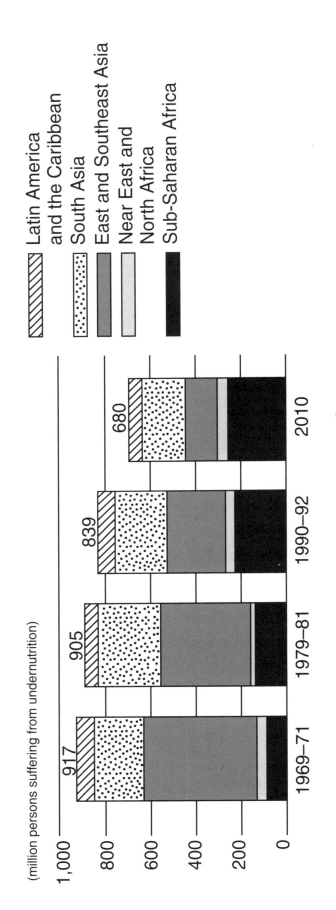

(million persons suffering from undernutrition)

Latin America and the Caribbean

South Asia

East and Southeast Asia

Near East and North Africa

Sub-Saharan Africa

917   905   839   680

1969–71   1979–81   1990–92   2010

1,000   800   600   400   200   0

Source:
Food and Agriculture Organization of the United Nations (FAO)

© Goodheart-Willcox

The Poverty Web

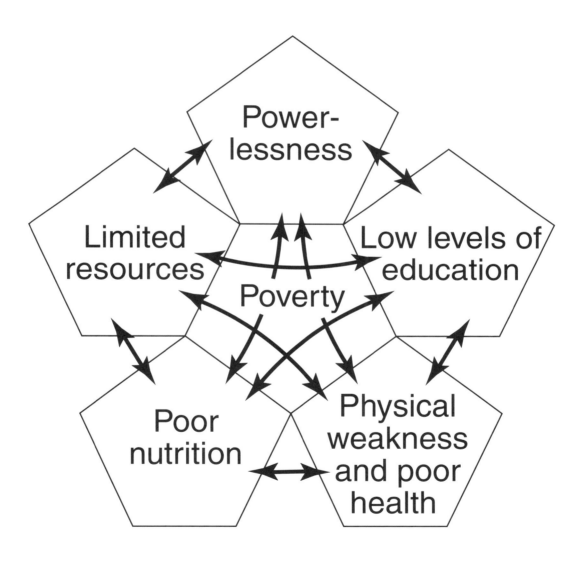

© Goodheart-Willcox

Emergency Food Assistance Survey

Name_____ **Date** _____ **Period** _____

Contact a local organization that provides for the emergency food needs of individuals and/or families. Use the following questions to interview a knowledgeable person about how the organization helps people in need.

Name of the organization_____

Address _____

Phone number _____

Contact person_____

1. Who is eligible to receive the emergency assistance? _____
   _____

2. About how many people do you serve each month?_____

3. How would you describe your typical client? _____
   _____

4. Do most of your clients rely on your services on a continual or a sporadic basis?_____

5. Approximately how much assistance do you provide each month?_____

6. How is the assistance provided to the people who need it? _____
   _____

7. What, if any, needs other than food needs do you address?_____
   _____

8. How do people find out about your services? _____
   _____

9. Where do your resources come from?_____
   _____

10. What are your sources of funding? _____
    _____

11. How can people help your organization?_____
    _____

12. What other comments or concerns can you share with me?_____
    _____

Student observations:

What did you learn about hunger issues by doing this interview? _____
_____
_____

© Goodheart-Willcox

Nutrition and Health: A Global Concern

Name_____

Date _____   Period _____   Score _____

Chapter 24 Test

Matching: Match the following terms and identifying phrases.

_____ 1. A weakened state caused by prolonged lack of food.

_____ 2. Eating too little food to maintain healthy body weight and normal activity levels.

_____ 3. Poor nutrition usually endured for a long period.

_____ 4. An extreme scarcity of food for an extended period, perhaps years.

_____ 5. Always having access to the food needed for a healthy life.

_____ 6. Having below-average height.

_____ 7. A death rate.

_____ 8. A population growth so rapid that it deteriorates the environment or the quality of life.

_____ 9. A crop that can be sold to an exporter.

_____ 10. A rule or regulation that affects food production, prices, or trade.

_____ 11. A system of highways, railroads, waterways, and other public works.

_____ 12. The wise use of natural resources to preserve them for later use.

A. cash crop
B. commodity food
C. environmental sustainability
D. famine
E. food policy
F. food security
G. hunger
H. infrastructure
I. malnutrition
J. mortality rate
K. overpopulation
L. stunted
M. undernutrition

True/False: Circle *T* if the statement is true or *F* if the statement is false.

T   F   13. The world's total population is expected to increase in the next 25 years.

T   F   14. In some developing nations, many families use nearly all their income to buy food.

T   F   15. Some nations have government policies that have allowed hunger to continue for years.

T   F   16. In developing nations, up to half of the children die before age five.

T   F   17. Babies born to malnourished women are generally just as healthy as babies born to well-nourished women.

T   F   18. An organization that analyzes the hunger conditions of people all over the world is the Food and Drug Administration (FDA).

T   F   19. Food scarcity only exists in developing nations.

T   F   20. People who feel compassion have a deep desire to provide hope as well as food for the world's hungry populations.

T   F   21. The main cause of hunger in the world is overpopulation.

T   F   22. A natural disaster usually results in short-term rather than long-term hunger problems.

T   F   23. Food can easily be grown in mountainous or desert areas.

T   F   24. Giving food to needy people will solve the world's hunger problems.

T   F   25. When steps are taken to solve a country's hunger issues, the economy of the nation is likely to improve.

(Continued)

© Goodheart-Willcox

Name_____

T F   26. Most of the known edible plants in the world are currently being used as food sources.

T F   27. An advocate is a person who is willing to speak out on an issue.

Multiple Choice: Choose the best response. Write the letter in the space provided.

_____28. The most common cause of famine in the world today is _____.
A. crop diseases
B. lack of compassion for the hungry
C. natural disasters
D. war

_____29. According to United Nation's figures, what percent of the world's population is undernourished?
A. 10 percent
B. 20 percent.
C. 30 to 40 percent.
D. 50 to 60 percent.

_____30. Which of the following nutrients are most often deficient in the diets of people in developing nations?
A. Phosphorus and magnesium.
B. Vitamin A and iron.
C. Vitamins C and D.
D. Vitamins E and K.

_____31. What type of reason for caring about hunger is the interdependence of countries in sharing resources?
A. Compassionate.
B. Economic.
C. Humanitarian.
D. Political.

_____32. How can culture impact hunger problems?
A. People may be missing nutrients because the only food sources are forbidden by the culture.
B. People may be unable to harvest available foods using traditional tools of the culture.
C. People may go hungry in a vegetarian culture.
D. People may not produce enough food when work is not valued by the culture.

_____33. Which food program is especially designed to offer food vouchers to low-income mothers with children up to age 5?
A. Commodity Distribution Program.
B. Congregate Meals Program.
C. National School Lunch Program.
D. Supplemental Food Program for Women, Infants, and Children (WIC).

_____34. Which statement represents a hunger myth?
A. Some groups of people profit from keeping people hungry.
B. Technology does not help poor people who lack the resources to buy it.
C. There is not enough food in the world to feed the hungry.
D. When people work together for solutions, hope brings change.

(Continued)

© Goodheart-Willcox

Name_____

_____ 35. A name used to describe scientific efforts in the 1970s and 1980s to improve seed quality, crop yields, and irrigation practices is _____.
A. environmental sustainability
B. farmland enhancement
C. green revolution
D. soil sciences

_____ 36. Which factor will most help slow the growth of the world population?
A. Effective infrastructure.
B. Goodwill.
C. Government food and nutrition programs.
D. Improved education.

_____ 37. What is the name of the day set aside each October to share information about world hunger?
A. Dare to Care Day.
B. Global Hunger Day.
C. U.N. Day.
D. World Food Day.

Essay Questions: Provide complete responses to the following questions or statements.

38. Provide an argument refuting the statement "Everyone wants hunger to end."

39. Describe the roles of two programs in the United States and one international organization in addressing hunger problems.

40. What are three actions a person can take to help fight hunger?

© Goodheart-Willcox

A Career for You in Nutrition and Fitness

25

Objectives

After studying this chapter, students will be able to

* list common job titles, responsibilities, and qualifications for people in the nutrition and fitness career areas.
* cite reasons for certification and license requirements for many jobs in the nutrition and fitness field.
* explain how interests, aptitudes, values, and goals can affect career decisions.
* describe steps to take during the teen years to help prepare for a career.
* use effective techniques to find, keep, and leave a job.
* explore opportunities for entrepreneurs.

Bulletin Board

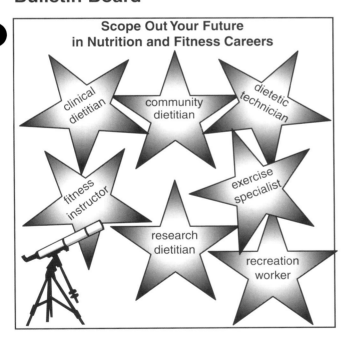

Scope Out Your Future in Nutrition and Fitness Careers

clinical dietitian
community dietitian
dietetic technician
fitness instructor
exercise specialist
research dietitian
recreation worker

Title: *Scope Out Your Future in Nutrition and Fitness Careers*

Place a cutout of a large telescope in the lower-left corner of the bulletin board. Scatter cutouts of stars around the bulletin board. Label each star with the name of a specific nutrition- or fitness-related career. You may also wish to attach pictures of nutrition and fitness professionals to the stars.

Teaching Materials

Text, pages 439-459
Learn the Language
Check Your Knowledge
Put Learning into Action
Explore Further

Student Activity Guide, pages 181-189
A. *Directions for Dietitians*
B. *Career Crossroads*
C. *Nutrition and Fitness—A Story of Opportunity*
D. *Career Preparation Checklist*
E. *Practicing Interview Questions*
F. *Backtrack Through Chapter 25*

Teacher's Resources
Get a Spin on a Career, reproducible master 25-1
Overlapping Career Areas, color transparency CT-25
Interview a Nutrition or Fitness Specialist, reproducible master 25-2
Is the Nutrition and Fitness Field for You? reproducible master 25-3
Networking That Works, transparency master 25-4
Interview Evaluation, reproducible master 25-5

Introducing the Chapter

1. Ask students to refer to Figure 25-1 on page 440 in the text, which illustrates a dietitian at work. Have students describe the physical environment in which the dietitian is working. Also have them describe the types of skills she must have to be effective, the materials and resources she is drawing upon, and the nature and characteristics of her clients. Have students compare this work setting to the setting in which the exercise leader in Figure 25-5 on page 444 is working. Ask students what features of each of these work settings they find desirable and undesirable.
2. Invite students to share their knowledge about people they know who work in health care or health promotion professions. What do these professionals say they like about their jobs? What problems do they face?
3. Ask students what factors might cause job opportunities in the fields of nutrition and fitness to grow. Relate their responses to text information.

Strategies to Reteach, Reinforce, Enrich, and Extend Text Concepts

Nutrition and Fitness Professionals

4. **RF** *Get a Spin on a Career,* reproducible master 25-1. Have each student use the Internet or library resources to complete the worksheet with information about a nutrition or fitness career that interests him or her.

5. **ER** Guest speakers. Invite a nutrition professional and a fitness professional to speak to the class about their career paths. Ask each speaker to discuss his or her educational and professional background. Ask students to note similarities and differences in the two career areas. Have the speakers describe licensing and/or certification requirements in their fields. Also ask the speakers to list criteria consumers should keep in mind when seeking help from a nutrition or fitness professional to avoid dealing with people who are not qualified to dispense accurate information.

6. **RT** *Overlapping Career Areas,* color transparency CT-25. Use the transparency to illustrate some of the tasks in which nutrition professionals and fitness professionals might be involved. Emphasize overlapping tasks that might be part of both areas.

7. **RF** Have students identify two-year and four-year colleges and universities within a 50-mile radius that offer accredited programs in nutrition and fitness areas. Ask students to share their findings in class.

8. **ER** *Interview a Nutrition or Fitness Specialist,* reproducible master 25-2. Have students use the questions on the handout to interview a nutrition or fitness professional about his or her career. After completing the interview, students are to answer a summary question at the bottom of the page.

9. **RF** *Directions for Dietitians,* Activity A, SAG. Students are to answer questions based on case situations about various types of dietitians.

10. **RF** *Nutrition and Fitness—A Story of Opportunity,* Activity C, SAG. Students are to use context clues and listed words to complete a story about teens who pursued nutrition and fitness careers.

Certification and License Requirements

11. **ER** Have students write to professional nutrition and fitness organizations to learn the requirements for becoming registered or certified. Have students contact local professionals and/or use the Internet to gather names and addresses of certifying agencies.

12. **RF** Have students make a set of flash cards with the initials that signify certification or licensing for nutrition and fitness professions on one side. Have students write out the appropriate certified or licensed titles on the backs of the cards. Students can use the cards to quiz themselves about labels and initials commonly used in nutrition and fitness professions.

Making a Positive Career Choice

13. **EX** *Is the Nutrition and Fitness Field for You?* reproducible master 25-3. Have students check the appropriate column on the handout to indicate whether each statement about characteristics typical of nutrition and fitness professionals applies to them. Then have students answer the questions at the bottom of the page.

14. **ER** Have students complete an aptitude test through the school guidance office. Discuss the aptitudes that would influence success in the nutrition and fitness fields.

15. **ER** Have each student draw pictures depicting three of his or her natural talents and/or abilities. Encourage students to share their pictures with one another in small group discussion. Ask students what new characteristics they learned about their fellow group members. Discuss why it is important for each person to recognize his or her talents and skills.

16. **RF** Define the term *values.* Slowly read the following list of value pairs to students: consistency/change, organization/chaos, predictability/uncertainty, risk avoidance/risk taking, personal rewards/financial rewards, career/family, people/tasks. On a sheet of paper, ask each student to write which item in each pair he or she values more. Discuss how the various values might relate to satisfaction with careers in the nutrition and fitness areas.

Career Preparation

17. **RF** Have students identify the specific school course offerings that feed into a nutrition and fitness career path. Invite teachers of identified courses to share their course outlines to help students more fully see the health/fitness connection.

18. **ER** Panel discussion. Invite a panel of officers from school clubs to describe the activities of their organizations. Ask panel members to highlight what they have gained from membership and participation.

19. **ER** Guest speaker. Invite a volunteer coordinator from your community to speak to the class about volunteer opportunities that are available for teens. Have the speaker describe the personal and community benefits of volunteering. Also ask the speaker to describe the commitments and

requirements involved in volunteer work. Provide details on how students can sign up for volunteer services.

20. **RF** Ask students how a volunteer position may be helpful in laying the foundation for a career in the areas of nutrition and fitness.

21. **RF** Have students brainstorm a list of employability skills needed in any career area. Then ask students to add to the list any specialized skills that would be needed in a nutrition or fitness career.

22. **RT** Draw a ladder on the chalkboard. Label the bottom rung with an entry-level position in a nutrition or fitness field. Label the other rungs with positions to illustrate a progression of jobs in a career. Discuss the skills a worker would learn in each job that would apply to the next job in the progression.

23. **RF** Review the list of items that might be included in a personal portfolio, as shown in Figure 25-12 on page 453 in the text. Ask students what an employer might be able to tell about a job applicant based on each item.

24. **ER** Have each student organize a personal portfolio. Divide the class into small groups. Have students share their portfolios with group members. Ask group members to evaluate portfolios and offer constructive criticism.

25. **RF** *Career Preparation Checklist,* Activity D, SAG. Students are to circle *yes* or *no* to indicate whether they have completed listed career planning steps and give details about their responses. Then students are to answer evaluation questions at the end of the activity.

Finding the Job You Want

26. **RF** *Networking That Works,* transparency master 25-4. Use the transparency to introduce a discussion of techniques students can use to find information about jobs, job skills, and job openings. Invite students to give additional suggestions.

27. **EX** Have students practice using electronic forms of communication, including e-mail, news groups, home pages, and faxes to begin a job search. Discuss the effectiveness of each form of electronic communication used.

28. **ER** Have students research the frequency of job-related accidents and injuries. Discuss the importance of recognizing and maintaining a safe work environment.

29. **EX** Have each student prepare a complete, up-to-date resume.

30. **ER** Ask students to list criteria for a well-written resume. Put this list in the form of a checklist students can use to evaluate their resumes.

31. **EX** Review with students appropriate format and content of a cover letter. Then have students write mock cover letters responding to a classified ad seeking teens for a variety of volunteer positions in a hospital.

32. **EX** Have students brainstorm a list of steps they might take to prepare for a job interview. List responses on the chalkboard. Then ask students to rank listed items in the order they should be done.

33. **RF** *Practicing Interview Questions,* Activity E, SAG. Students are to write their responses to frequently asked interview questions. After students have completed the worksheet, have pairs of students take turns asking and answering the questions in random order.

34. **ER** *Interview Evaluation,* reproducible master 25-5. Have students work in groups of three. Two students in each group will assume the roles of employer and job applicant. These students will role-play a job interview for a specified entry-level position in a nutrition or fitness career. The third student in each group will use the handout to evaluate the applicant's interview skills. Following the role-play, the three students should discuss the evaluation. Then group members should rotate roles and repeat the activity.

35. **ER** Have students practice writing follow-up letters to thank an employer who interviewed them. Discuss the features of a letter that makes a positive impact.

36. **ER** Have students investigate continuing education opportunities that are available for people working in nutrition and fitness areas. Have students share their findings in class. Discuss the skills workers can acquire and retain by participating in such educational activities and how this can help workers keep their jobs.

37. **EX** Have students role-play ethical situations they might face in the workplace, such as seeing a coworker steal office supplies or being asked to falsify records. Discuss how having a code of ethics can help workers know what to do when faced with these situations.

38. **RT** Asks students to list reasons a worker might choose to leave a job. List responses on the board and compare them with reasons mentioned in the text.

39. **ER** Have each student research one individual who is recognized as a successful entrepreneur in a nutrition or fitness area. Examples include Ray Kroc, Colonel Harland Sanders, Julia Child, Debbi Fields, and Richard Simmons. Ask each student to prepare a one-page brief on how the entrepreneur changed the food technology, nutrition, or fitness industry.

Chapter Review

40. **RF** *Career Crossroads,* Activity B, SAG. Students are to complete a crossword puzzle using terms from the chapter.
41. **RF** *Backtrack Through Chapter 25,* Activity F, SAG. Students are to provide complete answers to questions and statements that will help them recall, interpret, apply, and practice chapter concepts.
42. **RF** Have each student write one new fact he or she learned through the study of this chapter. Go around the room asking each student to share what he or she wrote.

Above and Beyond

43. **EX** Have each student shadow a professional for an extended period. Have students prepare notebooks describing the experience. Notebooks should include photographs, pamphlets, and a diary of daily activities and impressions. Contact a local newspaper to report program results to the community.
44. **EX** Have students plan a nutrition and fitness career fair. Students should work in pairs to prepare displays highlighting different careers. Students should also invite nutrition and fitness professionals to speak about their jobs and discuss opportunities in the field with interested students.
45. **EX** Have students invent and write nutrition and fitness job descriptions for the year 2030. Post these job descriptions on a bulletin board titled *Through the Looking Glass: What Could Be.*
46. **ER** Have students write to professional organizations related to the field of nutrition and fitness. Students should request career brochures, which they can place in a display for use by other members of the student body. Coordinate the setup of the display with the school guidance office.
47. **ER** As a class, develop a set of questions each student can use to interview a local entrepreneur in a food, nutrition, or fitness career area. Have students ask the entrepreneurs for permission to prepare audio- or videotapes of their interviews to share in class. After reviewing the tapes in class, ask students to summarize common characteristics of the entrepreneurs that appear to lead to successful businesses.

Answer Key

Text

Check Your Knowledge, pages 463-464

1. (List two:) greater general interest in nutrition and fitness, more seniors, more employee-sponsored fitness programs
2. analyzing a person's diet and performing diet treatment

3. (List five:) business, clinical, community, consultant, educator, management, and research dietitians
4. assists registered dietitians
5. false
6. (List and describe four. Student response.)
7. to make sure the person is qualified to do the job
8. people, information, material items
9. An aptitude is a natural talent. An ability is a skill developed through practice.
10. to help determine which career option will make the person happiest
11. (Student response.)
12. (List four:) taking appropriate courses, joining related clubs and school organizations, volunteering, acquiring employability skills, gaining work experience, talking with others, developing a portfolio
13. (List five:) problem-solving, leadership, teamwork, communication, creative thinking, organizational, technical
14. papers, letters, pictures, and projects that demonstrate job-related skills and achievements
15. (List four:) networking, reading want ads, checking bulletin boards, searching the Internet, attending job fairs and career days, contacting employment services
16. (List five:) adequate lighting, clear traffic ways, dry floors, sufficient ventilation, well-maintained equipment with safety guards and shields in place, clearly labeled and properly stored hazardous materials, safety gear and protective clothing, observable sanitation standards
17. to briefly outline a person's job qualifications
18. (List four. Student response.)
19. (List two each:) maintaining a job—exhibit traits that are key to job success, find a mentor and follow his or her example, stay up to date with new research and resources, apply professional ethics; leaving a job—give notice two weeks before leaving, give notice in writing, avoid angering the employer, thank the employer for opportunities
20. Market research helps entrepreneurs identify consumer needs and ways to meet those needs with new products or services. Through advances in technology, new research findings can be revealed and new products and services can be developed.

Student Activity Guide

Directions for Dietitians, Activity A

Case #1. A. clinical
B. Yes, he must be registered to plan diets for his patients.
Case #2. A. business
B. consultant

Case #3. A. educator and management
B. management, because she would need an advanced degree to become an educator dietitian
Case #4. A. community, because he likes working with people
B. speaking to community groups about nutrition

Career Crossroads, Activity B

Nutrition and Fitness—A Story of Opportunity, Activity C

1. dietitians
2. dietetic technicians
3. health
4. fitness
5. corporate
6. exercise leader
7. fitness
8. science
9. ergonomics
10. sports instructor
11. certified
12. registered
13. untrained
14. director
15. enhancement
16. exercise specialist
17. nutrition
18. entrepreneur

Backtrack Through Chapter 25, Activity F

1. bachelor's
2. (Student response. See pages 440-441.)
3. associate
4. (Student response. See pages 443-446.)

5. acceptable programs of study to complete, minimum level of education or degree required, internship and/or on-the-job experience, minimum grade required on a national exam
6. family, friends, life experiences
7. (List three:) They have a deadline. They are achievable. They are personal. They are stated in a positive way. They are specific.
8. family and consumer sciences, life management, health, foods and nutrition, business, management, communications, computers
9. Future Business Leaders of America; Family, Career and Community Leaders of America
10. (Student response. See page 459.)
11. dress as much like the employees there as possible
12. (List four:) positive attitude, good communication skills, creative, flexible, open to new ideas
13. innovative, willing to be risk takers, persistent
14. Unqualified people could hold important jobs and cause physical harm to those they advise.
15. An aptitude is a natural talent, whereas an ability is learned through practice.
16. Sports and athletics provide opportunities for a person to participate in physical activities and learn motivational techniques he or she can apply in a career in the fitness field.
17. You do not want to anger an employer you may need to list as a reference someday.
18. (Student response.)
19. (Student response.)
20. (Student response.)

Teacher's Resources

Chapter 25 Test

1. B	11. D	21. F	31. D
2. A	12. G	22. T	32. B
3. C	13. A	23. T	33. C
4. I	14. C	24. T	34. C
5. H	15. F	25. F	35. A
6. K	16. E	26. F	36. D
7. J	17. I	27. T	37. A
8. E	18. H	28. T	
9. G	19. T	29. F	
10. D	20. F	30. T	

38. (List five:) take appropriate courses; join related clubs and school organizations; volunteer; acquire employability skills; gain work experience; talk with others; develop a portfolio
39. ads in local newspapers and other publications; bulletin boards in public buildings; the Internet; job fairs and career days; public employment services
40. learn as much as possible about the employer and its business; prepare a resume and a portfolio; list questions to ask the employer about the job; practice answering questions orally

Get a Spin on a Career

Name_____   Date _____   Period _____

Use the Internet or library resources to complete the worksheet with information about a nutrition or fitness career that interests you.

Educational
Requirements

Job
Description

Future
Outlook

Job
Benefits

(career title)

Type of Work
Environment

Technical
Skills Needed

© Goodheart-Willcox

Interview a Nutrition or Fitness Specialist

Name_____   **Date** _____   **Period**_____

Use the questions below to interview a nutrition or fitness professional about his or her career. After completing the interview, answer the summary question at the bottom of the page.

1. Job title _____

2. Job description _____
   _____

3. How long have you been working in this field? _____

4. What other positions have you held in this career field? _____
   _____

5. Why did you select this occupation for your career? _____
   _____

6. What is your favorite part of your job? _____
   _____

7. What do you find most challenging about your job? _____
   _____

8. What educational requirements are necessary to enter a career such as yours? _____
   _____

9. What personal characteristics are necessary to be successful in a job like yours? _____
   _____

10. What experiences or coursework do you recommend for a teen who wants to enter a career path like yours?
   _____

11. What is the salary range for a person in your career area? _____

12. What do you see as the future for careers in your area in the next five years? _____
   _____

13. Describe how your time is divided during a typical day._____
   _____
   _____

14. How would you rate your level of satisfaction with your career? _____

Describe why you would or would not like a job like the one held by the person you interviewed.
_____
_____

© Goodheart-Willcox

Is the Nutrition and Fitness Field for You?

Name_____   Date _____   Period_____

The following statements relate to characteristics typical of professionals in the nutrition and fitness career areas. Check the appropriate column to indicate whether each statement applies to you. Then answer the questions at the bottom of the page.

Yes	No	
_____	_____	1. I enjoy working with people.
_____	_____	2. I express concern for others with a caring attitude.
_____	_____	3. I can communicate my ideas easily.
_____	_____	4. I am self-confident.
_____	_____	5. I enjoy solving complex problems.
_____	_____	6. I practice good health, nutrition, and fitness habits.
_____	_____	7. I keep my commitments to others.
_____	_____	8. I can keep information about other people to myself.
_____	_____	9. I easily adjust to changes at school and work.
_____	_____	10. I am very interested in food, fitness, and the preventive health care fields.
_____	_____	11. I am well organized.
_____	_____	12. I like to study chemistry, anatomy, physiology, and mathematics.
_____	_____	13. I like to learn new skills.
_____	_____	14. I have a positive attitude toward work.
_____	_____	15. I am ambitious.

Based on this analysis, how well do you feel you are suited for a career in the area of nutrition or fitness?_____

_____

Do you think you would enjoy working in a nutrition or fitness profession? Explain why or why not. _____

_____

_____

In what other career areas might the characteristics you have be important? _____

_____

Of these career areas, in which would you be most interested?_____

_____

What school organizations could you join now to help you prepare for these careers? _____

_____

© Goodheart-Willcox

Networking That Works

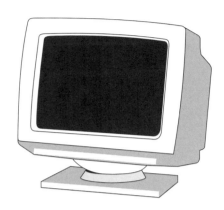

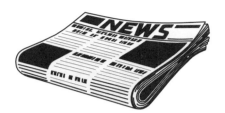

Volunteering—build relationships while providing a service to others

Community events—meet people and learn about resources

Advice from others—approach key contacts to critique your resume and portfolio; receive job search information

Newspaper—read want ads to learn about requirements for jobs of interest to you

Internet—get information from news groups, message boards, and career Web sites

Job fairs—learn more about specific companies from their representatives

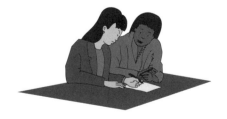

© Goodheart-Willcox

Interview Evaluation

Name _____ **Date** _____ **Period** _____

Work in groups of three. Role-play a situation in which a person is interviewing for a nutrition- or fitness-related job. One group member should play the applicant and another should play the employer. The third group member should evaluate the applicant's interview skills using the checklist below. Rotate roles and repeat the activity.

Name of job applicant: _____

Yes	No	
_____	_____	1. Was the applicant courteous to the employer?
_____	_____	2. Did the applicant offer a firm handshake of greeting?
_____	_____	3. Did the applicant introduce himself or herself to the employer?
_____	_____	4. Did the applicant maintain eye contact with the employer?
_____	_____	5. Was dress appropriate for the interview?
_____	_____	6. Did the applicant use good posture?
_____	_____	7. Did the applicant use positive body language?
_____	_____	8. Were the applicant's job skills stated clearly?
_____	_____	9. Were examples of the applicant's past accomplishments clearly described to the employer?
_____	_____	10. Was enthusiasm for the job expressed?
_____	_____	11. Did the applicant give information about his or her available work hours?
_____	_____	12. Did the applicant ask appropriate questions about the job?
_____	_____	13. Did the applicant thank the employer at the end of the interview?
_____	_____	14. Did the applicant ask when the decision about the position might be made?

What were the strengths of the applicant? _____

_____

_____

What were the weaknesses of the applicant? _____

_____

_____

List one suggestion that will help the applicant build interview skills. _____

_____

© Goodheart-Willcox

A Career for You in Nutrition and Fitness

Name_____

Date _____   Period _____   Score _____

Chapter 25 Test

Matching: Match the following terms and identifying phrases.

_____ 1. A natural talent.

_____ 2. A skill learned through practice.

_____ 3. A competency that individuals need for successfully obtaining and keeping a job.

_____ 4. An organized collection of papers, letters, pictures, and projects that shows what a person has accomplished.

_____ 5. Alerting a wide circle of people about an interest in a job.

_____ 6. An outline of a person's job qualifications.

_____ 7. The name of a person who will speak highly of an individual's skills and abilities.

_____ 8. A discussion between a job applicant and the person doing the hiring.

_____ 9. A coworker who has years of experience and can help a newer worker with questions and challenges in the workplace.

_____ 10. Someone who owns and operates his or her own business.

A. ability
B. aptitude
C. employability skill
D. entrepreneur
E. job interview
F. license
G. mentor
H. networking
I. portfolio
J. reference
K. resume

Matching: Match the following nutrition and fitness professionals with their descriptions.

_____ 11. Designs fitness programs to improve employees' state of wellness.

_____ 12. Supervises people who plan, prepare, and serve meals in schools and hospitals.

_____ 13. Assesses a patient's recovery goals and diet plans as part of a health care team.

_____ 14. Works under contract and offers dietetic advice to health care facilities, nursing homes, or athletic centers.

_____ 15. Manages fitness facilities; chooses equipment, hires staff, schedules programs, and handles finances.

_____ 16. Applies science and math principles to the structure of the body.

_____ 17. Conducts studies to find answers to nutrition questions.

_____ 18. Plans self-improvement and fitness programs in playgrounds, parks, and other public facilities.

A. clinical dietitian
B. community dietitian
C. consultant dietitian
D. corporate fitness specialist
E. exercise science specialist
F. health and fitness director
G. management dietitian
H. recreation worker
I. research dietitian

True/False: Circle *T* if the statement is true and *F* if the statement is false.

T   F   19. Job opportunities are growing faster in nutrition and fitness than for most other professions.

T   F   20. Registered dietitians need certificates but not bachelor's degrees.

(Continued)

© Goodheart-Willcox

Name_____

T F   21. Anyone can buy a license to practice nutrition counseling.

T F   22. Professional associations set standards for certification.

T F   23. A personal fitness trainer should be interested in interacting with people.

T F   24. People can use short-term goals to help them reach long-term goals.

T F   25. It is almost impossible to prepare for a career in nutrition and fitness areas until a person gets to college.

T F   26. Friends and relatives are not a good source of job information.

T F   27. Resumes should be written before a job interview.

T F   28. Ethics should guide every decision a worker makes.

T F   29. When leaving a job, a worker should tell his or her employer why he or she did not like the job.

T F   30. Advances in technology create new opportunities for entrepreneurs.

Multiple Choice: Choose the best response. Write the letter in the space provided.

_____31. Which job allows for the widest range of options in the nutrition area?
   A. Nutrition researcher.
   B. Dietetic technician.
   C. Community dietitian.
   D. Registered dietitian.

_____32. A dietetic technician _____.
   A. must have a master's degree
   B. can help people make food choices that fit into their diet plans
   C. works without guidance
   D. All the above.

_____33. Which describes the goal of preventive health care?
   A. To treat disease.
   B. To research the cause of disease.
   C. To preserve health now to prevent poor health later.
   D. To examine why quality of life is important.

_____34. What is one main difference between certification and a license?
   A. A license is less valued than a certificate.
   B. Qualifications are less rigid for licensing than certification.
   C. Standards of performance are regulated by a government agency for a license but not for certification.
   D. There are no differences; a license and certification are the same.

_____35. How will participating in school organizations help your career?
   A. You will develop leadership and team building skills.
   B. Your personal image will be boosted.
   C. You will not have to get a license.
   D. You are guaranteed a job after graduation.

_____36. Which of the following activities would support nutrition career development?
   A. Waiting on tables.
   B. Serving in the cafeteria.
   C. Preparing family meals.
   D. All the above.

(Continued)

© Goodheart-Willcox

Name_____

_____37. Which of the following would be included on a resume?
  A. Work experience.
  B. Personal likes and dislikes.
  C. Medical history.
  D. Family background.

Essay Questions: Provide complete responses to the following questions or statements.

38. List five ways a person can start preparing for a career during high school.

39. Name five information sources a person might check to find job openings.

40. List four ways to prepare for a job interview.

© Goodheart-Willcox